# Handbook of Capsule Endoscopy

Zhaoshen Li · Zhuan Liao
Mark McAlindon

Editors

# Handbook of Capsule Endoscopy

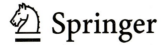 Springer

*Editors*
Zhaoshen Li
Zhuan Liao
Department of Gastroenterology
Changhai Hospital
Shanghai
China

Mark McAlindon
Gastroenterology
Royal Hallamshire Hospital
Sheffield
UK

ISBN 978-94-017-9228-8     ISBN 978-94-017-9229-5   (eBook)
DOI 10.1007/978-94-017-9229-5
Springer Dordrecht Heidelberg New York London

Library of Congress Control Number: 2014943402

Printed on acid-free paper

Springer is part of Springer Science+Business Media (www.springer.com)

# Contents

# Contributors

**Samuel Adler** Department of Gastroenterology, Shaare Zedek Medical Center, Jerusalem, Israel

**Peter Baltes** Clinic for Internal Medicine, Bethesda Hospital Bergedorf, Hamburg, Germany

**Nigel Beejay** Institute of Medicine, Sheikh Khalifa Medical City Hospital, Abu Dhabi, United Arab Emirates. London Independent Hospital, London, UK

**Dan Carter** Department of Gastroenterology, Sheba Medical Center, Sackler School of Medicine, Tel-Aviv University, Tel-Aviv, Israel

**Hoon Jai Chun** Division of Gastroenterology and Hepatology, Department of Internal Medicine, Korea University Anam Hospital, Korea University College of Medicine, Seongbuk-Gu, Seoul, South Korea

**Joo Won Chung** Division of Gastroenterology, Department of Internal Medicine, National Medical Center, 245 Euljiro, Jung-gu, Seoul 100-799, Korea

**Stanley Cohen** Children's Center for Digestive Health Care, Atlanta, GA, USA

**Carolyn Davison** South Tyneside NHS Foundation Trust, Tyne and Wear, UK

**Edward J. Despott** Royal Free Unit for Endoscopy, Royal Free Hospital, University College London, Institute for Liver and Digestive Health, London, UK

**Sarah Douglas** The Royal Infirmary of Edinburgh, Centre for Liver and Digestive Disorders, Edinburgh, UK

**Xiaodong Duan** Department of Gastroenterology, Changhai Hospital, Second Military Medical University, Yangpu District, Shanghai, China

**Rami Eliakim** Department of Gastroenterology, Sheba Medical Center, Sackler School of Medicine, Tel-Aviv University, Tel-Aviv, Israel

**Anton Emmanuel** GI Physiology Unit, University College London, London, UK

**Chris Fraser** Wolfson Unit for Endoscopy, St Mark's Hospital and Academic Institute, Imperial College London, London, UK

**Zhaotao Gong** Chongqing Jinshan Science and Technology Co., Ltd., Chongqing, China

**Qiang Guo** Department of Gastroenterology, The First People's Hospital of Yunnan Province, Kunming, China

**Melissa F. Hale** Directorate of Gastroenterology, Royal Hallamshire Hospital, Sheffield Teaching Hospitals NHS Trust, Sheffield, UK

**Qiong He** Department of Gastroenterology, The Third Affiliated Hospital of Southern Medical University, Guangzhou, ChinaDepartment of Gastroenterology, Nanfang Hospital, Southern Medical University, Guangzhou, China

**Rahul Kalla** Gastrointestinal Unit, Institute of Genetics and Molecular Medicine, University of Edinburgh, Edinburgh, England

**Martin Keuchel** Clinic for Internal Medicine, Bethesda Hospital Bergedorf, Hamburg, Germany

**Anastasios Koulaouzidis** The Royal Infirmary of Edinburgh, Centre for Liver and Digestive Disorders, Edinburgh, Scotland, UK

**Niehls Kurniawan** Clinic for Internal Medicine, Bethesda Hospital Bergedorf, Hamburg, Germany

**Zhaoshen Li** Department of Gastroenterology, Changhai Hospital, Second Military Medical University, Yangpu District, Shanghai, China

**Zhuan Liao** Department of Gastroenterology, Changhai Hospital, Second Military Medical University, Yangpu District, Shanghai, China

**Mark McAlindon** Directorate of Gastroenterology, Royal Hallamshire Hospital, Sheffield Teaching Hospitals NHS Trust, Sheffield, UK

**Peter Mooney** Directorate of Gastroenterology, Royal Hallamshire Hospital, Sheffield Teaching Hospitals NHS Trust, Sheffield, UK

**Salvatore Oliva** Pediatric Gastroenterology and Liver Unit, Sapienza University of Rome, Rome, Italy

**Simon Panter** South Tyneside NHS Foundation Trust, Tyne and Wear, UK

**Sung Chul Park** Division of Gastroenterology and Hepatology, Department of Internal Medicine, Kangwon National University Hospital, Kangwon National University School of Medicine, Chuncheon, Kangwon-do, South Korea

**Clare Parker** South Tyneside NHS Foundation Trust, Tyne and Wear, UK

**Praful Patel** Gastrointestinal Department, University Hospital Southampton Foundation Trust, Southampton, UK

**Marco Pennazio** 2nd Division of Gastroenterology, Department of Medicine, San Giovanni Battista University Teaching Hospital, Torino, Italy

**John N. Plevris** Centre for Liver and Digestive Disorders, The Royal Infirmary of Edinburgh, Edinburgh, Scotland

**Imdadur Rahman** Gastrointestinal Department, University Hospital Southampton Foundation Trust, Southampton, UK

**Emanuele Rondonotti** Ospedale Valduce, Gastroenterology Unit, Como, Italy

**David Sanders** Directorate of Gastroenterology, Royal Hallamshire Hospital, Sheffield Teaching Hospitals NHS Trust, Sheffield, UK

**Reena Sidhu** Gastroenterology and Liver Unit, Royal Hallamshire Hospital, Sheffield Teaching Hospitals NHS Trust, University of Sheffield, Sheffield, England

**Si Young Song** Division of Gastroenterology, Department of Internal Medicine, Yonsei University College of Medicine, Brain Korea 21 Project for Medical Science, 250 Seongsanno, Seodaemun-gu, Seoul, Korea

**Cristiano Spada** Digestive Endoscopy Unit, Catholic University, Rome, Italy

**Min Tang** Department of Gastroenterology, The First People's Hospital of Yunnan Province, Kunming, China

**Bangmao Wang** Department of Gastroenterology, General Hospital Affiliated to Tianjin Medical University, Tianjin, China

**Jinshan Wang** Chongqing Jinshan Science and Technology Co., Ltd., Chongqing, China

**Xinhong Wang** Department of Gastroenterology, Changhai Hospital, Second Military Medical University, Yangpu District, Shanghai, China

**Hao Wu** Department of Gastroenterology, Changhai Hospital, Second Military Medical University, Yangpu District, Shanghai, China

**Guohua Xiao** Department of Gastroenterology, Changhai Hospital, Second Military Medical University, Yangpu District, Shanghai, China

**Fachao Zhi** Department of Gastroenterology, Nanfang Hospital, Southern Medical University, Guangzhou, China

**Zhizheng Ge** Department of Gastroenterology and Hepatology, Digestive Endoscopy Centre, Renji Hospital, School of Medicine, Shanghai Jiao Tong University, Shanghai, China

**Wenbin Zou** Department of Gastroenterology, Changhai Hospital, Second Military Medical University, Yangpu District, Shanghai, China

# The History of Wireless Capsule Endoscopy: From a Dream to a Platform of Capsules

Rami Eliakim

Direct visualization of the gastrointestinal tract by traditional endoscopy was introduced and developed over the last 50 years or so. Fairly fast gastroenterologists moved from rigid esophago-gastroscopes to flexible scopes and to high-definition videoscopes, daily used for the upper and lower GI endoscopies as well as for the biliary tract. The small intestine posed a problem as no direct visualization of its whole course was available, push enteroscopy allowing visualization of about 50 % of its length.

In the early 1980s, 1981 to be exact, two Israelis, an electro-optical engineer, Gabi Iddan, on sabbatical from Rafael Ltd and a gastroenterologist, Eitan Scapa, also on sabbatical, living in the same neighborhood in Boston, met and discussed their respective fields of work and interest. Through this neighborly chat, Iddan learned what gastroenterology was all about, about fiber-optic endoscopes, their use as well as limitations, one of which was their inaccessibility to visualize most of the small intestine. It was Scapa that challenged Iddan into finding a method to view the entire small bowel. The idea was there, but there were no good solutions nor advanced technology.

The two became friends, and 10 years later, in 1991, Scapa visited Iddan who was again on sabbatical and rechallenged him with the same problem. By that period of time, small-format image sensors (CCD) were developed (for usage in video cameras) and were starting to be used in the new-generation endoscopes replacing the fiberscope method.

This led Gabi to think of cutting the camera tip of the endoscope and letting it move naturally through threw GI tract, connected to the endoscope via a thin "umbilical" cable. This idea was dropped very fast, knowing the actual length of the small bowel.

The next step/thought was to replace the cable with a transmitter. This idea of a transmitter-equipped camera was continuously developed. Apart from the apparatus itself, other basic questions arose: How would the camera lens be kept clean? How long will it take for it to move through the small bowel and will the physician be available for like 8 h? Will the existing miniature batteries operate for longer than 10–15 min, without taking into account energy needed for transmission and for illumination. These overwhelming challenges almost caused Iddan to abandon the project. Then, he decided to tackle each obstacle at a time.

His first assumption regarded the shape of the camera's optic dome; he fabricated an axicon optic window assuming this shape will continuously be cleaned while moving. He added a miniature CCD and a light source and experimentally showed that this produced reasonable

R. Eliakim (✉)
Department of Gastroenterology, Chaim Sheba Medical Center, 2nd Sheba Road, 52621 Ramat-Gan, Israel
e-mail: abraham.eliakim@sheba.health.gov.il

Z. Li et al. (eds.), *Handbook of Capsule Endoscopy*,
DOI: 10.1007/978-94-017-9229-5_1, © Springer Science+Business Media Dordrecht 2014

**Fig. 1.1** Historical prototypes of the capsule. Reprint with permission from Gastrointest Endosc Clin N Am [2]

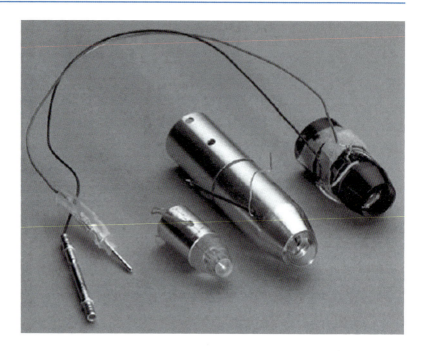

images. Some of these first models are shown in Fig. 1.1.

One of the first experiments Iddan recalls was using a store-bought chicken to test and understand what power and frequency required for transmission from the GI tract. They learned that with proper tuning of the frequency, microwatt level of power was needed to transmit clear video images, which was very encouraging.

A big step forward was done a year later, in 1993, when a new-generation CCD imager was developed and reported on [1], requiring much less energy than the old ones. Another breakthrough, though conceptual, was to separate the device into 3 parts: an imager + transmitter, recorder, and a workstation, a solution that will enable the physician to interpret the results independently from the workstation, without constant real-time viewing. A multiple antenna array system was added to guarantee proper reception and was the basis of the later-on-incorporated localization system. In 1995, Iddan presented his idea to Gavriel Meron, at the time the CEO of Applitec Ltd., a company developing small cameras for fiberscopes. In 1997, a new start-up company headed by Meron and

Iddan (Given Imaging) was initiated. By that time, they were aware of the development of the complementary metal oxide semiconductor imaging (CMOS camera) that allowed good-quality images with substantially less energy than the CCD, crucial for the development of a capsule endoscope.

Practically at the same time, as early as 1981, another group of researchers led by a gastroenterologist, Paul Swain, and his colleagues were working on laser devices and radio frequency to treat bleeding in the GI tract. Later on, they developed a wireless pH capsule which was sewn to the stomach wall and started to use that technology. In the early 1990s, they started to explore wireless technology for endoscopy and acquired tiny video cameras and transmitters from various sources including security cameras and sport video equipment firms.

In 1994, Paul Swain brought up the possibility of a wireless endoscope in a lecture given during the world congress of gastroenterology. Later on, in 1966, Swain's group started testing transmission of video images through the human body, when they surgically inserted a large prototype device with video camera and

**Fig. 1.2** Time line of the development of the different capsules in the given platform

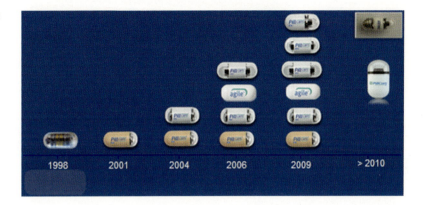

**Fig. 1.3** Various small bowel capsule endoscopes in use

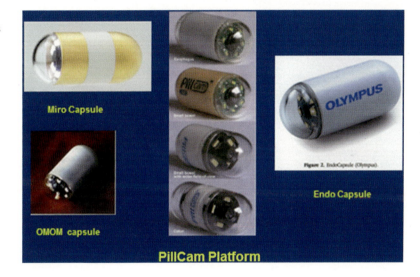

microwave transmission, a light source, and a battery into a pig stomach. This allowed acquiring images at 30 frames per second for about 20 min.

In 1997, the two groups met for the first time, and in 1998, the groups agreed to collaborate. Experiments with working prototypes were conducted in the beginning of 1999 in Israel, followed by the first human experiment of swallowing a 11 × 33 mm capsule by Paul Swain in Eitan Scapa's private clinic, the battery of which lasted for 2 h. Gastroscopy was done to sure the capsule has passed the pylorus. Swain swallowed a second capsule the next day in his hotel room which transmitted good-quality images for 6 h in which the capsule reached the cecum.

The initial findings were presented in Digestive Disease Week in 2000, the first patient trial was initiated, the invention was published in Nature [3], and FDA approve that same year.

Since then a platform of capsules was introduced by Given Imaging including a second and third generation of small bowel capsules (PillCam SB3) in which the light source, battery time, angle of view, and frame rates per second were improved, two generations of a two-sided esophageal capsule (PillCam Eso2), two generations of colon capsule (PillCam Colon2) with adapted frame rate and a much wider angle of view, and two generations of a patency capsule (Agile) allowing to test whether a regular capsule will pass were developed (Fig. 1.2). Human studies on an upper GI magnetic capsule have been published by both Given Imaging and Olympus, and there are many self-propelling capsules that are being developed and tested in animals. Moreover, competitive small bowel capsules have been manufactured by Korean, Japanese, Chinese, and American companies (Fig. 1.3). Small bowl capsule endoscopy is in routine use all over the globe for many indications—a dream come true.

# References

1. Fossum ER. Active image sensors: are CCDs dinosaurs? Int Soc Opt Eng (SPIE). 1993;1900:2–14.
2. Iddan GV, Swain P. History and development of capsule endoscopy. Gastrointest Endosc Clin N Am. 2004;14:1–9.
3. Iddan G, Meron G, Glukhovsky A, Swain P. Wireless capsule endoscopy. Nature. 2000;405:417.

# The Current Main Types of Capsule Endoscopy

**2**

Zhaoshen Li, Dan Carter, Rami Eliakim,
Wenbin Zou, Hao Wu, Zhuan Liao, Zhaotao Gong,
Jinshan Wang, Joo Won Chung, Si Young Song,
Guohua Xiao, Xiaodong Duan and Xinhong Wang

Z. Li (✉) · W. Zou (✉) · H. Wu · Z. Liao (✉) ·
G. Xiao  X. Duan · X. Wang
Department of Gastroenterology, Changhai
Hospital, Second Military Medical University, 168
Changhai Road, Yangpu District, Shanghai, 200433
China
e-mail: shanghailizhaoshen@gmail.com

W. Zou
e-mail: zwbpeak@gmail.com

Z. Liao
e-mail: liao.zhuan@gmail.com

D. Carter
Department of Gastroenterology, Chaim Sheba
Medical Center, 2nd Sheba Road, 52621
Ramat-Gan, Israel
e-mail: dan.carter@sheba.gov.il

Z. T. Gong · J. S. Wang
Chongqing Jinshan Science and Technology Co.,
Ltd., Chongqing, China

J. W. Chung
Division of Gastroenterology, Department of
Internal Medicine, National Medical Center, 245
Euljiro, Jung-gu, Seoul, 100-799 Korea
e-mail: drbeatrix@hanmail.net

S. Y. Song (✉)
Division of Gastroenterology, Department of
Internal Medicine, Yonsei University College of
Medicine, Brain Korea 21 Project for Medical
Science, 250 Seongsanno, Seodaemun-gu, Seoul,
Korea
e-mail: sysong@yuhs.ac

R. Eliakim (✉)
Head Department of Gastroenterology, Chaim
Sheba Medical Center, 2nd Sheba Road, 52621
Ramat-Gan, Israel
e-mail: Abraham.eliakim@sheba.health.gov.il

## 2.1 The Given Imaging Capsule Endoscopy Platform: Clinical Use in the Investigation of Small Bowel, Esophageal and Colonic Diseases

### 2.1.1 Introduction

The first video capsule endoscope was introduced in 2001 by Iddan as a new tool for the investigation of the small bowel [1]. Initially called mouth to anus (M2A), its goal was small bowel visualization. Since then, various studies have shown the potential of this minimally invasive technique to improve diagnostic outcomes among a variety of gastrointestinal (GI) conditions. Later on, the esophageal and colonic capsules [2, 3] were launched into the market, and the patency capsule was introduced as well. The introduction of the second or even third generation of capsules enabled broadening the horizon for its possible medical use (Fig. 2.1, Table 2.1). To date, multiple capsule endoscopy (CE) systems are available (Fig. 2.2), mostly for the small bowel. As mentioned, the first capsule endoscopy system was manufactured by Given Imaging (Yokneam, Israel). To date, the Given Imaging platform of capsule endoscopes includes the PillCam SB2 and SB3 for the small intestine, the PillCam ESO2 for esophageal imaging, PillCam Colon2 for the large

**Fig. 2.1** PillCam small
bowel 3 capsule endoscope
system

**PillCam® SB 3**

**PillCam SB 3**

**PillCam Recorder DR 3**

**PillCam Sensor Belt SB 3**

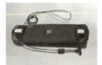

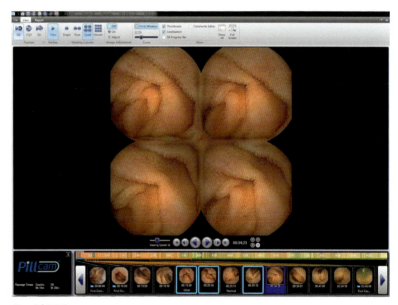

**Rapid 8 View screen**

bowel, as well as the Agile Patency capsule (second generation) (Fig. 2.3). Additional small bowel capsule systems include the Olympus EndoCapsule (Olympus, Japan) [4], the Chinese OMOM pill (Jinshan science and technology, Chongqing, China) [5], the Korean Miro pill [6], and the American CapsoCam SV-1. Comparative studies between the PillCam SB1 and the Olympus EndoCapsule or the Korean Miro Capsule did not show significant differences. Currently, only the Given PillCam SB system and the Olympus EndoCapsule are FDA- and CE-approved.

**Table 2.1** Indications for the use of capsule endoscopy according to anatomic site

*Esophagus*

Gastroesophageal reflux disease

Barrett's esophagus

Esophageal varices

*Small Bowel*

Obscure gastrointestinal bleeding

Suspected Crohn's disease

Suspected small bowel tumor

Evaluation of any abnormal small bowel imaging

Evaluation of partially responsive celiac disease

Surveillance of inherited polyposis syndromes

Evaluation of drug-induced small bowel injury

Evaluation of mucosal response to medications

*Colon*

Polyp screening

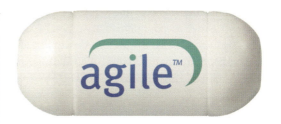

**Fig. 2.3** The Agile patency capsule system

The PillCam SB3 video capsule endoscopy system consists of (a) a 2 × 11 mm capsule containing the video camera, illumination, and batteries; (b) a sensing system comprising an array of sensor pads, a data recorder, and a battery pack; and (c) a workstation, based on a commercially available personal computer (Fig. 2.1). The new data recorders (DR3) also contain a portable real-time viewer that allows direct monitoring of the images received during

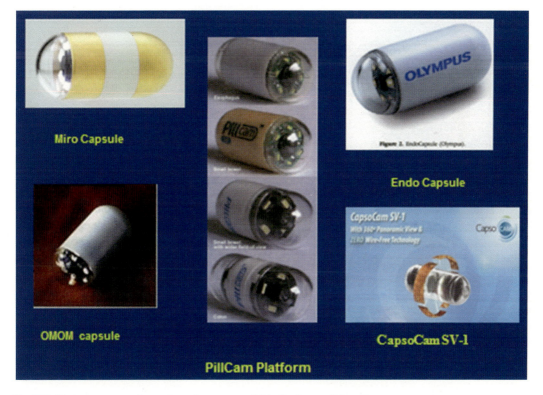

**Fig. 2.2** Various systems of capsule endoscopes available for the small bowel

the examination. While the PillCam captures images using a complementary metal-oxide semiconductor (CMOS) sensor, the EndoCapsule, MiroCam, and OMOM capsule use a charge-coupled device camera (CCD). The four capsules also differ with regard to dimensions, image acquisition frame rate, field of view, and recording duration.

Almost all of the information provided in the literature is regarding the Given Imaging PillCam SB, as it dominated the market for a few years by itself, later on joined by the other small bowel capsules, and thus is the one on which most of the literature is written.

### 2.1.2 Small Bowel Video Capsule Endoscopy

Until the introduction of the small bowel video capsule endoscopy (SBCE), the small bowel was an organ that was very difficult to explore with the available techniques. Since its development, SBCE provided a reliable, noninvasive, and well-accepted and well-tolerated procedure, which has revolutionized the study of the small bowel.

PillCam SB3 video capsule endoscope is a wireless capsule (11 × 26 mm) comprised of a light source, lens, CMOS imager, battery, and a wireless transmitter. A slippery coating allows easy ingestion and prevents adhesion of bowel contents, as it moves via peristalsis from the mouth to the anus (Figs. 2.1, 2.4). The battery provides >11 h of work in which the capsule photographs using an adaptive frame rate technique two to six images per second (>80,000 images all together), in a 156° field of view and 8:1 magnification. The pictures are transmitted via a newly developed 'no attachments' sensor belt, to a small data recorder (DR3) which also allows real-time imaging. The recorder is downloaded into a Reporting and Processing of Images and Data computer workstation (RAPID 8) and seen as a continuous video film. Support systems have been added since the first prototype of the RAPID system, including a localization system, a blood detector, a double and quadric

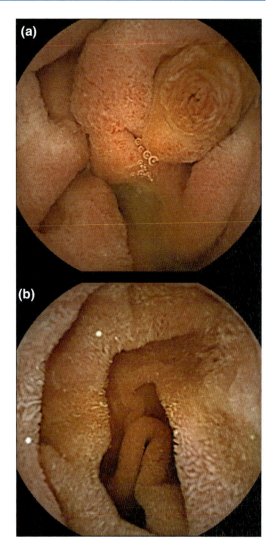

**Fig. 2.4** Small bowel pictures taken with PillCam SB3: **a** Ampulla of Vater. **b** Small bowel normal mucosa

picture viewer, a 'quick viewer,' single picture adjustment mode, incorporation of the Fuji Intelligent Color Enhancement (FICE) system, an inflammation (Lewis) scoring system, and an atlas, all meant to assist the interpreter.

**The procedure**: The patient is on clear liquids the day prior to the procedure and swallows the capsule with water after a 12-h fast. Drinking clear fluids is allowed 2 h after ingestion as is a light lunch after 4 h. During the procedure, he is free to do his daily activities.

A few grading scales have been developed to assess the quality of bowel preparation in video capsule endoscopy, the most recent being a computer-assisted cleansing score (CAC) [7]. The impact of bowel preparation on the image quality and transit time was assessed in two meta-analyses. Preparation was found to improve the quality of visualization, but had no effect on transit times or percentage of capsules reaching the cecum, and no consensus was reached as to the effects on the diagnostic yield of the study [8, 9]. Another attempt to improve the small bowel diagnostic yield was attempted by using a capsule with two cameras (one on each side), which resulted in diagnosis of more lesions [10].

**The main indications for SBCE include the following**:
1. Obscure gastrointestinal bleeding
2. Crohn's disease (suspected/known)
3. Suspected small bowel tumor
4. Evaluation of abnormal small bowel imaging
5. Partially/non-responsive celiac disease
6. Surveillance of inherited polyposis syndromes
7. Evaluation of drug-induced small bowel injury and response to medications

**Contraindications include the following**:
1. History of or suspected small bowel obstruction
2. Swallowing disorders
3. Pregnancy
4. Non-compliance

**Relative contraindications are as follows**:
1. Major abdominal surgery in the previous 6 months.
2. Cardiac devices—pacemaker/defibrillator.

Although the capsule is easily ingested and swallowed by most individuals, patients with severe dysphagia, large Zenker's diverticulum, pill phobia, significant gastroparesis, and small children may have problems ingesting the device. For these situations, a capsule-loading device (AdvanCE, US Endoscopy, Mentor, Ohio, USA) is available to directly deliver the capsule into the stomach or duodenum.

In case of suspected small bowel obstruction, the use of a patency capsule (the AGILE capsule, Given Imaging, Yokneam, Israel) has been shown to provide evidence of the functional patency of the gastrointestinal tract [10] (Fig. 2.3). This system consists of a self-disintegrating capsule without a camera that contains radio frequency identification (RFID) tag and a RFID scanner. In a case of obstructive small bowel pathology, the AGILE capsule disintegrates within 30 h, and the remnants can pass through even small orifices [11]. The radio-opaque capsule can be detected by plain abdominal X-ray.

### 2.1.3 Occult GI Bleeding

Occult GI bleeding accounts for up to two-thirds of SBCE studies performed [12]. It was shown that 20–38 % of patients with normal upper and lower endoscopy have significant intestinal lesions [13, 14] (Fig. 2.5). SBCE has been shown to be superior to push enteroscopy, abdominal computed tomography, abdominal magnetic resonance and angiographic studies [15–18], and as good as balloon-assisted small bowel enteroscopy [19], with diagnostic yield between 39 and 90 % [20]. Moreover, the rate of rebleeding in patients with occult GI bleeding and negative SBCE was found to be significantly lower (4.6 %) compared with those with a positive SBCE (48 %) [21].

**This information will be covered in detail in the chapter on PillCam small bowel**.

### 2.1.4 Crohn's Disease

SBCE is an important tool both in the diagnosis and in the follow-up of Crohn's disease. It is used to establish the diagnosis, to assess disease extent, severity, and disease activity, and to assess mucosal healing post-therapy (Fig. 2.6).

SBCE has a high diagnostic yield in suspected Crohn's disease. Moreover, for both known and suspected Crohn's disease, SBCE was found to

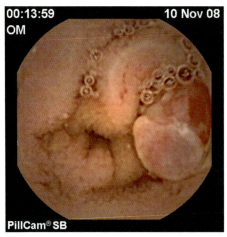

Panel A: Active bleeding

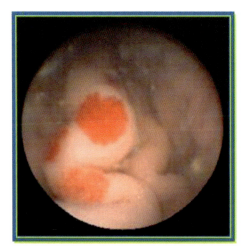

Panel B: Angioectasia

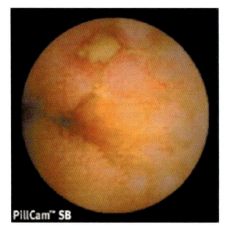

Panel C: Small bowel ulceration

**Fig. 2.5** Causes for small bowel obscure bleeding

have a better incremental yield (ranging between 15 and 44 %) compared with other modalities, including small bowel follow-through, computed tomography, MRI, ileo-colonoscopy, and push enteroscopy [21]. Increase in the diagnostic yield of SBCE can be achieved by selecting patients with high pretest probability such as those with perianal disease and negative work-up, using the international conference on capsule endoscopy (ICCE) selection criteria and/or patients with high fecal calprotectin level.

SBCE may alter disease management of patients with known Crohn's, by assessing mucosal healing after medical therapy. SBCE is the only method, except for double-balloon enteroscopy, to accurately assess small bowel mucosal healing. SBCE was also found to be clinically useful for categorizing patients with indeterminate colitis, although negative SBCE study did not exclude further diagnosis of Crohn's.

The rate of SBCE retention in patients with suspected Crohn's disease is similar to the general population (1.4 %), but retention rates of more than 8 % were reported in patients with established Crohn's disease.

## 2.1.5 Small Bowel Tumors

The introduction of SBCE had resulted in doubling the rate of diagnosis of small bowel tumors to 6–9 % of patients undergoing SBCE for various indications, obscure GI bleeding being the most common indication. More than half of the tumors diagnosed were malignant. Adenocarcinoma is the most common malignant tumor, followed by carcinoids, lymphomas, sarcomas, and hamartomas [22]. Gastrointestinal stromal tumors are the most frequent benign neoplasm (32 % of all cases). Melanoma is the most common tumor metastasizing to the small bowel, although metastases derived from colorectal cancer and hepatocellular carcinoma have also been reported. Tumors are located most frequently in the jejunum (40–60 %), followed by the ileum (25–40 %), and the duodenum (15–20 %). Small bowel tumors can be easily missed due to the predominant submucosal and extraluminal

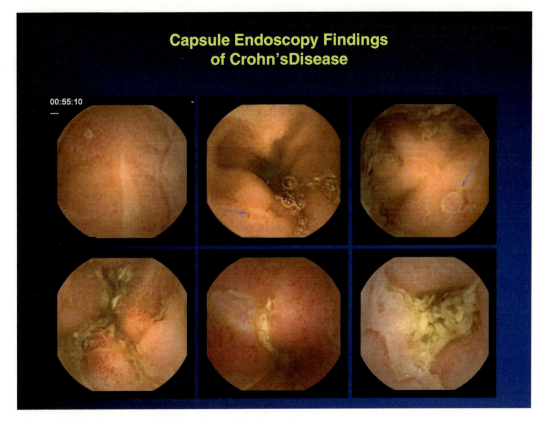

**Fig. 2.6** Small bowel Crohn's disease

location of the tumors. Specific indexes and scales were developed for improving the detection rate of small bowel tumors, including the Smooth Protruding Index on Capsule Endoscopy (SPICE score) and an automated scale using multiscale wavelet-based analysis [23, 24].

**More details will be provided in the chapter on PillCam SB**.

### 2.1.6   Celiac Disease

SBCE has a role in both the diagnosis of celiac disease and in the evaluation of gluten refractory celiac disease (Fig. 2.7). SBCE provides high-resolution magnified view of the mucosa, easily identifying the endoscopic changes found in celiac such as scalloping, mosaic pattern, flat mucosa, loss of folds, and nodularity. In a recent published meta-analysis, SBCE had an overall pooled sensitivity of 89 % and specificity of

95 % for identifying celiac disease [25]. In gluten non-responsive celiac disease, SBCE can be used for investigating the small bowel for tumors (enteropathy-associated T-cell lymphoma and adenocarcinoma) and ulcerative jejuno-ileitis (Fig. 2.7).

### 2.1.7   Inherited Polyposis Syndromes

SBCE was shown to be effective tool in detecting small bowel polyps in Peutz–Jegher syndrome. It is especially effective in demonstrating small- and medium-size polyps. However, large polyps are sometimes only demonstrated partially, and polyp location is not accurate [26]. The duodenum is a potential pitfall as the capsule passes it very fast and thus may give false-negative results. The new SB3 SBCE may improve that with its six frames per second mode. Coupling of SBCE with double-balloon

**Fig. 2.7** Typical PillCam SB findings in celiac disease

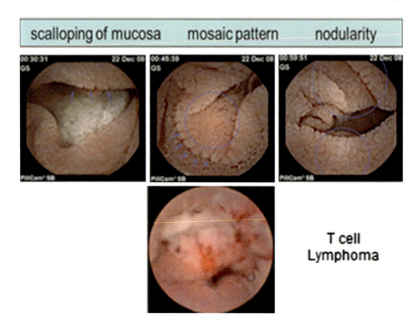

enteroscopy and polypectomy may offer an ideal method of follow-up and treatment of these patients, possibly avoiding surgery.

Another indication for SBCE in this setting is familial adenomatosis polyposis (FAP) in which one may find patients with duodenal polyps, as well as small bowel polyps. However, the major papilla is not demonstrated effectively, and complementary examination with a side-view duodenoscope is mandatory.

### 2.1.8 Monitoring Effects and Side Effects of Drugs

SBCE can be used to monitor deleterious effects of drugs such as NSAIDs on small bowel mucosa. Lesions that can be found in these patients include erythema, erosions, small ulcerations, and weblike strictures. SBCE can be used to monitor the effect of drugs used to protect against NSAIDs-induced small bowel injury, to monitor the small bowel mucosal appearance in transplanted patients, to manage graft versus host disease, and, possibly, to monitor mucosal healing of small bowel Crohn's disease after various medical treatments.

### 2.1.9 Capsule Retention

Capsule retention is the major complication of SBCE. Very rarely this may end in bowel obstruction/perforation. High risk of retention occurs in patients on NSAIDs, with known Crohn's, with radiation enteritis, or with small bowel tumors. Normal prior radiological examination does not always protect from having capsule retention. Once retention is diagnosed (capsule not excreted 2 weeks after ingestion), endoscopic (balloon-assisted enteroscopy) or surgical removal was shown to be effective. The intervention not only allows removal of the capsule, but also allows the offending abnormality.

### 2.1.10 Esophageal Video Capsule Endoscopy

In 2004, Given Imaging developed an esophageal video capsule (PillCam ESO) as a noninvasive device for the examination of the esophagus. The second-generation esophageal capsule, the Pill-Cam ESO2 (Given Imaging, Yokneam, Israel), was FDA-approved for marketing in 2007

**Fig. 2.8** PillCam ESO capsule endoscope

**PillCam Eso 2**

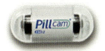

- 11mm x 26mm
- 2 cameras
- 18 frames/second
- Advanced optics / 3 lenses
- Advanced ALC
- Extra-wide AOV  169°

(Fig. 2.8). The esophageal capsule endoscope (ECE) is a 26 × 11 mm capsule that differs from the SBCE in a few parameters: It has optical domes on both sides, the frame rate is much faster (9 frames from each side versus 2), a wider angle of view (169 vs. 156°), more advanced optics (3 lenses), and a shorter battery life of up to 30 min, all aimed to address the very short time (<2 s) of esophageal transit as well as the necessity to demonstrate the esophageal–gastric junction, where most of the esophageal pathology is located. It works for approximately 30 min and then shuts off and passed through the intestine via peristalsis and is naturally excreted. As in PillCam SB 3 system, or PillCam Colon2, real-time viewing is feasible.

**Procedure**: Prolongation of the transit time of the capsule has been achieved by an alteration of the capsule ingestion technique, using the simplified ingestion procedure (SIP) (Fig. 2.9), where the patient swallows the capsule after at least 3 h of fasting, lying in the right lateral position while sipping 15 mL of water every 30 s through a straw [27]. The procedure requires up to 5 min in an unsedated patient. Thus far, no other esophageal capsules are in the market. Competition includes attempts to attach a string to a Given Imaging small bowel capsule, the Given Imaging magnetic capsule, and the Olympus gastric capsule which are maneuvered with a joystick (Fig. 2.10).

**Indications for ECE**:
- Screening for Barrett's esophagus
- Surveillance of esophageal varices in patients with portal hypertension.

ECE is safe, well tolerated, and reported to be preferred by patients to unsedated EGD. ECE was found to have variable sensitivity and specificity for the detection of GERD-related complications. Few studies reported very high specificity and sensitivity for the detection of erosive esophagitis and Barrett's esophagus (Fig. 2.11) [28, 29], while others found much lower rates of sensitivity and specificity. A recent meta-analysis of seven studies involving 446 patients, ECE was found to have a sensitivity of 86 % and specificity 81 % in detecting esophageal varices (Fig. 2.12) [30].

**Further details will be given in the chapter on Esophageal Capsule Endoscopy**.

ECE may be used as an alternative to conventional upper GI endoscopy for the diagnosis of varices in complex patients with portal hypertension. It is most useful in certain patient groups: patients who poorly tolerate endoscopy or who have significant comorbidity, thus increasing the risks of repeated endoscopy, and patients with high risk of variant Creutzfeldt–Jakob disease.

Although the major innovations and technological advancement, at this point of time, ECE is not recommended as initial screening tool for the mentioned conditions, mainly due to the lower cost and higher availability of upper endoscopy.

### 2.1.11 Colon Capsule Endoscopy

Colon capsule endoscopy (CCE) (Given Imaging Ltd., Yokneam, Israel) was introduced in 2006 for the diagnosis of colonic pathologies, mainly polyps and tumors. In 2009, it went through major upgrading when the second generation of the capsule was introduced (Fig. 2.13). The second-generation capsule is slightly larger than the SBCE (31 × 11 mm) and has two camera domes with an adaptive frame rate of 4–35 frames per second, a 172° view angle for each camera, and longer life of up to 11 h due to the addition of a third battery and advanced engineering techniques. As mentioned, the frame rate can reach up to 35 frames

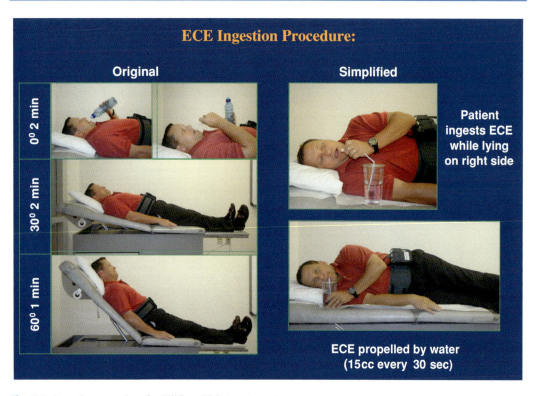

**Fig. 2.9** Ingestion procedure for PillCam ESO capsule endoscope

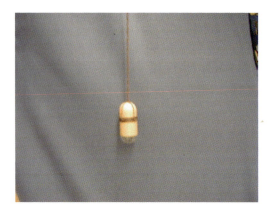

**Fig. 2.10** String capsule device. Reprint with permission from Ramirez et al. [32]

per second depending on the capsule movement speed in the colon and is determined using the revolutionized adaptive frame rate technique via a cross talk between the capsule and the data recorder (DR3). This new recorder is endowed with artificial intelligence that communicates with the capsule, as well as with the patient by beeping and vibrating when the capsule leaves the stomach and displaying on the LCD screen a message that informs the patient to ingest a booster laxative which will accelerate the passage of the capsule through the small bowel.

**Procedure**: As in colonoscopy, bowel preparation is compulsory in order to achieve adequate mucosal visualization. This is done using a strict preparation that includes liquid diet on the day prior to capsule ingestion, two doses of 2 l of PEG solution (on the evening prior to ingestion and on the morning of the capsule ingestion), as well as propulsive agents to enhance capsule movement in the small bowel and advance it to and through the colon, while the battery is still working.

The main indication for CCE is colonic polyp detection (Table 2.1, Fig. 2.14). Colonic screening programs in moderate- and high-risk groups reduced the incidence, morbidity, and mortality due to colorectal carcinoma. However,

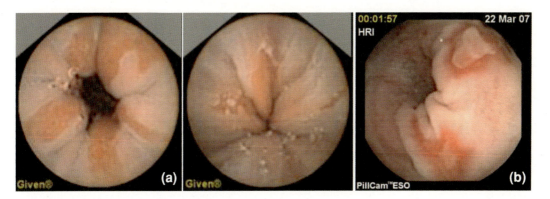

**Fig. 2.11** PillCam ESO pictures of Barrett's (**a**) and esophagitis (**b**)

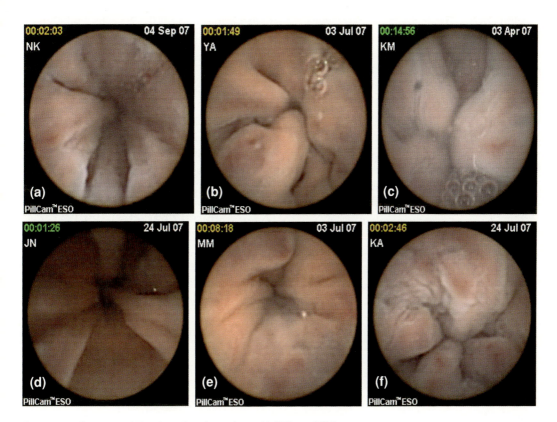

**Fig. 2.12** **a–f** Images of Esophageal varices taken with Pillcom ESO

compliance rates to colonoscopy screening programs are hampered due to fear of the invasiveness and possible complications. CCE allows visualization of colonic mucosa with a minimally invasive procedure using no sedation, insufflation, or radiation and a practically complication-free method for colorectal screening.

Because noninvasive colorectal imaging tests cannot provide a histological diagnosis, morphological criteria (i.e., polyp/mass ≥6 mm in size, or ≥3 polyps) are accepted as surrogate markers of advanced neoplasia. The average sensitivity of the first generation of CCE for significant findings (≥6 mm size, or ≥3 polyps

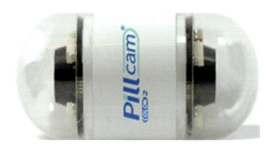

**Fig. 2.13** PillCam Colon2 capsule endoscope

irrespective of size) was relatively low, but it significantly improved with the use of the second-generation CCE (49).

**Indications**: The latest guidelines published in 2012 by the European Society of Gastrointestinal Endoscopy (ESGE) [31] state that:

- CCE is feasible and safe and appears to be accurate when used in average-risk individuals.
- In patients with high risk for colorectal carcinoma in whom colonoscopy is not possible or not feasible, CCE could be a possible study.
- CCE is also a feasible and safe tool for visualization of the colonic mucosa in patients with incomplete colonoscopy and without stenosis.

Another possible indication for CCE is in the diagnostic work-up or in the surveillance of patients with suspected or known inflammatory bowel disease (IBD), especially ulcerative colitis. Further details can be found in the chapter on Colonic Capsule Endoscopy.

## 2.1.12 Summary

Since its introduction almost 13 years ago, the clinical indications for the use of capsule endoscopy have widened considerably. Capsule endoscopy has been proven to be a useful minimally invasive tool in the exploration of the entire gastrointestinal tract, allowing visualization of previously inaccessible parts and achieving worthy satisfaction from both physicians and patients. New indications and future possibility to control the capsule movement enabling new possibilities for diagnosis and targeted therapy will evolve with the future technologic advancement.

## 2.2 EndoCapsule

The EndoCapsule (Olympus, Tokyo, Japan) is a video capsule endoscopy for the small intestine using a charge-coupled device sensor instead of a CMOS to acquire images (Fig. 2.15). Launched in Europe in 2005, EndoCapsule obtained FDA clearance in 2007 [33]. The EndoCapsule consists of a camera, light source, transmitter, and batteries. Once the capsule is activated and swallowed by the patient, it begins transmitting images of the digestive system to a receiver worn by the patient. After the examination, the patient returns the receiver to the physician or a nurse who can download all images to a computer and find the abnormalities in small intestine (Fig. 2.16).

### 2.2.1 Special Characteristics [34]

1. High-resolution CCD
2. Smart Recorder: It combines a receiver and viewer in a compact and easy-to-handle unit, allowing the physician to playback and capture images any time during the procedure.
3. 3D Track Function: That function offers intuitive operation, showing capsule location to help you decide what approach should be taken for subsequent procedures.

### 2.2.2 Preparation

The bowel preparation of Endocapsule examination includes a 12-h fast prior to the procedure, the administration of 2 l of polyethylene glycol (PEG) solution in the evening and 1 l 30 min before the procedure.

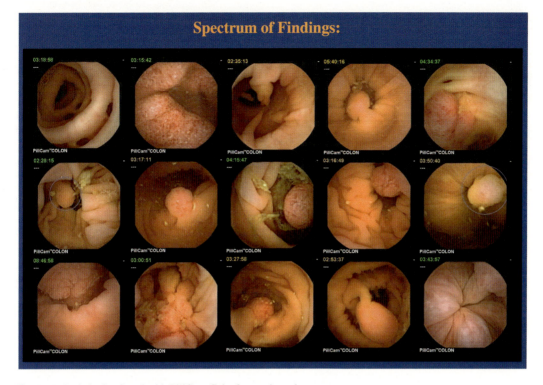

**Fig. 2.14** Pathologies found with PillCam Colon2 capsule endoscope

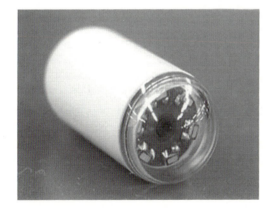

**Fig. 2.15** The Endocapsule. Reprint with permission from Ogata et al. [38]

### 2.2.3   Clinical Studies

In a British retrospective cohort study, 70 patients performed Endocapsule examination using either overview with express-selected (ES) or overview with auto-speed-adjusted (ASA) modes. The ES-mode software eliminates

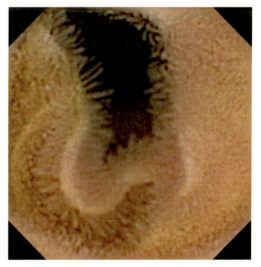

**Fig. 2.16** Small intestinal villi detected by the Endocapsule. Reprint with permission from Cave et al. [36]

images with no significant changes (compared with the previous frames) in the video. And the ASA-mode software speeds up the fps of the CE video when detecting repetitive images. Among 40 (57 %) patients found with clinically significant findings, 32 (80 %) were recognized with overview function alone, while 39 (97.5 %) were recognized with overview function plus ES or ASA modes. The average reading time for overview with ES mode (19 ± 5 min) was significantly less than for overview with ASA mode (34 ± 10 min) ($p = 0.001$). These new playback systems can efficaciously reduce reading times of CE but need further evaluation in prospective multicenter studies [35].

Cave et al. carried out a multicenter randomized comparison of the Endocapsule and the PillCam SB in the USA. Results showed the positive percent agreement of 70.6 % and a negative percent disagreement of 82.4 % with an overall agreement of 74.5 %. The overall agreement was 74.5 % (38/51) with a $\kappa$ of 0.48 and $P = 0.008$. The study demonstrated that Endocapsule had a similar diagnostic yield and better image quality compared with PillCam SB [36].

In another randomized head-to-head comparison study in Austria, 50 patients were randomly assigned to swallow either the MiroCam first, followed by the EndoCapsule 2 h later, or vice versa. The MiroCam and EndoCapsule devices were not statistically different with regard to their rates of complete small bowel examinations (96 vs. 90 %) or diagnostic yield (50 vs. 48 %). However, the findings were concordant in 68 % only (kappa = 0.50). The combined diagnostic yield was 58 % [37].

## 2.3 OMOM Capsule Endoscopy Platform

### 2.3.1 Overview

The creation of capsule endoscopy provides a new method for the visualized diagnosis of digestive diseases. It fixes the deficiency of the visualized diagnosis of small bowel diseases and brings a development direction of noninvasive, convenient, safe, and comfort diagnosis.

OMOM capsule endoscopy system is developed by Chongqing Science and Technology (Group) Co. Ltd. Comparing with other similar products, the unique feature of duplex multichannel communication mode has largely increased the controllability and convenience in its clinical use. Through the verification of clinical application, the product has equal validity and yield rate comparing with other similar products from overseas in the diagnosis of small bowel diseases, such as obscure GI bleeding, Crohn's disease, small bowel tumor, and small bowel polyp [39–41].

Since the first generation of OMOM capsule endoscopy successfully created in 2004, Chongqing Jinshan Science and Technology has been dedicated to provide comprehensive solutions in the diagnosis of digestive diseases. Based on the first generation of capsule endoscopy, the company has developed various new capsule endoscopy products according to different clinical uses, such as controllable capsule endoscopy, storable capsule endoscopy, and CCE, in which it can provide safe, noninvasive, comfort, and convenient visualized diagnosis for the whole digestive tract.

After nearly 10 years of development, Chongqing Jinshan Science and Technology in the field of digestive medical area has launched a series of high-end products according to different clinical uses, in which they are able to provide accurate diagnosis of digestive tract disease with comprehensive and personalized solutions. The following article will describe in detail about the application range, product formation, functions, and features of the products.

### 2.3.2 Small Bowel Capsule Endoscopy

OMOM small bowel capsule endoscopy is mainly used for visualized diagnosis of small bowel diseases. It is a new diagnosis method which is noninvasive, painless, safe, and comfort. After swallowing the capsule, it will pass through esophagus, stomach, duodenum, jejunum, ileum, and colon and finally expel from human body naturally by digestive tract

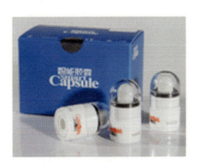
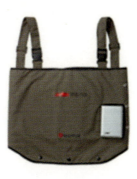
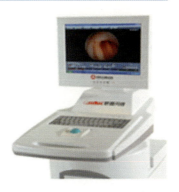

Capsule          Image recorder          Image workstation

**Fig. 2.17** Small bowel capsule endoscopy system formation

peristalsis. The capsule will continuously capture images of the GI tract during its movement process and transmit real-time image data wirelessly to the external image recorder. After the monitoring process, doctors can replay and analyze the saved images through the image workstation and finally make diagnosis of the gastrointestinal illness.

Small bowel capsule endoscopy system is mainly comprised of three parts: capsule, image recorder, and image workstation (Fig. 2.17), and functions of each part are described below:

**Capsule**: Capturing real-time image of GI tract and transmitting image wirelessly to the external image recorder; meanwhile, it is able to receive control signal from the image recorder to adjust working parameter.

**Image recorder**: Receiving and saving digital images from the capsule; also, it is able to send control signal to adjust the working parameter of the capsule.

**Image workstation**: Man–machine interactive operation platform can monitor the working condition of the capsule in real time and adjusting its working status. It is able to download and replay image data from the image recorder, assisting doctors to make diagnosis.

**Indications**:
1. GI hemorrhage, with no positive finding in upper and lower GI tract endoscopic examination;
2. Small intestine imaging anomaly suggested by other examinations;
3. Any type of IBDs, excluding bowel obstruction;
4. Unexplained abdominal pain and diarrhea;
5. Small intestine tumor (benign, malignant, carcinoid, etc.);
6. Unexplained iron-deficient anemia.

**Contradictions**:
1. Patients who are confirmed (or suspected) to suffer from digestive tract malformation, gastrointestinal obstruction, gastrointestinal perforation, stenosis, or fistula;
2. Patients implanted with pacemaker or other electronic devices;
3. Patients suffering from severe dysphagia;
4. Patients suffering from acute enteritis or severe iron deficiency, for example, bacillary dysentery at active phase and ulcerative colitis at acute phase, particularly for patients suffering from fulminant diseases;
5. Patients allergic to polymer material;
6. Use with caution for patients below 18 and above 70 and for psychopath;
7. Pregnant woman.

### 2.3.2.1 Features
- Pioneer of duplex communication

It supports duplex data transmission between the capsule and the image recorder. The real-time monitoring function, which can check the captured images in real time during the

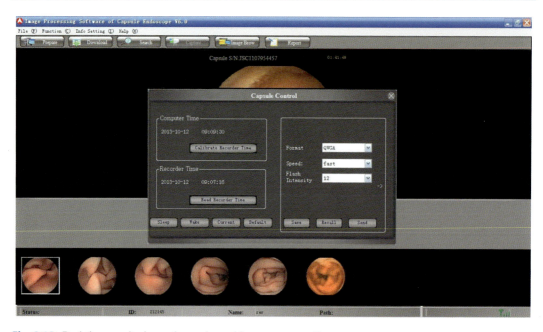

**Fig. 2.18** Real-time monitoring and capsule working parameter adjustment

examination, can able to make intuitive judgment about the location of the capsule within the GI tract. At the same time, it can control the parameters of the capsule, such as capture frequency, brightness, and exposure, in order to extend the monitoring time (Fig. 2.18). This function has been widely spread in clinical use, and it can increase the completion rate of small bowel examination up to 100 % [42, 43].

• Unique multichannel mode

OMOM capsule endoscopy system supports simultaneous activation of multiple capsules at the same place, without interference between each of the capsules. Currently, OMOM capsule has 10 channels, which means it can undertake 10 patients simultaneously at the same location in the hospital without interference between each other. The image workstation can simultaneously monitor images from four capsules in real time (Fig. 2.19).

• Unique wireless USB monitoring

The wireless USB monitor is a convenient tool. It enables wireless communication, real-time monitoring, and capsule working parameter adjustment between the image recorder and the image workstation.

### 2.3.2.2 Clinical Application

Since 2005, OMOM capsule endoscopy has been used in clinic for over 8 years, and it has completed over 1 million samples. Clinical contrast study shows that OMOM capsule endoscope comparing with PillCam SB by Israeli company Given Imaging has no significant differences in the diagnosis of small bowel diseases, such as obscure GI bleeding, vascular malformation, small bowel tumor, small bowel polyp, and Crohn's disease [44]. In addition, during the clinical use of OMOM capsule, its special feature of duplex communication function that enables real-time adjustment of image capture frequency can achieve 100 % completion rate of small bowel examination [42].

In 2,400 patients who had OMOM capsule examination [45], the diagnostic yield of small bowel diseases was 47.7 %. In all findings of small bowel, 28.1 % was vascular malformation, 18.9 % small bowel tumor, 10.4 % polyp, 7.9 % Crohn's disease, 15 % mucosa injury and ulcers, 5.2 % bleeding, 11.3 % parasite, diverticulum, and so on. Comparing with traditional clinical methods such as GI radiography and CT, OMOM capsule endoscopy can provide more

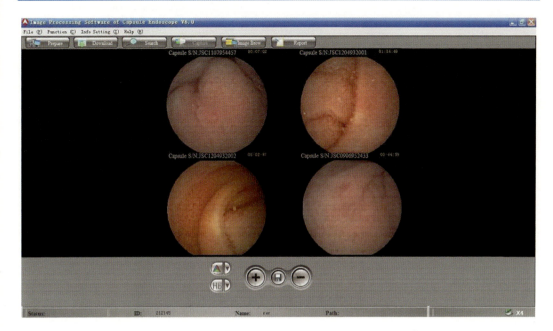

**Fig. 2.19** Real-time monitoring of four capsules

intuitive and clear images of small bowel, which is able to significantly increase the complete small bowel examination rate (CSER) and yield rate, and also, it provides more safety and reliability [46, 47]. At the same time, OMOM capsule endoscopy can incorporate other diagnostic methods such as double-balloon endoscopy in clinical use. It can further improve the CSER and yield rate, and it can help to confirm the lesion position and features prior to the small bowel surgery which is efficient to lower the risk and difficulty of the surgery, thus improving the surgery succession rate [48, 49].

### 2.3.3   Controllable Capsule Endoscopy

OMOM controllable capsule endoscopy is developed based on the small bowel capsule endoscopy. It can not only be used for visual diagnosis of small bowel, but can also achieve movement and angle control within the stomach. After swallowing the controllable capsule into the stomach, an external controller can control

the capsule movement, posture, and angle from outside the body, which makes stomach examination controllable and comprehensive. After the stomach examination, the capsule will enter duodenum, jejunum, and ileum through GI tract peristalsis, and after the complete visualized examination of small bowel, it will pass through colon and be expelled from the body naturally. The capsule will continuously capture images within the stomach and small bowel during the examination, and the images will be transmitted and stored into the external image recorder wirelessly. After the examination, doctors can analyze the images and make diagnosis through the image workstation. The controllable capsule endoscope has solved the problems of ordinary capsule when undertaking stomach examination, such as large blind spot, insufficient observation, and high misdiagnose rate. It provides a painless, noninvasive, safe, and comfort method for stomach examination. Clinical study shows that the controllable capsule can achieve comprehensive examination of stomach fundus, stomach antrum, stomach corner, and stomach body

**Fig. 2.20** Controller

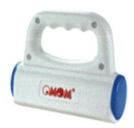

Controller

with high detection rate and low misdiagnose rate [50, 51].

Controllable capsule endoscopy system is comprised of four parts: capsule, image recorder, image workstation, and controller (Fig. 2.20).

### 2.3.4 Storable Capsule Endoscope

Storable capsule endoscope uses a large capacity storage module instead of traditional data transmission module. The captured images will be stored within the internal capsule memory module.

The advantages of storable capsule endoscopes are as follows: Patients do not need to wear an image recorder after swallowing the capsule, and they only need to be aware of the time of expelling the capsule from the body and collecting it. Then, a unique data reading and image viewing tool is used to process the images in order to make an analysis.

The storable capsule endoscope is disposable. The large capacity storage module contains 8 GB of memory which can store over 120,000 images. The working duration of the capsule reaches 15 h.

Storable capsule endoscope system is comprised of three parts: capsule, data reader, and image workstation.

Storable capsule endoscope is mainly used for the diagnosis of small bowel diseases such as unknown abdominal pain, GI hemorrhage, small bowel tumor, and Crohn's disease.

### 2.3.5 Colon Capsule Endoscope

Colon capsule endoscope is a painless, noninvasive, safe, and comfortable diagnose method specially designed for colon disease. According to the physiological structure of colon and based on traditional capsule endoscope, it augmented more features such as capsule controlling, position measurement, posture measurement, and adjustment. It can achieve to control the movement, posture, and position of the capsule within the whole colon. Colon capsule can be entered to the colon through swallowing or anus insertion. The movement of the capsule can be fully controlled by the external controlling device. The capture images will be transmitted to the control panel in real time wirelessly, and adjust the capsule posture and angle to ensure the comprehensiveness and reliability of the examination. Therefore, comprehensive diagnosis of the whole colon can be achieved.

Colon capsule endoscope system is comprised of three parts: colon capsule, controlling device, and control panel (Fig. 2.21).

Colon capsule endoscope system is mainly used for the diagnosis of various colon diseases such as colon inflammation, ulcer, diverticulum, polyp, and tumor.

### 2.3.6 pH Capsule Wireless Monitoring System

Gastroesophageal reflux disease (GERD) is a common digestive disease which affects 10–20 % of European and American population [52], and this ratio is relatively lower in Asia, but it has an increasing trend [53]. Clinical research shows that continuous pH monitoring within esophagus is the most effective way of diagnosing GERD [54]. OMOM pH capsule wireless monitoring system is mainly used to monitor the pH value inside the esophagus and make diagnosis of GERD through detecting the change in pH value.

**Fig. 2.21** Colon capsule endoscope system formation

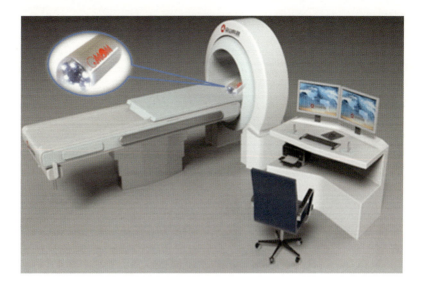

The pH capsule is sent and fixed on the mucosa of the esophagus through the catheter, and it will monitor the pH value within the esophagus with the sensor through 96 h of continuous examination. The monitored data will be transmitted to the external data recorder wirelessly, and the doctor can make diagnosis by analyzing the continuously monitored pH data parameter through the workstation after the examination is completed. The capsule will naturally drop off from the mucosa and finally expel from the body.

Clinical application research shows that OMOM pH capsule wireless monitoring system is safe and efficient for diagnosing GERD. Long continuous monitoring time can reflect the status of the gastroesophagus reflux, which leads to high GERD positive detection rate, and it can effectively evaluate the frequency and severity of the reflux [55]. Comparing with traditional pH monitoring method such as catheter-based monitoring and endoscopy, it has similar diagnosis effect, but with easier and more convenient clinical operation [56, 57]; also, long monitoring time of 96 h is not only effective for GERD diagnosis in the early stage, but also effective for assisting therapeutic decision in the later stage, and it evaluates the effectiveness of medical treatment.

pH capsule wireless monitoring system is mainly comprised of three parts: pH capsule (including the catheter), data recorder, and data analyzing software.

**Indications**:

1. Patients have classic symptoms of acid reflux or heartburn and are considered as GERD patients;
2. Patients suffer from unexplained chronic pharyngitis, hoarseness, trachitis, or asthma and are considered as those having extra-esophageal symptoms of GERD;
3. Patients who are considered as GERD patients and are positive in PPI therapeutic test;

**Contradictions**:

1. Patients who are confirmed (or suspected) to suffer from upper esophageal or nasopharyngeal obstruction;
2. Patients who are confirmed (or suspected) to suffer from esophageal varices according to gastroscopy, clinical radiology, or other examinations;
3. Patients who are confirmed to suffer from esophageal mucosa erosion according to gastroscopy or other examinations;
4. Patients who are confirmed (or suspected) to suffer from congenital digestive tract malformation, gastrointestinal obstruction, and perforation, stricture, or fistula of digestive tract according to clinical radiology or other examinations;
5. Patients who had bleeding tendency or gastrointestinal bleeding in the recent 6 months or have taken anticoagulant drugs for a long period of time;

6. Patients who suffer from heart disease and are not stable;
7. Patients implanted with pacemaker or other medical devices;
8. Patients who had history of allergy to polymer material.

### 2.3.7 Impedance–pH Monitoring System

Impedance–pH monitoring system is used for the diagnosis of GERD, which is an alternative method of pH capsule wireless monitoring system. The principle of this product is that it integrated both pH sensor and impedance sensor. The sensors are sent to the esophagus through nose by using a catheter, they will continuously monitor the patient's pH data and impedance data within the esophagus, and the data will be transmitted to the external data recorder. Doctors can analyze the changes of pH data and impedance data through the workstation, in order to make the final diagnosis. Through clinical study, the added impedance monitoring can not only increase the reliability of diagnosing GERD, but also detect alkaline reflux, which is valuable for comprehensive GERD monitoring and evaluation in clinical use [58, 59].

Impedance–pH monitoring system consists of three parts: catheter, data recorder, and data analyzing workstation.

### 2.3.8 Conclusion

Capsule endoscope has provided a new method of diagnosing GI diseases in clinical use. The medical field calls it as the development trend of GI endoscopy in twenty-first century, and it brings the third revolution in GI endoscopy development history. Its existence has made the development trend of GI disease diagnosis toward noninvasive, convenient, safe, and comfort.

OMOM capsule endoscope has entered for clinical use since 2005, and in 8 years of clinical use and research, it has verified this product as

an effective method of visualized diagnosis for GI diseases. Comparing with similar products such as PillCam by Given Imaging, EndoCapsule by Olympus, and MiroCam by Intromedic, OMOM capsule endoscope has same diagnosis effect with lower price which is more acceptable and affordable for patients. Based on OMOM capsule endoscope, Chongqing Jinshan Science and Technology has developed a series of new products according to the clinical use of visualized diagnosis in GI diseases, such as controllable capsule endoscope and colon capsule endoscope. At the same time, it has developed products for diagnosing GI function disorders, such as pH capsule wireless monitoring system and impedance–pH monitoring system which is able to provide comprehensive solutions for GI disease diagnosis.

With the development of new technologies and applications in the field of medical application, the future research and application of the GI diagnostic technology will mainly carry out in three directions: (1) the application of multisensing and detection technology for more comprehensive diagnostic information; (2) the development direction from minimal invasive to noninvasive; and (3) the development direction from diagnosis to diagnosis–treatment combined. The capsule endoscope will eventually develop from a diagnostic tool to a diagnosis–treatment-combined intelligent robot.

## 2.4 MiroCam

### 2.4.1 Background of Development

Since the first development of a wireless capsule endoscope, M2A, the prototype of PillCam (Given Imaging Yokneam, Israel) in 2000 [60], it has been widely applied in clinical practice for the investigation of small bowel disease. Capsule endoscopy is easily performed only by swallowing the pill-sized capsule and so overcomes the limitations of conventional endoscopy such as highly uncomfortable process, the necessity for skilled physician, and varied quality or outcome of examination depending on the physician's skill. Followed by M2A, other companies competitively released new capsule endoscopes in the market: Endocapsule EC type 1 (Olympus Ltd., Tokyo, Japan) in Japan [61] and OMOM (Jinshan Science and Technology Company, Chongqing) in China [62]. Even though there is a little difference in detail specs, these capsule endoscopes adopted the same transmission system, radio frequency (RF), for exporting imaging data to the receiver. RF system made wireless capsule endoscopes possible, but this system is energy-consuming, which limits the operation time of capsule endoscopes and complete examination up to cecum.

MiRo capsule endoscope, which was introduced in Korea in 2007 [63] and prototype of MiroCam, is the smallest and lightest capsule endoscope with the longest operation time up to 11 h by using distinctly different transmission system and human body communication. Miro-Cam was approved for general clinical use in Europe in August 2007 and by the US Food and Drug Administration (FDA) in June 2012.

### 2.4.1.1 Specifications of MiroCam

Generally, capsule endoscope systems have three components: a capsule endoscope body, an external receiving antenna with attached portable hard disk drive (data recorder), and a customized PC work station with dedicated software for review and interpretation of images [64]. Miro-Cam capsule is a pill-sized endoscopic body consisting of lens, imaging sensor, light source, power source, and telemetry device (Fig. 2.22).

### Characteristics of MiroCam

The MiroCam is $10.8 \times 24$ mm, smaller than PillCam at $11 \times 24$ mm and weighed 3.3 g [65]. It has an image field of 150° and resolution power of $320 \times 320$ pixels, which is a significant improvement over the $256 \times 256$ pixels in the PillCam. It includes a sensitive, low-power CMOS image sensor converting the optical rays to electrical voltages and a white-light-emitting

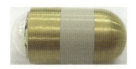

**Fig. 2.22** MiroCam (MC1000)

diode (LED) as the illumination source. Two serial silver oxide batteries are used as a power source and operate for 9–11 h.

### A Novel Transmission System and Human Body Communication with Electric Field Propagation

For imaging transmission, conventional endoscopes have a direct signal path, such as a conductive wire between the camera and data recorder. But capsule endoscope systems need wireless transmitter that delivers the imaging data to a receiver outside of the body. The basic telemetry system of capsule endoscope is composed of three elementary components [65]. The transmitter, at some location in space, converts the message signal produced by a source of information into a form suitable for transmission over a channel. The channel, in turn, transports the message signal and delivers it to a receiver at some other location in space [67].

For the wireless transmission, the standard capsule endoscope uses RF communication technology. But RF system has a drawback of severe power consumption as follows. A local oscillator makes a very-high frequency carrier, and an amplifier lets signal transport high power. In addition most energy generated from transmitter is lost because of radiation characteristics of RF energy [65]. Instead of this power-consuming technology, MiroCam adopted novel human body communication technology known as electric field propagation, which is patent in the USA [67]. This technology uses the human body as a semiconductor for data transmission, and an elective field can be induced and consequently generates drift current, even though the body has poor conductivity compared with a metal wire [65]. A space-occupying additional antenna or high-frequency circuit for remote communication is useless in MiroCam, and only

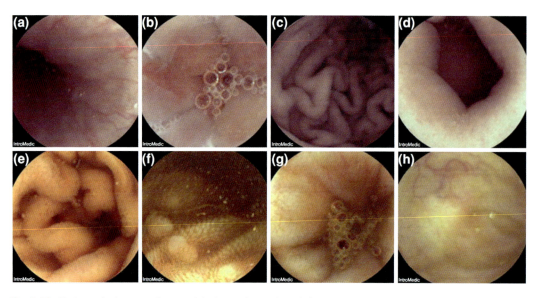

**Fig. 2.23** Endoscopic images of normal lesions taken by MiroCam. **a** Esophagus. **b** Esophageal–gastric junction. **c** Body of stomach. **d** Pylorus of stomach. **e** Small bowel. **f** Lymphoid hyperplasia of terminal ileum. **g** Ileocecal valve. **h** Appendiceal orifice of Cecum

simple physical structure as a pair of gold plates coated on the surface of the capsule is enough for transmission.

## Advantages of MiroCam

MiroCam overcomes inferior image quality of conventional capsule endoscopes that is inevitably caused by data compression for efficient data transmission under RF module. Blurring at edges of objects and of small or thin objects may hinder detection of mucosal lesion [64]. However, MiroCam with human body communication does not need data compression, which results in more precise images (Figs. 2.23, 2.24). In the first clinical trial, the fine structures of the bowel mucosal surface, including villi and vasculature of the entire small bowel lumen, could be observed without blurring or distortion in more than 90 % of cases [65].

MiroCam dramatically reduced power consumption in various ways. Firstly, human body communication consumes less power compared with RF by making the high-frequency modulation process unnecessary. Secondly, the CMOS image sensor was designed to minimize power consumption, and thirdly, the telemetry chip and image sensor were combined on one chip to reduce the current required for fan-out between chips. With this advantage, the capsule operation time prolonged up to 11 h only with two usual silver oxide batteries, and thereby, MiroCam improves the complete ratio to explore the entire small bowel [68].

Other functional equipments could be put in place where the additional antenna and high-frequency circuit of RF had been occupied, because these devices became unnecessary in human body communication. Capsule endoscope with the function of biopsies, drug delivery, or locomotive guidance will soon be realized.

### 2.4.1.2 Clinical Studies of MiroCam

## Clinical Studies for the Diagnostic Feasibility and Safety
- **First clinical study of diagnostic feasibility and safety of the prototype of MiRo capsule**

The first clinical study for safety and diagnostic feasibility of MiRo capsule endoscope was reported in 2009 [65]. This study verified the safety of the MiRo capsule in human beings, especially with regard to the cardiac and neuromuscular systems, and evaluating the validity in the diagnosis of human small bowel. All 45

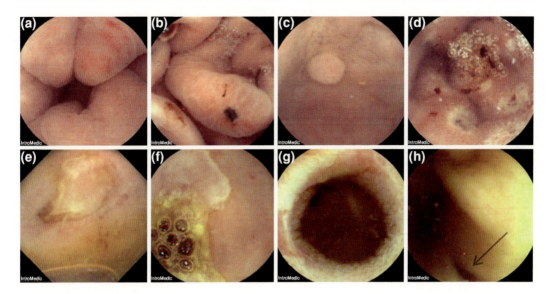

**Fig. 2.24** Endoscopic images of abnormal lesions taken by MiroCam. **a** Gastritis. **b** Gastric erosion with adherent blood clot. **c** Duodenal polyp. **d** Duodenitis with erosions. **e** Small bowel ulcer. **f** and **g** Small bowel ulcer with stricture. **h**, Colonic diverticuli (*arrow*)

volunteers experienced no adverse effects, and there was no disturbance on one's daily life. All capsule endoscopes were expelled within 2 days, and the mean total duration of image transmission was 9 h 51 min (5 h 35 min–11 h). Complete exploration of the entire small bowel was achieved in all 45 volunteers. In 68.9 %, the images were fine and sophisticated and revealed microstructures over more than 75 % of the entire small bowel. The image quality was graded as good or better in 91 %.

- **Safety of MiroCam in patients with cardiac devices**

Patients with cardiac pacemakers or implantable cardiac defibrillators always require their attention to environmental electromagnetic interference (EMI) which may cause serious cardiac device dysfunction. By the same reason, capsule endoscopy should be performed carefully in these patients due to EMI produced by electrical signals of capsule endoscope when the capsule wirelessly transmits endoscopic images to a receiver outside the patient's body. For this reason, the US FDA considers the presence of a cardiac pacemaker or ICD as a relative contraindication for CE.

When capsule endoscope operates, EMI with cardiac devices may occur by oversensing or undersensing the electric signal. Oversensing may be developed by the radio frequencies of 434 MHz pulsed with 2 or 4 Hz used in capsule endoscopy as a transmission method, because the frequency is equivalent to a heart rate of 120 or 420 beats/min that represents slow ventricular tachycardia to ventricular fibrillation [69]. Therefore, cardiac devices may recognize it as nonexisting heart signals and inhibit ventricular pacing, which may cause bradycardia and symptomatic dizziness or syncope. Moreover, inappropriate shock or antitachycardia pacing could occur if an ICD detects an electric signal originating from a capsule endoscope. On contrary, undersensing may result in competition with native QRS complexes. If cardiac device cannot recognize the actual heart signal, it fails to deliver an appropriate therapy with potential induction of asynchronous ventricular or noise-mode function and tachyarrhythmia will continue. However, these effects have not been observed to this time in vitro or clinical studies of conventional capsule endoscope [69–76]. Because, the vector of RF transmission with capsule endoscope is mostly within the abdomen, where is far from the location of the cardiac devices [71].

MiroCam equipped other transmission systems instead of RF, and it may be affected by an additional source of interference. Because this method uses the human body as a conductive medium for transmission of endoscopic images, an actual electric current flows directly into the heart and skews the signals of cardiac devices. However, energy generated from MiroCam is only 0.0225 J, which is weaker than $0.5 \sim 360$ J of cardiac device. Power of mobile phone that caused significant disturbance of cardiac devices was 2 W, and it is $2 \times 10^6$ times stronger than 1uW of MiroCam. Moreover, frequency of cardiac devices, $0.5 \sim 5$ Hz, is quite different to $1.5 \sim 3$ MHz of MiroCam.

Based on these theories, clinical study was conducted in six patients with three pacemakers and three implantable cardiac defibrillators [77]. No disturbance in cardiac devices or arrhythmia was detected on telemetry monitoring during capsule endoscopy. No significant changes in the programmed parameters of the cardiac devices were noted after capsule endoscopy. There were no imaging disturbances from the cardiac devices on capsule endoscopy. Capsule endoscope with human body communication was safely completed in patients with cardiac devices in this study, however, in which, only small number of patients and limited types of cardiac devices were included. Therefore, it is recommended that capsule endoscope should be performed under continuous ECG monitoring in a hospital setting after cardiac assessment by cardiologists. And further study is in need of verifying the safety of capsule endoscopy in a large number of patients with various types of cardiac devices.

## Comparative Studies with the Conventional Capsule Endoscopes

Several studies were conducted to compare the diagnostic yield and complete examination rate between MiroCam and other capsule endoscopes. While studies showed no statistical significance in difference of performance between MiroCam and other capsule endoscopes, a trend for the MiroCam to detect more small bowel lesions than with the other capsule endoscopes was observed.

The pilot study of sequential capsule endoscopies using MiroCam and PillCam showed complete examination rate 83.3 % in MiroCam and 58.3 % in PillCam ($p = 0.031$) [68]. Diagnostic yields for MiroCam and PillCam were 45.8 % and 41.7 % ($p > 0.05$), respectively. The agreement rate between the two capsules was 87.5 % with a $\kappa$ value of 0.74.

In French multicenter study, 83 patients with obscure GI bleeding were enrolled and ingested the two capsules at a one-hour interval [78]. After analyzing 73 cases (10 technical issues), there were 30 concordant positive cases (41.1 %), and the diagnostic concordance between the two systems was satisfactory ($\kappa = 0.66$). The final diagnosis was different in 12 patients (16.4 %) with nine positive findings only on MiroCam, two positive findings only on PillCam, and one different diagnosis in one patient. MiroCam and PillCam identified 95.2 and 78.6 % of positive cases, respectively ($p = 0.02$). The significant difference may be explained in part by the longer transit time and the higher number of images produced. But there was no significant difference on image quality, field depth, and lightening between MiroCam and PillCam.

Another multicenter comparative study was performed in six academic hospitals in USA and enrolled 105 patients with obscure GI bleeding [79]. The result showed an overall agreement of 78.7 % (95 % CI, $68.7 \sim 86.6$ %), a positive agreement of 77.4 % (95 % CI, $58.9 \sim 90.4$ %), and negative agreement of 79.3 % (95 % CI, $66.7 \sim 88.8$ %). Twelve abnormal findings were observed only in MiroCam, and seven were observed only in PillCam. MiroCam had a 5.6 % higher rate of detecting small bowel lesions ($p = 0.54$). On average, MiroCam took 6.6 h to reach the cecum, which is longer than the time taken by PillCam, i.e., 5.2 h ($P < 0.0001$). This difference in small bowel transit time may be explained by the difference of the dimension of two capsules (10.8 vs. 11.0 mm). It was assumed that the smaller MiroCam may be sufficiently large to ultimately be propelled through the small bowel; However, there may be some slippage with each peristalsis that causes the MiroCam to have a longer transit time in small bowel [79]. Despite longer transit time, the MiroCam achieved higher complete ratio than PillCam (93.3 vs. 84.3 %, $P = 0.1$)

To compare MiroCam and Endocapsule, a total of 50 patients with obscure GI bleeding, chronic diarrhea, and anemia of unknown origin participated in the clinical study in Austria [80]. Complete small bowel examination was achieved in 96 % patients using MiroCam and 90 % patients using EndoCapsule (odds ratio 2.67, 95 % CI, 0.49–14.45, $p = 0.38$). Diagnostic yield in the small bowel was 50 % in MiroCam and 48 % in EndoCapsule without statistical significance (OR 1.08, 95 % CI, 0.49–2.37, $P > 0.99$). The diagnostic concordance rate between the two different capsule endoscopes was 68 % ($\kappa = 0.50$).

Summarizing these comparative studies, MiroCam detects small bowel abnormalities at a rate that is at least comparable to that of other capsule endoscopes (Table 2.2). The longer operational time of the MiroCam resulted in a higher rate of complete small bowel examination. Although statistical insignificance, the larger numbers of images generated at three frames per second increased the detection rate of small bowel lesions [79].

### 2.4.1.3 Upgraded MiroCam and Advanced Capsule Endoscope

Upgraded model of the MiroCam (MC1000-W) has plans to market. The field of view of new model is improved to 170° compared with 150° of previous model (MC1000) (Table 2.3). The size is minimally changed from 10.8 × 24 mm to 10.8 × 24.5 mm, and the weight is reduced from 3.3 to 3.25 g. Resolution power of 320 × 320 pixels and frame rate of three frames per second are identical with previous model. Operating time over 11 h is maintained, and transmission method is same as human body communication using E-field propagation.

External receiver was upgraded to wire–wireless real-time viewer, and data transmission rate was two times higher. MiroView software was also upgraded from version 1.0 to 2.0 (Fig. 2.25). Rapid detection of bleeding focus by map view became available, and reading time could be markedly decreased by reading many images at a time using range view. Software system divided by sever, client, and operator makes reading easier anywhere and anytime via internal network of the hospital. Exporting program of the final report to the hospital image program such as PACS was also improved.

**Capsule Endoscopes with Active Movement**
The movement of capsule endoscopes entirely depends on the natural peristalsis of GI tract, which might be a main reason to prolong the gastrointestinal transit time. The uncontrollable movement of capsule endoscope might be obstacles to reach the cecum within capsule operating time and to make accurate diagnosis. Therefore, techniques for active control of the capsule movement have been being developed, such as a magnetic steering mechanism by external manipulation [81–87] and a locomotive mechanism by internal manipulation [88–91].

- **Magnetic steering capsule endoscope (MiroCam Navi)**

  MiroCam Navi (MC1000-WM) is one of the magnetic steering capsule endoscope, which was approved for clinical use in Europe. Observing the images on real-time viewer, magnetic capsule endoscope could be manipulated to move up and down by MiroCam Navi controller outside the body (Fig. 2.26). With MiroCam Navi, gastric transit time might be shortened, and the small bowel lesion could be observed in more detail. Moreover, targeted drug delivery will be realized with this ability to operate freely in the near future.

- **Paddling-based locomotive capsule endoscope**

  For internal locomotive devices, paddling-based capsule endoscope has been developed. When a locomotive robot was suggested by Hirose [92], Pratt [93], and Ryu [94], it was

**Table 2.2** Comparative studies of MiroCam to other capsule endoscopes

| | | Patients (n) | Diagnostic yield | Agreement rate | Rate of complete examination | Small bowel transit time | Operating time |
|---|---|---|---|---|---|---|---|
| Kim et al. [68] | MiroCam | 24 | 45.8 % | 87.5 %, $\kappa$ = 0.74 | 83.3 %* | – | 702 ± 60 min* |
| | PillCam | | 41.7 % | | 58.3 %* | – | 446 ± 28 min* |
| Pioche et al. [78] | MiroCam | 73 | 56.2 % | $\kappa$ = 0.66 | – | 268.1 min (58 – 538)* | – |
| | PillCam | | 46.6 % | | – | 234.5 min (51 – 502)* | – |
| Choi et al. [79] | MiroCam | 105 | – | 78.7 %, | 93.3 % | 6.6 ± 2.2 h | 11.1 ± 1.5 h* |
| | PillCam | | – | $\kappa$ = 0.547 | 84.3 % | 5.2 ± 1.4 h | 7.8 ± 0.8 h* |
| Dolak et al. [80] | MiroCam | 50 | 50 % | 68 %, $\kappa$ = 0.50 | 96 % | 319 ± 113 min | 704 ± 56 min* |
| | EndoCapsule | | 48 % | | 90 % | 316 ± 100 min | 578 ± 53 min* |

* $P < 0.05$

**Table 2.3** Comparisons of MiroCam (MC1000) to upgraded MiroCam (MC1000-W)

| | MC1000 | MC1000-W |
|---|---|---|
| Image | 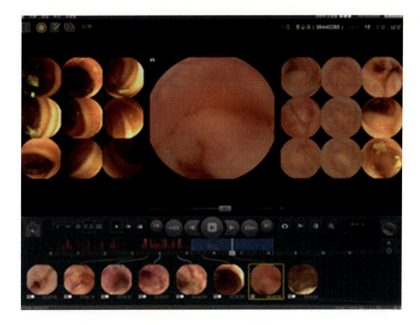 | |
| Size (mm) | 10.8 × 24 | 10.8 × 24.5 |
| Weight (g) | 3.45 | 3.25 |
| Pixels | 320 × 320 | 320 × 320 |
| Frames per second | 3 | 3 |
| Field of view (°) | 150 | 170 |
| Operation time (h) | Over 11 | Over 11 |
| Communication mechanism | Electric field propagation | Electric field propagation |

**Fig. 2.25** Updated MiroView (2.5)

**Fig. 2.26** MiroCam Navi (MC1000-WM)

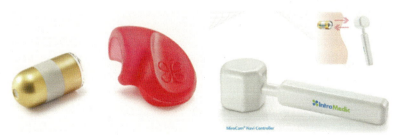

difficult to miniaturize the proposed legged mechanisms, and thus, that was not applied to capsule locomotion. In 2004, Menciassi proposed a legged locomotion in gastrointestinal tract [95], and with this 8-legged capsule, a full colonic passage was successfully demonstrated in the ex vivo phantom model [90]. However, the multilegged locomotion capsule needs multiple actuators and controllers, which limited miniaturization and energy conservation.

An inchworm-like microrobot comprising actuation modules and clamping modules for capsule endoscopes has been proposed in Korea in 2004 [96]. However, spring-type SMA actuators in this inchworm-like microrobot were not enough to get over resistance force of small bowel and to realize long stroke with high efficacy [97–100]. In order to solve this problem, a new paddling-based locomotive mechanism was developed in 2006 [101]. This locomotive mechanism is originated from paddling a canoe. The paddle of a canoe is embodied as the legs of our microrobot, and the canoeist is replaced by the linear actuator which is composed of a reliable commercialized micromotor and a lead screw. And the more enhanced paddling-based locomotive CE was presented in 2010 and demonstrated its efficacy in vitro and in vivo experiments [102].

1. Concept design of the microrobot

At first, the paddling-based locomotive microrobot consists of a linear actuator which comprises micromotor and lead screw, an inner cylinder, an outer cylinder, multiple legs, and robot outer body [101]. The functions of this novel microrobot are illustrated as follows [101]: (1) The linear actuator moves the inner cylinder backward and forward. (2) The inner cylinder has grooves, and there is some clearance between the grooves and the legs. Owing to the clearance, the inner cylinder makes the legs rotate and moves the legs and the outer cylinder. (3) The outer cylinder is connected with the multilegs by wire-type pin and is moved inside of the robot outer body. (4) The multilegs are protruded out of the robot body and are folded in the robot body. The microrobot has six legs which are radially positioned and are in contact

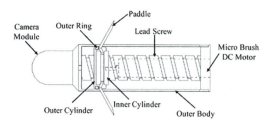

**Fig. 2.27** Concept design of paddling-based locomotive capsule endoscope (Reprint with permission from Kim et al. [102])

with the intestinal surface. (5) Finally, in order to reduce the frictional force between the robot outer body and the intestinal surface, the head of the microrobot is designed as a semisphere and the robot outer body is coated with lubricant such as silicon oil. And for the protruding and folding the legs, the microrobot outer body has the lateral slits.

In the modified locomotive capsule endoscope, outer ring is added to generate continuous friction between the outer body and the outer cylinder and to provide robustness in the kinematic configuration, such as the positional difference between the inner and the outer cylinders for protruding or folding paddles [102] (Fig. 2.27). As a result, the capsule endoscope can satisfactorily move inside the GI tract during repetitive movements. Moreover, this CE is teleoperated by the automatic controller, with which a reciprocating cycle for the cylinders of the capsule endoscope can be moderated by setting desired cycle time using a microprocessor on the controller [102]. This automatic control mechanism reduces power consumption and accelerates locomotion compared with the manual switching for the control used in the previous locomotive capsule endoscope [101].

2. Locomotive mechanism of the proposed microrobot

Locomotive mechanism is illustrated in Fig. 2.28. By repeating paddling motion, this capsule moves forward in the GI tract [102]. For this, the paddles linked to the outer cylinder are protruded and folded according to the direction of linearly actuating the inner and the outer cylinders along the lead screw. The clearance between inner and outer cylinders causes

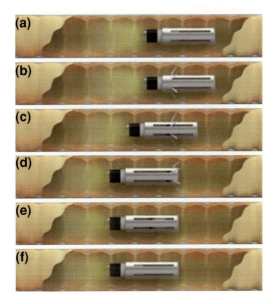

Fig. 2.28 Locomotive mechanism of the paddling-based locomotive capsule endoscope (Reprint with permission from Kim et al. [102]). **a** Initial state of the capsule-type microrobot in the intestine. **b** When the linear actuating mechanism starts to move the inner cylinder backward, the paddles linked to the outer cylinder are stretched, due to the kinematic relationship between the inner and the outer cylinders, and clamp the intestinal surfaces. **c** While the actuator moves the inner cylinder farther, the outer body of the capsule endoscope advances forward. **d** End of the stroke of the linear actuating mechanism. At this point, when the actuating mechanism is about to move the inner cylinder forward, the paddles fixed to the intestine are released and folded into the capsule body as the above kinematic relationship works inversely. **e** The cylinders and folded paddles return without the movement of the capsule body. **f** The locomotion principle returns to the same state in step A

relative position delay of the outer cylinder to the inner one during linear motion. As a result, the paddles rotate on pivotal points for protruding or folding when multiple grooves inner cylinder relatively push the end of paddles to right or left, as shown.

3. Specification of modified paddling-based locomotive capsule endoscope

The locomotive capsule endoscope is 15 × 43 mm in size and weighs 14 g. The length of the slit, meaning an actual stroke length of paddles for advancing, is 33 mm. A camera module is located in front of the

locomotive capsule endoscope and had a field of view of 125 and resolution power of 320 × 320 pixels. The capsule endoscope transmits video images at 10 frames per second to outside receiver. Two cables are connected to the end of the locomotive capsule endoscope for power supply and locomotion control, and four cables transmit image data from a camera. The cables are extended to the external controller and the recorder, twisted as a bundle with a length of 2 m from the end of the capsule endoscope.

The active movement of this novel capsule endoscope with paddling-based locomotion was demonstrated in in vivo test with an anesthetized pig [102]. The movement was fast and stable with a regular velocity (17 cm/min over 40 cm lengths) set by the automatic controller. And there were no serious complications during its active movement.

Even this paddling-based locomotive capsule endoscope has several advantages, such as long stoke, simple structure and control, and fast locomotion, the present external controller should be miniaturized and embedded in the capsule endoscope. Moreover, a wireless telemetry system should be equipped for actual operation and transmission of acquired images to recorder. A novel communication technology using human body communication [65] is a very suitable method for developing a wireless locomotive capsule endoscope due to its capability of energy conservation.

In the in vivo study, peristalsis seldom occurred in colon of the general anesthetized pigs. Actually, peristalsis might disturb the active movement of the capsule endoscope because the direction of capsule endoscope is opposite to that of peristalsis. Further study is needed to investigate the forward movement against provoked peristalsis by cholinergic drugs. Study about actual movement at anatomic obstacles, such as acute angles of recto-sigmoid junction or feces, should be evaluated. And further technologic improvement should be achieved to use in humans. A miniaturized steering module should be developed to change a direction of CE and to view at specific directions.

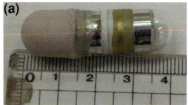 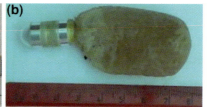

**Fig. 2.29** Concept design of self-stabilizing capsule endoscope (Reprint with permission from Filip et al. [105]). **a** Modified MiroCam capsule endoscope with stabilizing component. **b** Fully expanded self-stabilizing capsule endoscope

- **Self-stabilizing colonic capsule endoscopy**

The smaller capsule is the better to swallow. However, small bowel capsule endoscope tends to tumble in larger-lumen organs such as stomach or colon [68, 103], which limits the visual field causing failure to catch significant lesions or grossly distorting the perceived dimensions of polyps [104]. Therefore, self-expanding capsule endoscope after it enters into the bowel was developed to visualize the colon without tumbling [105].

Self-stabilizing capsule endoscope is modified from MiroCam capsule endoscope coupled to stabilizing component (Fig. 2.29). This stabilizing component was a thermally treated, woven, biodegradable, liquid-permeable, flexible polyglactin 910 mesh (vicryl, Ethicon Inc., Somerville, NJ) filled with super-absorbent polymer granules (Favor PAC, Evonik Industries, Stockhausen, Germany) [106]. The expandable material was salt granules of hydrophilic, non-toxic, cross-linked polyacrylate polymer. These granules can absorb several hundred times their weight in water, but cannot dissolve because of their 3D polymeric network structure, and only the formation of a gel takes place [107]. The advantages of this super-absorbent polymer as an expandable material for the device are as follows; it is biocompatible, swells extensively, swells in a relatively short period of time, exerts a reasonable swelling pressure on the walls of the lumen, and withstands the pressure in the colon by remaining attached to the imaging component while keeping its consistency [105]. Moreover, the increased viscosity of the surrounding liquid in water allows the capsule to move smoothly in the colon, and its flexibility is enough to pass through sharp colonic turns such as the hepatic and splenic flexures [108]. This bending capability should be uniform up to the base of the expandable component that is attached to the rigid but relatively small imaging component.

In living dogs, the study was conducted to evaluate the efficacy of this self-stabilizing capsule endoscopy by quantitatively comparing the detection rate of intraluminal suture marker lesions for colonoscopy [109]. Four mongrel dogs underwent laparotomy and the implantation of 5 to 8 suture markers to approximate colon lesion. Each dog consecutively administered both unmodified capsule endoscope and self-stabilizing capsule endoscopy in random order by endoscopic insertion into the proximal lumen of the colon. After capsule endoscopy, blinded standard colonoscopy was performed. The average percentage of the marker detection rates for unmodified capsule endoscope, self-stabilizing capsule endoscope, and colonoscopy, respectively, was 31.1, 86, and 100 % ($P < 0.01$). Self-stabilizing endoscope delivered a significant improvement in detection rates of colon suture marking when compared with the unmodified capsule endoscope, but there were no comparisons of small bowel transit time. Further studies are needed for the safety and efficacy of the self-stabilizing capsule endoscope in human. The worrisome problem is a premature expansion or obstruction in the small intestine or stomach. And timed launching in the cecum, detection of colon polyps, and imaging qualities should be investigated.

## 2.5 The Ankon Magnetic-Controlled Capsule Endoscopy Platform in the Clinical Investigation of Stomach Diseases

**Abstract** Gastric diseases are great burden not only in China but also worldwide. Capsule endoscopy is a noninvasive tool in the exploration of the entire gastrointestinal tract. However, conventional capsule endoscopies have shown that observation of the stomach is highly variable because of the impossibility of thorough exploration of the gastric cavity with a passive power. The steerable capsules with external magnetic field may be the most viable approaches for active control, and several explorations have showed promising benefits. We have developed a novel magnetic-controlled capsule endoscopy system (MCE) with magnetic field generated by an external industry robot (provided by Ankon Technologies Inc.), which has been demonstrated to be safe and feasible in the examination of human stomach. For the main diagnostic outcomes, MCE and gastroscopy had very similar results (the overall agreement was more than 90 %). The acceptability of MCE was much higher than gastroscopy, and most patients could tolerate ingestion of the large amount of water. This comparative study showed that MCE is a promising alternative for noninvasive screening of gastric diseases.

### 2.5.1 Introduction

Gastric diseases are great burden not only in China but also worldwide [110–112]. The prevalence of peptic ulcer disease confirmed endoscopically could reach to 17.2 % [113] in China, substantially higher than in Western populations. Gastric cancer remains the fourth most common malignancy and the second leading cause of cancer mortality in the world [114]. It is important to screen, diagnose, or exclude gastric diseases at an early stage. Gastroscopy is the reference method for the detection of gastric mucosal lesions. Unfortunately, it is widely regarded as uncomfortable and invasive for gastroscopy examination, thus with low patient compliance [115]. Conscious sedation in endoscopy could have potential drug-related side effects and increase medical cost, which limits its use in certain population [116]. Capsule endoscopy (CE) might offer a more patient-friendly alternative without discomfort or need for sedation. Since the first brief communication published in Nature in 2000 introducing CE, it has rapidly become the criterion standard for small intestine examination [117–119]. However, for a large organ like stomach, the random movement of passive capsule can let it observe only a small part of the whole gastric mucosa.

Since the first case report of maneuverable capsule system, published by Paul Swain et al in 2010, endoscopy companies such as Given Imaging, Olympus, Siemens, and OMOM have done some early-stage researches on this field. Capsule with propellers [120], paddles [121], and legs [122] has been studied with some success; however, a lot of work is still required for these to become clinical reality. Through recent years of efforts, the steerable capsules with external magnetic field may be the most viable approaches for active control [123, 124], and several explorations (external magnet paddle or special MRI machine) have showed promising benefits [120, 125–128]. However, these systems still have some limitations. The magnetic force generated by handheld external magnet appeared to be insufficient to prevent accidental emptying of the capsule from strong retraction of pylori [125]. The equipment derived from magnetic resonance imaging procedures provided adequate force and acceptable performance but indicated possibly fairly high cost [126].

Robotic control on magnetic capsule endoscopy based on industry robot may provide a much more cost-effective solution. An in vivo animal trial demonstrated that robotic control on magnetic steering capsule was more precise and reliable than manual operation [127]. We have developed a novel MCE system with magnetic field generated by an external industry robot,

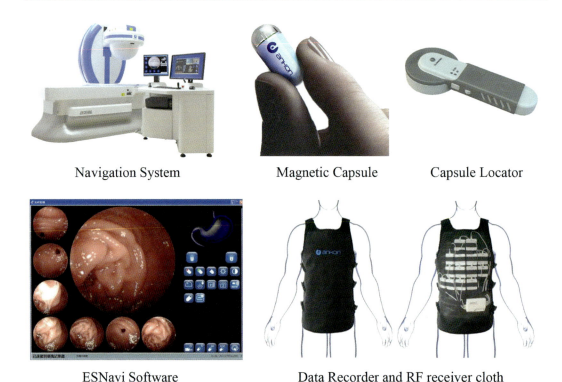

Navigation System          Magnetic Capsule          Capsule Locator

ESNavi Software          Data Recorder and RF receiver cloth

**Fig. 2.30** The NaviCam MCE system

which has been demonstrated to be safe and feasible in the examination of human stomach by a pilot study of 34 healthy volunteers [129].

### 2.5.2 The ANKON MCE System

Ankon Technologies Inc. began its MCE research in 2009, and its NaviCam got SFDA's approval in China in 2013. The ANKON MCE system consisted of capsule endoscopy, a guidance magnet robot, a data recorder, and a computer workstation with software for real-time view and control (Fig. 2.30).

The capsule endoscopy in stomach was performed well and safe in simulator model and porcine model. The capsule has a size of $28 \times 12$ mm, which consisted of CMOS camera, LED, batteries, the magnet, RF transmitter, and magnetic and acceleration sensor. It has a view angle of 140° and a resolution of $480 \times 480$. The guidance magnet robot provides five degrees of control freedom: two rotational and three translational. The capture rate of MCE is two frames per second from a single CMOS sensor. It transmits images to the data recorder via a set of sensors placed on the patient's skin. The images are viewed in real time on monitor and stored into workstation simultaneously.

The guidance magnet robot is of C-arm type with five degrees of freedom. The complete working area on the MCE is more than $50 \times 50 \times 50$ cm$^3$. The magnetic field generated by guidance robot system can be adjusted during the examination and reach 200 mT at maximum, which is much less than that from standard 1.5T MRI. Actual strength of magnetic field used to control the navigation of MCE is about 5 to 30 mT, which is 60 to 300 times greater than the Earth's magnetic field and generates magnetic force in the order of the capsule's weight. With permanent magnet, the

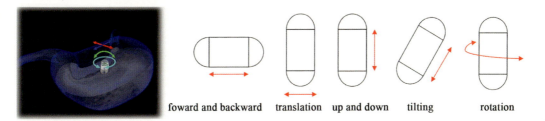

foward and backward    translation   up and down    tilting        rotation

Fig. 2.31  Movements of the capsule

guidance magnet robot runs very quiet and consumes low electric power requiring no cooling system at all.

During examination, the doctor sits in front of the workstation with dual monitors. The left monitor displays the real-time view of stomach from the capsule and the view of patients from cameras. The right monitor is the operating interface collecting the information about strength of magnetic field, attitude of capsule, and so on. The ESNavi can also show the real-time location of capsule in the three-dimensional mode. The attitude information of capsule is obtained through simulation on the basis of the magnetic field generated by the guidance system. MCE can be controlled by the magnet guidance robot through a joystick or automatic mode by which the MCE can make linear movement or rotation without manual control (Fig. 2.31). The capsule could reach from the lower to the upper side of gastric wall, no matter what content the stomach is full of (water, air, or the mixture). When the stomach is partially filled with water, the capsule can float stably at the water level (Fig. 2.32).

### 2.5.3  Procedure

The patient arrived at the hospital between 8:00 am and 10:00 am after fasting overnight (>8 h). All subjects drank 500 ml of clear water and 5 ml simeticone about 1 h before capsule ingestion, another 500 ml of clear water 15 min before ingestion, and 6 g air-producing power (Tianzhili Biological Technology, Fuzhou, China) with 5 ml of water 5 min before ingestion. The air-producing powder served to distend the stomach through releasing about 540 ml $CO_2$ every 6 g. After swallowing the MCE together with 5 ml of water, the patient immediately lies down on the bed attached to the guidance robot. The position of the bed was adjustable for optimal gastric imaging and maximal magnetic force for capsule navigation.

During the examination, the patient lies down on the bed and kept minimum movement. After the MCE reached stomach, the doctor moves the joystick to control the movement of the magnetic head based on the real-time images and parameters displayed on the operating interface (Fig. 2.33). The doctor performed the following

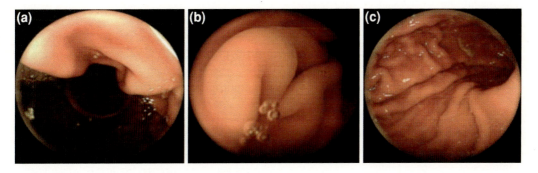

Fig. 2.32  **a** Floating view; **b** capsule under the water; and **c** capsule in the air

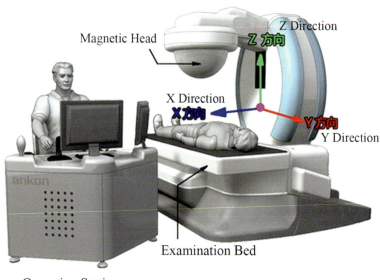

**Fig. 2.33** Capsule navigation system operation

steps: lifting the capsule away from the posterior wall, rotating and advancing the capsule to the fundus and cardiac region, then rotating capsule to observe stomach body, and finally observing the angulus, antrum, and pylorus. If the distension was insufficient, ingestion of additional air-producing powder or water was repeated. The whole examination duration lasted for about 30 min.

### 2.5.4 Indications

1. Patients with upper gastrointestinal symptoms, including abdominal discomfort, pain, acid reflux, dysphagia, belching, and hiccups.
2. Screening for gastric cancer.
3. Follow-up examination for gastric ulcer, atrophic gastritis, and precancerous lesions.

### 2.5.5 Contraindications

1. Patients with impaired bowel movement from ileus or organic digestive diseases
2. Patients with known large and obstructing tumors of the upper GI tract

3. Patients after upper GI surgery or abdominal surgery altering GI anatomy
4. Patients under full anticoagulation
5. Patients in poor general condition
6. Patients using equipment that may be affected by magnetic field, such as pacemakers and defibrillators
7. Pregnancy or suspected pregnancy
8. Patients allergic to materials or drugs involved
9. Patients mentally ill or unable to cooperate.

In our pilot study of 34 healthy volunteers, the cleanliness was evaluated as good in 88 % subjects [129]. The distention of gastric cavity was evaluated as good in the 85 % subjects. Maneuverability of the MCE to movements of the guidance magnet robot was graded as good in 85 % subjects. More than 75 % gastric mucosa was visualized in 79 % subjects and 50 % to 75 % in 20 % subjects. Visualization of the gastric cardia, fundus, body, angulus, antrum, and pylorus was subjectively assessed as complete in 82, 85, 100, 100, 100, and 100 %, respectively. No entire gastric mucosa was observed in all subjects for three reasons: (1) small amounts of fluid blocked the view of the most apical parts of the fundus; (2) insufficiency of gastric distention; and (3) difficult for guidance MCE in the cardiac region. The removal of mucus by drugs will need further researches because it is a critical issue with regard to capsule navigation and visibility.

In another double-center comparative trial of MCE and standard gastroscopy, both of them had very similar results of the main diagnostic outcomes (the overall agreement was more than 90 %). The acceptability of MCE was much higher than gastroscopy, and most patients could tolerate ingestion of the large amount of water. This study also showed that MCE is a promising alternative for noninvasive screening of gastric diseases.

In spite of initial and encouraging advancement in different kinds of MCE, there were many concerns in its practical value at present [130]. The drawbacks of current MCE comparing with the standard gastroscopy are clear: (1) complicated gastric preparation; (2) lack of biopsy capacity; and (3) long examination time. However, in our view, all these drawbacks may be solved in the future with the advancement of technology. As pointed by Rey, after balancing the pros and cons of standard gastroscopy and MCE, the latter might be a more cost-effective use of medical and social resources [126]. In the future, MCE may be adopted as the screening examination tool for gastric disease, especially for the elderly with sedation contraindications.

## 2.6 CapsoCam

Two of limitations of capsule endoscopy are as follows: (1) incomplete examination of the small intestine due to inadequate battery life and (2) the inability to observe some areas on the side wall because the camera is located at the end of the capsule [131]. The CapsoCam (Capsovision, Saratoga, CA, USA) was a recently developed 11 × 31 mm capsule endoscopy, which represents a new concept of detecting lesions in the small intestine: 360° panoramic lateral view with four cameras [132]. CapsoCam SV-1 capsule consisted of lens, imaging sensor, light

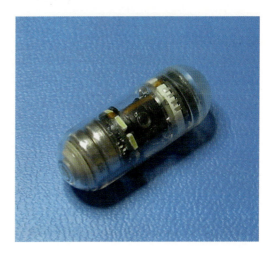

**Fig. 2.34** The CapsoCam SV1. Reprint with permission from Friedrich et al. [132]

source, power source, and flash memory (Fig. 2.34). It has a high frequency of 20 frames per second during the first 2 h and thereafter 12 frames per second, with a battery life of 15 h.

### 2.6.1 Special Characteristics

1. 360° Panoramic View: The CapsoCam employs four cameras facing the sides of the capsule that together image a full 360° about the capsule's circumference and capture high-resolution images of the mucosa including surfaces hidden behind folds.
2. Wire-Free Technology: There is no generation and transfer of RF signals, and all the images captured are stored on board with CapsoCam. The patient does not need any form of external devices, and the clinician is free of the receiver equipment and other accessories for data retrieval. However, because of not including the recording system, the capsule has to be retrieved by the patient after expulsion in order for the video to be downloaded.
3. Smart Motion Sense Technology: The Smart Motion Sense Technology allows the cameras to be activated to capture images only during capsule motion. When the capsule does not move and is stationary, the sensor

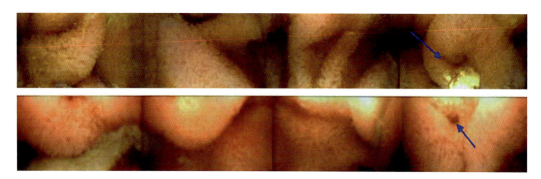

**Fig. 2.35** Images of the duodenal papilla detected by CapsoCam SV1. Reprint with permission from Friedrich et al. [132]

goes into the monitoring mode before switching to active mode during motion, which also helps to conserve battery power.

comparable efficiency of the CapsoCam and PillCam SB2 capsule systems in terms of diagnostic yield and image.

## 2.6.2 Clinical Studies

Friedrich et al. firstly carried out a prospective dual-center study of CapsoCam in Germany [132]. The study evaluated the feasibility and completeness of small bowel examination together with secondary end points of duodenal papilla detection in 33 patients. Small bowel examination was complete in all procedures. Mean time to pass the small bowel was $258 \pm 136$ min. The duodenal papilla was identified in 71 % of the patients (Fig. 2.35). No adverse effect was observed. It demonstrated that CapsoCam is a safe and efficient tool in small bowel examination.

To evaluate diagnostic concordance of the PillCam SB2 and CapsoCam capsules in the same patients, a prospective comparative study was conducted in four French referral endoscopy units [133]. Seventy-three patients ingested the two capsules 1 h apart and in a randomized order. Results showed that concordant positive diagnosis was 38.3 % and a negative diagnosis 43.3 %. The kappa value is 0.63, indicating that the concordance was good. In a per lesion analysis, the CapsoCam capsule detected significantly more lesions (108 vs. 85 lesions, $P = 0.001$). Reading time was longer for CapsoCam procedures (32.0 vs. 26.2 min, $P = 0.002$). This study shows

## References

1. Iddan G, Meron G, Glukhovsky A, Swain P. Wireless capsule endoscopy. Nature. 2000;455:417–8.
2. Eliakim R, Yassin K, Shlomi I, et al. A novel diagnostic tool for detecting oesophageal pathology: the PillCam oesophageal video capsule. Aliment Pharmacol Ther. 2004;20:1083–9.
3. Eliakim R, Fireman Z, Gralnek IM, et al. Evaluation of the PillCam Colon capsule in the detection of colonic pathology: results of the first multicenter, prospective, comparative study. Endoscopy. 2006;38:963–70.
4. Cave DR, Fleischer DE, Leighton JA, et al. A multicenter randomized comparison of the EndoCapsule and the PillCam SB. Gastrointest Endoscop. 2008;68:487–94.
5. Liao Z, Gao R, Li F, et al. Fields of application, diagnostic yield and findings of OMOM capsule endoscopy in 2400 Chinese patients. World J Gastroenterol. 2010;16:2669–76.
6. Bang S, Park JY, Jeong S, et al. First clinical trial of the 'Miro' capsule endoscope by using a novel transmission technology: electric field propagation. Gastrointest Endoscop. 2009;69:253–9.
7. Van Weyenberg JB, De Leest HTJI, Mulder CJJ. Description of a novel grading system to assess the quality of bowel preparation in video capsule endoscopy. Endoscopy. 2011;43:406–11.
8. Niv Y. Efficiency of bowel preparation for capsule endoscopy examination: a meta-analysis. World J Gastroenterol. 2008;14:1313–7.
9. Rokkas T, Papaxoinis K, Triantafyllou K, et al. Does purgative preparation influence the diagnostic

yield of small bowel video capsule endoscopy? A meta-analysis. Am J Gastroentereol. 2009;104:219–27.

10. Herrerias JM, Leighton JA, Costamagna G, et al. Agile patency system eliminates risk of capsule retention in patients with known intestinal strictures who undergo capsule endoscopy. Gastrointest Endosc. 2008;67:902–9.

11. Postgate AJ, Burling D, Gupta A, et al. Safety, reliability and limitations of the given patency capsule in patients at risk of capsule retention: a 3-year technical review. Dig Dis Sci. 2008;53:2732–8.

12. Fry LC, Carey EJ, Shiff AD, et al. The yield of capsule endoscopy in patients with abdominal pain or diarrhea. Endoscopy. 2006;38:498–502.

13. Annibale B, Capurso G, Baccini F, et al. Role of small bowel investigation in iron deficiency anaemia after negative endoscopic/histologic evaluation of the upper and lower gastrointestinal tract. Dig Liver Dis. 2003;35:784–7.

14. Fry LC, Bellutti M, Neumann H, et al. Incidence of bleeding lesions within reach of conventional upper and lower endoscopes in patients undergoing double-balloon enteroscopy for obscure gastrointestinal bleeding. Aliment Pharmacol Ther. 2009;29:342–9.

15. Triester SL, Leighton JA, Leontiadis GI, et al. A meta-analysis of the yield of capsule endoscopy compared to other modalities in patients with obscure gastrointestinal bleeding. Amer J Gastroenterol. 2005;100:2407–18.

16. Hara AK, Leighton JA, Sharma VK, et al. Small bowel: preliminary comparison of capsule endoscopy with barium study and CT. Radiology. 2004;230:260–5.

17. Costamagna G, Shah SK, Riccioni ME, et al. A prospective trial comparing small bowel radiographs and video capsule endoscopy for suspected small bowel disease. Gastroenterology. 2002;123:999–1005.

18. Leung WK, Ho SSM, Suen B-Y, et al. Capsule endoscopy or angiography in patients with acute overt obscure gastrointestinal bleeding: a prospective, randomized study with long-term follow-up. Amer J Gastroenterol. 2012;107:1370–6.

19. Pasha SF, Leighton JA, Das A, et al. Double balloon enteroscopy and capsule endoscopy have comparable diagnostic yield in small bowel disease: a meta-analysis. Clin Gastroenterol Hepatol. 2008;6:671–6.

20. Pennazio M, Santucci R, Rondonotti E, et al. Outcome of patients with obscure gastrointestinal bleeding after endoscopy: report of 100 consecutive cases. Gastroenterology. 2004;126:643–53.

21. Lai LH, Wong GI, Chow DK, et al. Long term follow-up of patients with obscure gastrointestinal bleeding after negative capsule endoscopy. Am J Gastroenterol. 2006;101:1224–8.

22. Rondonotti E, Pennazio M, Toth E, et al. Small-bowel neoplasms in patients undergoing video capsule endoscopy: a multicenter European study. Endoscopy. 2008;40:488–95.

23. Girelli CM, Porta P, Colombo E, et al. Development of a novel index to discriminate bulge from mass on small bowel capsule endoscopy. Gastointest Endosc. 2011;74:1067–74.

24. Barbosa DC, Roupar DB, Ramos JC, et al. Automatic small bowel tumor diagnosis by using multiscale wavelet-based analysis in wireless capsule endoscopy images. Biomed Eng Online. 2012;11:3.

25. Rokkas T, Niv Y. The role of video capsule endoscopy in the diagnosis of celiac disease: a meta-analysis. Eur J Gastroenterol Hepatol. 2012;24:303–8.

26. Caspari R, von Falkenhausen M, Krautmacher C, et al. Comparison of capsule endoscopy and magnetic resonance imaging for the detection of polyps of the small intestine in patients with familial adenomatous polyposis or with Peutz–Jeghers syndrome. Endoscopy. 2004;36:1054–9.

27. Gralnek IM, Rabinovitz R, Afik D, Eliakim R. A simplified ingestion procedure for esophageal capsule endoscopy: initial evaluation in healthy volunteers. Endoscopy. 2006;38:913–8.

28. Eliakim R, Sharma VK, Yassin K, et al. A prospective study of the diagnostic accuracy of PillCam ESO esophageal capsule endoscopy versus conventional upper endoscopy in patients with chronic gastroesophageal reflux diseases. J Clin Gastroenterol. 2005;39:572–8.

29. Gralnek IM, Adler SN, Yassin K, et al. Detecting esophageal disease with second-generation capsule endoscopy: initial evaluation of the PillCam ESO 2. Endoscopy. 2008;40:275–9.

30. Lu Y, Gao R, Liao Z, Hu LH, Li ZS. Meta-analysis of capsule endoscopy in patients diagnosed or suspected with esophageal varices. World J Gastroenterol. 2009;15:1254–8.

31. Spada C, Hassan C, Galmiche JP, et al. Colon capsule endoscopy: European Society of Gastrointestinal Endoscopy (ESGE) Guideline. Endoscopy. 2012;44:527–36.

32. Ramirez FC, Hakim S, Tharalsonet EM, et al. Amer J Gastroenterol. 2005;100:1065–71.

33. Moglia A, Menciassi A, Dario P, et al. Capsule endoscopy: progress update and challenges ahead. Nat Rev Gastroenterol Hepatol. 2009;6(6):353–62.

34. Rey JF, Kuznetsov K, Vazquez-Ballesteros E. Olympus capsule endoscope for small and large bowel exploration. Gastrointest Endosc. 2006;63:AB176.

35. Subramanian V, Mannath J, Telakis E, et al. Efficacy of new playback functions at reducing small-bowel wireless capsule endoscopy reading times. Dig Dis Sci. 2012;57(6):1624–8.

36. Cave DR, Fleischer DE, Leighton JA, et al. A multicenter randomized comparison of the

Endocapsule and the Pillcam SB. Gastrointest Endosc. 2008;68(3):487–94.

37. Dolak W, Kulnigg-Dabsch S, Evstatiev R, et al. A randomized head-to-head study of small-bowel imaging comparing MiroCam and EndoCapsule. Endoscopy. 2012;44(11):1012–20.

38. Ogata H, Kumai K, Imaeda H, et al. Clinical impact of a newly developed capsule endoscope: usefulness of a real-time image viewer for gastric transit abnormality. J Gastroenterol. 2008;43(3):186–92.

39. Zhang QL, Nian WD, Wang HH, et al. Preliminary clinical evaluation of OMOM capsule endoscope. Chin J Dig Endosc. 2005;22:86.

40. Geng Y, Wang A, Gao W. The value of OMOM capsule endoscope in small bowel disease diagnosis. Chin J Clin Gastroenterol. 2011; 22(1).

41. Yuan JH, Xin L, Liao Z, et al. Advances in complete small-bowel examination by capsule endoscopy. ShijieHuaren Xiaohua Zazhi 2010;18(34):3662–6

42. Liao Z, Li ZS, Xu C. Reduction of capture rate in the stomach increases the complete examination rate of capsule endoscopy: a prospective randomized controlled trial. Gastronintest Endosc. 2009;69(3):418–25.

43. Liao Z, Xu C, Li ZS. Completion rate and diagnostic yield of small-bowel capsule endoscopy: 1 vs. 2 frames per second. Endoscopy. 2010;42(5):360–4.

44. Li CY, Zhang BL, Chen CX, Li YM. OMOM Capsule Endoscopy in diagnosis of small bowel disease. J Zhejiang Univ SCI B. 2008;9(11):857–62.

45. Liao Z, Gao R, Xu C, et al. Fields of applications, diagnostic yields and findings of OMOM capsule endoscopy in 2400 Chinese patients. World J Gastroenterol. 2010;16(21):2669–76.

46. Xin L, Liao Z, Li ZS. The diagnosis of Crohn's disease of the small bowel: comparing CT enterography, capsule endoscopy. World Chin J Digestol. 2009;17(19):1972–7.

47. Lu X, Qin M, Wen X. The comparison between capsule endoscope, small bowel CT, small bowel enterography and colonoscopy in the diagnosis the Crohn's disease. Chin J Intern Med. 2010; 49(9).

48. Li XB, Ge ZZ, Dai J, et al. The role of capsule endoscopy combined with double-balloon enteroscopy in diagnosis of small bowel diseases. Chin Med J (Engl). 2007;120(1):30–5.

49. Zhang Y, Han S, Zhou X, et al. Double-balloon endoscopy and capsule endoscopy for small intestinal bleeding. Chin J Dig Endosc. 2010;27(8):402–5.

50. Rey JF, Ogata H, Hosoe N, et al. Feasibility of stomach exploration with a guided capsule endoscope. Endoscopy. 2010;42(7):541–5.

51. Fan Du, Huiqiong Cao, Tieyi Yang. Preliminary research of controllable capsule endoscopy. Chin J Dig Endosc. 2012;29(3):133–6.

52. Vakil N, van Zanten SV, Kahrilas P, et al. The Montreal definition and classification of gastroesophageal reflux disease: a global evidence-based consensus. Am J Gastroenterol. 2006;101:1900–20.

53. He J, Ma X, Zhao Y, et al. A population-based survey of the epidemiology of symptom-defined gastroesophageal reflux disease: The Systematic Investigation of Gastrointestinal Diseases in China. BMC Gastroenterol. 2010;10:94.

54. Domingues GR, Moraes-Filho JP, Domingues AG. Impact of prolonged 48-h wireless capsule esophageal pH monitoring on diagnosis of gastroesophageal reflux disease and evaluation of the relationship between symptoms and reflux episodes. Arq Gastroenterol. 2011;48(1):24–9.

55. Li JN, Liu CL, Tao XH. Clinical utility and tolerability of JSPH-1 wireless esophageal ph monitoring system. BMC Gastroentrol. 2013;13:10.

56. Azzam RS, Sallum RA, Brandao JF. Comparative study of two modes of gastroesophageal reflux measuring: conventional esophageal pH monitoring and wireless pH monitoring. Arq Gastroenterol. 2012;49(2):107–12.

57. Feng G, Zhao L, Liu Y. pH monitoring of normal and abnormal GERD positive patients with endoscopy tests in esophageal dynamics. World Chin J Dig. 2008; 01.

58. Fang WJ, Xu SC, Chen Y. Evaluation about the Reflux Symptom of GERD Patients Signed with Chronic Cough by 24-hour Impedance-pH Monitoring System. Gastroenterology. 2011; 16(10).

59. Xiao YL, Lin JK, Huang YJ. The application of joint test-tube multichannel intracavity impedance-pH monitoring in heartburn patients. The seventh national digestive epidemiology conference proceedings.

60. Iddan G, Meron G, Glukhovsky A, et al. Wireless capsule endoscopy. Nature. 2000;405:417.

61. Gheorghe C, Iacob R, Bancila I. Olympus capsule endoscopy for small bowel examination. J Gastrointestin Liver Dis. 2007;16:309–13.

62. Li CY, Zhang BL, Chen CX, et al. OMOM capsule endoscopy in diagnosis of small bowel disease. J Zhejiang Univ Sci B. 2008;9:857–62.

63. Kim TS, Song SY, Jung H, et al. Micro capsule endoscope for gastro intestinal tract. Conf Proc IEEE Eng Med Biol Soc. 2007;2007:2823–6.

64. Cave DR. Reading wireless video capsule endoscopy. Gastrointest Endosc Clin N Am. 2004;14:17–24.

65. Bang S, Park JY, Jeong S, et al. First clinical trial of the "MiRo" capsule endoscope by using a novel transmission technology: electric-field propagation. Gastrointest Endosc. 2009;69:253–9.

66. Haykin S, Moher M. Introduction to Analog and Digital Communications. 2nd ed. New Jersey: Wiley; 2007. p. 498–500.

67. Kim T, Park J, Moon S, et al. inventors; Korea Institute of Science and Technology, assignee. Method and apparatus for communication between inside and outside of transmission medium using

transmission medium as communication line. US patent US 7,307,544 B2. December 11, 2007.

68. Kim HM, Kim YJ, Kim HJ, et al. A Pilot Study of Sequential Capsule Endoscopy Using MiroCam and PillCam SB Devices with Different Transmission Technologies. Gut Liver. 2010;4:192–200.

69. Bandorski D, Irnich W, Bruck M, et al. Do endoscopy capsules interfere with implantable cardioverter-defibrillators? Endoscopy. 2009;41:457–61.

70. Leighton JA, Sharma VK, Srivathsan K, et al. Safety of capsule endoscopy in patients with pacemakers. Gastrointest Endosc. 2004;59:567–9.

71. Leighton JA, Srivathsan K, Carey EJ, et al. Safety of wireless capsule endoscopy in patients with implantable cardiac defibrillators. Am J Gastroenterol. 2005;100:1728–31.

72. Payeras G, Piqueras J, Moreno VJ, et al. Effects of capsule endoscopy on cardiac pacemakers. Endoscopy. 2005;37:1181–5.

73. Dubner S, Dubner Y, Rubio H, et al. Electromagnetic interference from wireless video-capsule endoscopy on implantable cardioverter-defibrillators. Pacing Clin Electrophysiol. 2007;30:472–5.

74. Bandorski D, Irnich W, Bruck M, et al. Capsule endoscopy and cardiac pacemakers: investigation for possible interference. Endoscopy. 2008;40:36–9.

75. Bandorski D, Lotterer E, Hartmann D, et al. Capsule endoscopy in patients with cardiac pacemakers and implantable cardioverter-defibrillators - a retrospective multicenter investigation. J Gastrointestin Liver Dis. 2011;20:33–7.

76. Bandorski D, Jakobs R, Bruck M, et al. Capsule Endoscopy in Patients with Cardiac Pacemakers and Implantable Cardioverter Defibrillators: (Re)evaluation of the Current State in Germany, Austria, and Switzerland 2010. Gastroenterol Res Pract. 2012;2012:717408.

77. Chung JW, Hwang HJ, Chung MJ, et al. Safety of capsule endoscopy using human body communication in patients with cardiac devices. Dig Dis Sci. 2012;57:1719–23.

78. Pioche M, Gaudin JL, Filoche B, et al. Prospective, randomized comparison of two small-bowel capsule endoscopy systems in patients with obscure GI bleeding. Gastrointest Endosc. 2011;73:1181–8.

79. Choi EH, Mergener K, Semrad C, et al. A multicenter, prospective, randomized comparison of a novel signal transmission capsule endoscope to an existing capsule endoscope. Gastrointest Endosc. 2013;78:325–32.

80. Dolak W, Kulnigg-Dabsch S, Evstatiev R, et al. A randomized head-to-head study of small-bowel imaging comparing MiroCam and EndoCapsule. Endoscopy. 2012;44:1012–20.

81. Wang X, Meng MQ. A magnetic stereo-actuation mechanism for active capsule endoscope. Conf Proc IEEE Eng Med Biol Soc. 2007;2007:2811–4.

82. Carpi F, Galbiati S, Carpi A. Controlled navigation of endoscopic capsules: concept and preliminary experimental investigations. IEEE Trans Biomed Eng. 2007;54:2028–36.

83. Carpi F, Pappone C. Magnetic robotic manoeuvring of gastrointestinal video capsules: preliminary phantom tests. Biomed Pharmacother. 2008;62:546–9.

84. Swain P, Toor A, Volke F, et al. Remote magnetic manipulation of a wireless capsule endoscope in the esophagus and stomach of humans (with videos). Gastrointest Endosc. 2010;71:1290–3.

85. Ciuti G, Donlin R, Valdastri P, et al. Robotic versus manual control in magnetic steering of an endoscopic capsule. Endoscopy. 2010;42:148–52.

86. Rey JF, Ogata H, Hosoe N, et al. Feasibility of stomach exploration with a guided capsule endoscope. Endoscopy. 2010;42:541–5.

87. Keller J, Fibbe C, Volke F, et al. Inspection of the human stomach using remote-controlled capsule endoscopy: a feasibility study in healthy volunteers (with videos). Gastrointest Endosc. 2011;73:22–8.

88. Zuo J, Yan G, Gao Z. A micro creeping robot for colonoscopy based on the earthworm. J Med Eng Technol. 2005;29:1–7.

89. Kwon J, Park S, Park J, et al. Evaluation of the critical stroke of an earthworm-like robot for capsule endoscopes. Proc Inst Mech Eng H. 2007;221:397–405.

90. Quirini M, Menciassi A, Scapellato S, et al. Feasibility proof of a legged locomotion capsule for the GI tract. Gastrointest Endosc. 2008;67:1153–8.

91. Wang K, Yan G, Ma G, et al. An earthworm-like robotic endoscope system for human intestine: design, analysis, and experiment. Ann Biomed Eng. 2009;37:210–21.

92. Hirose S. walking and group robots for super mechano-system. In: IEEE International Conference on Systems, Man, and Cybernetics. IEEE SMC'99 Conference Proceedings. 1999; 129–33.

93. Pratt GA. Legged robots at MIT: what's new since Raibert? IEEE Robot Autom Mag. 2000;7:15–9.

94. Ryu J, Jeong Y, Tak Y et al. A ciliary motion based 8-legged walking micro robot using cast IPMC actuators. In: Proceedings of 2002 International Symposium on Micromechatronics and Human Science. MHS. 2002; 85–91.

95. Menciassi A, Stefanini C, Gorini S, et al. Locomotion of a legged capsule in the gastrointestinal tract: theoretical study and preliminary technological results. Conf Proc IEEE Eng Med Biol Soc. 2004;4:2767–70.

96. Kim B, Lee S, Park JH et al. Inchworm-like microrobot for capsule endoscope. In: IEEE International Conference on Robotics and Biomimetics. ROBIO. 2004; 458–63.

97. Fung Y. Biomechanics: mechanical properties of living tissues. Berlin: Springer; 1993.

98. Rosen J, Hannaford B, MacFarlane MP, et al. Force controlled and teleoperated endoscopic grasper for minimally invasive surgery–experimental performance evaluation. IEEE Trans Biomed Eng. 1999;46:1212–21.

99. Pioletti DP, Rakotomanana LR. Non-linear viscoelastic laws for soft biological tissues. Eur J Mech A Solids. 2000;19:749–59.

100. Tanaka E, Del Pozo R, Sugiyama M, et al. Biomechanical response of retrodiscal tissue in the temporomandibular joint under compression. J Oral Maxillofac Surg. 2002;60:546–51.

101. Park S, Park H, Park S, et al. A paddling based locomotive mechanism for capsule endoscopes. J Mech Sci Technol. 2006;20:1012–8.

102. Kim HM, Yang S, Kim J, et al. Active locomotion of a paddling-based capsule endoscope in an in vitro and in vivo experiment (with videos). Gastrointest Endosc. 2010;72:381–7.

103. Eliakim R, Fireman Z, Gralnek IM, et al. Evaluation of the PillCam Colon capsule in the detection of colonic pathology: results of the first multicenter, prospective, comparative study. Endoscopy. 2006;38:963–70.

104. Lieberman D. Progress and challenges in colorectal cancer screening and surveillance. Gastroenterology. 2010;138:2115–26.

105. Filip D, Yadid-Pecht O, Andrews CN, et al. Self-stabilizing colonic capsule endoscopy: pilot study of acute canine models. IEEE Trans Med Imaging. 2011;30:2115–25.

106. Filip D, Yadid-Pecht O, Mintchev MP. Progress in self-stabilizing capsules for imaging of the large intestine. In: 17th IEEE International Conference on Electronics, Circuits, and Systems (ICECS). 2010; 231–4.

107. Haselbach J, Hey S, Berner T. Short-term oral toxicity study of FAVOR PAC in rats. Regul Toxicol Pharmacol. 2000;32:310–6.

108. Nakaji S, Fukuda S, Iwane S, et al. New method for the determination of fecal consistency and its optimal value in the general population. J Gastroenterol Hepatol. 2002;17:1278–82.

109. Filip D, Yadid-Pecht O, Muench G, et al. Suture marker lesion detection in the colon by self-stabilizing and unmodified capsule endoscopes: pilot study in acute canine models. Gastrointest Endosc. 2013;77:272–9.

110. Everhart JE, Ruhl CE. Burden of digestive diseases in the United States part I: overall and upper gastrointestinal diseases. Gastroenterology. 2009;136:376–86.

111. Li Z, Zou D, Ma X, et al. Epidemiology of peptic ulcer disease: endoscopic results of the systematic investigation of gastrointestinal disease in China. Am J Gastroenterol. 2010;105:2570–7.

112. Matsuda T, Marugame T, Kamo K, et al. Cancer incidence and incidence rates in Japan in 2006: based on data from 15 population-based cancer registries in the monitoring of cancer incidence in Japan (MCIJ) project. Jpn J Clin Oncol. 2012;42:139–47.

113. Bai Y, Li ZS, Zou DW, et al. Alarm features and age for predicting upper gastrointestinal malignancy in Chinese patients with dyspepsia with high background prevalence of Helicobacter pylori infection and upper gastrointestinal malignancy: an endoscopic database review of 102,665 patients from 1996 to 2006. Gut. 2010;59:722–8.

114. Ferlay J, Shin HR, Bray F, et al. Estimates of worldwide burden of cancer in 2008: GLOBOCAN 2008. Int J Cancer. 2010;127:2893–917.

115. Abraham N, Barkun A, Larocque M, et al. Predicting which patients can undergo upper endoscopy comfortably without conscious sedation. Gastrointest Endosc. 2002;56:180–9.

116. Vargo JJ, Delegge MH, Feld AD et al. Multisociety Sedation Curriculum for Gastrointestinal Endoscopy. Am J Gastroenterol. 2012.

117. Faigel DO, Baron TH, Adler DG, et al. ASGE guideline: guidelines for credentialing and granting privileges for capsule endoscopy. Gastrointest Endosc. 2005;61:503–5.

118. Ladas SD, Triantafyllou K, Spada C, et al. European Society of Gastrointestinal Endoscopy (ESGE): recommendations (2009) on clinical use of video capsule endoscopy to investigate small-bowel, esophageal and colonic diseases. Endoscopy. 2010;42:220–7.

119. Liao Z, Gao R, Xu C, et al. Indications and detection, completion, and retention rates of small-bowel capsule endoscopy: a systematic review. Gastrointest Endosc. 2010;71:280–6.

120. Morita E, Ohtsuka N, Shindo Y, et al. In vivo trial of a driving system for a self-propelling capsule endoscope using a magnetic field (with video). Gastrointest Endosc. 2010;72:836–40.

121. Kim HM, Yang S, Kim J, et al. Active locomotion of a paddling-based capsule endoscope in an in vitro and in vivo experiment (with videos). Gastrointest Endosc. 2010;72:381–7.

122. Quirini M, Menciassi A, Scapellato S, et al. Feasibility proof of a legged locomotion capsule for the GI tract. Gastrointest Endosc. 2008;67:1153–8.

123. Ciuti G, Menciassi A, Dario P. Capsule endoscopy: from current achievements to open challenges. IEEE Rev Biomed Eng. 2011;4:59–72.

124. Volke F, Keller J, Schneider A, et al. In-vivo remote manipulation of modified capsule endoscopes using an external magnetic field. Gastrointest Endosc. 2008;67:AB121–2.

125. Keller J, Fibbe C, Volke F, et al. Inspection of the human stomach using remote-controlled capsule

endoscopy: a feasibility study in healthy volunteers (with videos). Gastrointest Endosc. 2011;73:22–8.

126. Rey JF, Ogata H, Hosoe N, et al. Blinded nonrandomized comparative study of gastric examination with a magnetically guided capsule endoscope and standard video endoscope. Gastrointest Endosc. 2012;75:373–81.

127. Ciuti G, Donlin R, Valdastri P, et al. Robotic versus manual control in magnetic steering of an endoscopic capsule. Endoscopy. 2010;42:148–52.

128. Rey JF, Ogata H, Hosoe N, et al. Feasibility of stomach exploration with a guided capsule endoscope. Endoscopy. 2010;42:541–5.

129. Liao Z, Duan X-D, Xin L, et al. Feasibility and safety of magnetic-controlled capsule endoscopy system in examination of human stomach: a pilot study in healthy volunteers. J Interv Gastroenterol. 2012;2:155–60.

130. Bjorkman DJ. Maneuverable Video capsule Gastroscopy: Not Ready for Prime Time. Journal Watch Gastroenterology, March 2 2012. http://gastroenterology.jwatch.org/cgi/content/full/2012/302/5.

131. Ghoshal UC. Small bowel endoscopy in 2013: the reality and the potential. Nat Rev Gastroenterol Hepatol. 2014;11(2):86–7.

132. Friedrich K, Gehrke S, Stremmel W, et al. First clinical trial of a newly developed capsule endoscope with panoramic side view for small bowel: a pilot study. J Gastroenterol Hepatol. 2013;28(9):1496–501.

133. Pioche M, Vanbervliet G, Jacob P et al. Prospective randomized comparison between axial- and lateral-viewing capsule endoscopy systems in patients with obscure digestive bleeding. Endoscopy, 27 Nov 2013. [Epub ahead of print].

# Small Bowel Capsule Endoscopy

**3**

Imdadur Rahman, Praful Patel, Emanuele Rondonotti,
Anastasios Koulaouzidis, Marco Pennazio, Rahul Kalla,
Reena Sidhu, Peter Mooney, David Sanders,
Edward J. Despott, Chris Fraser, Niehls Kurniawan,
Peter Baltes, Martin Keuchel, Carolyn Davison, Nigel Beejay,
Clare Parker and Simon Panter

## Abbreviations

| | |
|---|---|
| AVM | Arterio-venous malformation |
| CE | Capsule endoscopy |
| CNSU | Chronic non-specific multiple ulcers of the small intestine |
| CMUSE | Cryptogenic multifocal ulcerous stenosing enteritis |
| CT | Computed tomography |

I. Rahman (✉) · P. Patel
Gastrointestinal Department, University Hospital
Southampton Foundation Trust, Southampton,
SO16 6YD, UK
e-mail: imdi81@hotmail.com

P. Patel
e-mail: praful.patel@uhs.nhs.uk

E. Rondonotti
Gastroenterology Unit, Ospedale Valduce,
via Dante 11, 22100 Como, Italy
e-mail: ema.rondo@gmail.com

A. Koulaouzidis
Endoscopy Unit, The Royal Infirmary of Edinburgh,
51 Little France Crescent, Edinburgh, EH16 4SA,
UK
e-mail: akoulaouzidis@hotmail.com

M. Pennazio (✉)
2nd Division of Gastroenterology, Department of
Medicine, San Giovanni Battista University
Teaching Hospital, Via Cavour 31,
10123 Torino, Italy
e-mail: pennazio.marco@gmail.com

R. Kalla
Gastrointestinal Unit, Institute of Genetics and
Molecular Medicine, University of Edinburgh,
Edinburgh, EH4 2XU, England
e-mail: rahul.kalla@ed.ac.uk

R. Sidhu (✉)
Gastroenterology and Liver Unit,
Royal Hallamshire Hospital, Sheffield Teaching
Hospitals NHS Trust, University of Sheffield,
Glossop Road, Sheffield, S10 2JF, England
e-mail: reena_sidhu@yahoo.com

P. Mooney (✉) · D. Sanders
Directorate of Gastroenterology,
Royal Hallamshire Hospital, Sheffield Teaching
Hospitals NHS Trust, Glossop Road, Sheffield,
S10 2JF, UK
e-mail: peter.mooney@sth.nhs.uk

D. Sanders
e-mail: david.sanders@sth.nhs.uk

E. J. Despott (✉)
Royal Free Unit for Endoscopy, Royal Free
Hospital, University College London, Institute for
Liver and Digestive Health, London, UK
e-mail: edespott@doctors.org.uk

C. Fraser
Wolfson Unit for Endoscopy, St Mark's Hospital
and Academic Institute, Imperial College London,
London, UK
e-mail: chris.fraser@imperial.ac.uk

N. Kurniawan · P. Baltes · M. Keuchel (✉)
Clinic for Internal Medicine, Bethesda Hospital
Bergedorf, Glindersweg 80, 21029 Hamburg,
Germany
e-mail: keuchel@bkb.info

Z. Li et al. (eds.), *Handbook of Capsule Endoscopy*,
DOI: 10.1007/978-94-017-9229-5_3, © Springer Science+Business Media Dordrecht 2014

| DAE | Device-assisted enteroscopy |
| DY | Diagnostic yield |
| GI | Gastrointestinal |
| GIST | Gastrointestinal stromal tumours |
| IBD | Inflammatory bowel disease |
| IDA | Iron-deficiency anaemia |
| IOE | Intra-operative enteroscopy |
| NaP | Sodium phosphate |
| NSAID | Non-steroidal anti-inflammatory drug |
| NET | Neuroendocrine tumours |
| OGIB | Obscure gastrointestinal bleeding |
| PE | Push enteroscopy |
| PEG | Polyethylene glycol |
| PHE | Portal hypertensive enteropathy |

## 3.1 Preparation for Small Bowel Capsule Endoscopy

### 3.1.1 Introduction

Although optical technology in the gastrointestinal tract has much improved in the last decade, image quality is only as good as the preparation achieved. As current capsule technology does not allow suctioning or flushing of fluid from the surface of the small bowel mucosa, there is consequently a greater imperative for adequate preparation to optimise detection of any potential lesion by the capsule endoscope.

Opinions are divided regarding the best cleansing regimen but most would agree some sort of bowel preparation is better than none. Currently the preparation type, dose and time of administration differ amongst centres across the world.

There is ample data to show that good preparation for colonoscopy, and more recently for gastroscopy, improves visualisation of lesions, speed of procedure and patient outcomes [1–3].

### 3.1.2 Pre-capsule Ingestion Preparation

There is now very little doubt that fasting and allowing clear fluid alone yield inferior small bowel visibility compared to that achieved with bowel preparation [4–6]. The evidence clearly shows that bowel preparation significantly improves visualisation of the small bowel mucosa. However, this improved visualisation does not always translate to an increased diagnostic yield (although the lack of association may be for other reasons, as mentioned later).

The best bowel regimen should be one that is both efficacious and acceptable to patients. Unfortunately, there is unlikely to be an optimal regimen as undoubtedly the effect will differ amongst patient groups. On a practical level, it is

N. Kurniawan
e-mail: Kurniawan@bkb.info

P. Baltes
e-mail: baltes@bkb.info

C. Davison (✉) · C. Parker · S. Panter
South Tyneside NHS Foundation Trust, Harton Lane, South Shields, Tyne and Wear, England NE34 0PL, UK
e-mail: carolyn.davison@stft.nhs.uk

C. Parker
e-mail: clare.e.parker@doctors.org.uk

S. Panter
e-mail: simon.panter@stft.nhs.uk

N. Beejay
Institute of Medicine, Medical City Hospital, Abu Dhabi, United Arab Emirates; London Independent Hospital, London, UK
e-mail: nigelbeejay@gmail.com

useful to adopt one regimen for the capsule service being offered with an additional regimen for those with poor preparation or an incomplete examination.

Several studies have looked into small bowel preparation based mainly on polyethylene glycol (PEG) and sodium phosphate (NaP). Some have combined the use of a prokinetic (mainly erythromycin or metoclopramide), to evaluate their impact on small bowel cleansing, diagnostic yield and rate of completeness of capsule endoscopy examination. Unfortunately, there has been a wide heterogeneity between trials with the type of purgatives used, dosage and scheduling.

There is consensus that a period of fasting, but allowing clear fluids (i.e. allowed water, clear lemonade, milk-less tea), for a period of around 12–24 h before ingestion is important. The safety profile of PEG seems to favour its use over NaP, which has associated potential nephrotoxicity [7, 8]. Two litres of PEG solution (e.g. Klean Prep) appears to be as efficacious as 4 L, when taken the evening before the study [9].

Most studies have looked into preparation taken the day before ingestion of the capsule, and only a handful have looked into taking the bowel preparation soon after ingestion [10–12]. Ito et al. used a regimen where, in addition to a 12-h fast and simethicone taken at the time of capsule ingestion, the intervention group drank a small volume of 500 ml of PEG solution 30 min to 2 h after ingestion of the capsule [10]. There was significant improvement in capsule image quality compared with the control group. Unfortunately, they did not have a comparison group taking PEG solution before ingestion. This regimen does potentially appear to have some scientific rationale. The PEG solution is completely transparent, so views may be clearer than that through intestinal fluid. PEG solution has also been shown to move through the intestine much faster than the capsule, so it may well have been completely cleared from an area of the intestine by the time the capsule reaches that area despite being ingested afterwards [13].

The administration of simethicone combined with fasting and purgatives does appear to improve small bowel visual quality; however, the exact dosage and time for this to be administered has differed considerably amongst studies (80–600 mg taken evening before or shortly before procedure) [14–18]. As side effects are seldom, it has the potential to be used as an adjunct to a regimen whether this be ad hoc or regularly.

Routine bowel preparation with prokinetics cannot be recommended, as the current data does not support its use due to conflicting outcomes and potential side effects, albeit occurring rarely. However, a recent meta-analysis has shown that the use of prokinetics as an adjunct to concurrent purging, when real-time monitoring is used, could be effective in improving the completion rate [19]. This effect seems to be more evident with metoclopramide. However, as the pharmacokinetics and peak onset of action differ with different modes of administration, timing of administration should be taken into account (onset of action 1–3 min for IV, 10–15 min for IM and 30–60 min for oral) [20].

The main reason for intolerability of bowel preparation is the associated nausea and inevitable diarrhoea. Recently, Niv et al. approached the concept of small bowel preparation with the notion that the small bowel is not a reservoir for faeces (concept of colonic preparation) but an area for digestion and absorption. With this in mind, they conducted a two centre prospective study with a liquid, fibre-free formula (ensure) taken the day before the procedure compared with 3 other regimens; 2 dietary restrictions and one PEG solution group. All patients observed an overnight 12-h fast [21]. Results showed similar efficacy (defined by cleanliness) to PEG but without the side effects. Unfortunately, the intervention group was small and there were some differences in the baseline patient characteristics. Nevertheless, this has the potential to be a fall back regimen for patients unable to tolerate purgatives.

### 3.1.3 Cleanliness Score

One of the contributors to the controversy about bowel preparation is the varying number of grading systems used to define the varying degrees of mucosal visualisation and cleanliness. Some are purely subjective with an overall operator consensus (good, fair, poor), and others are more objectively measured in a more systematic way either by assigning a single overall score or a composite score comprising assessments obtained at different points in the small bowel. The main use to date for a small bowel cleanliness scores has been for research purposes, but it has potential clinical value in commenting on the validity of the examination. The most useful and practical method is probably the one devised by Park et al., which is relatively simple, as well as having a good inter-observer and intra-patient agreement [22].

The scoring system uses a 4-step scale in 2 visual parameters; the proportion of mucosa visualised and the degree to which debris/bile/bubbles obscures visualisation (see Table 3.1; Fig. 3.1). Images from the small bowel are selected at 5-min intervals and reviewed. A score is allocated by summing the score from each selected frame and dividing it by the

**Table 3.1** CE image score system

| *The proportion of visualised mucosa* | |
| --- | --- |
| Score 3 (%) | ≥75 |
| Score 2 (%) | 50–75 |
| Score 1 (%) | 25–50 |
| Score 0 (%) | <25 |
| *The degree of bubbles, debris and bile* | |
| Score 3 | <5 %, not obscured |
| Score 2 | 5–25 %, mildly obscured |
| Score 1 | 25–50 %, moderately obscured |
| Score 0 | ≥50 %, severely obscured |

number of examined frames. The representative value from each parameter is then averaged to give an overall average. A score greater than 2.25 (as extrapolated from the studies ROC curve) is deemed as being satisfactorily sensitive (85 %) and specific (87 %) (Table 3.1).

### 3.1.4 Post-capsule Ingestion Preparation

Some accommodation needs to be made for differences between sensors and receivers of different manufacturers with regards to pre- and post-

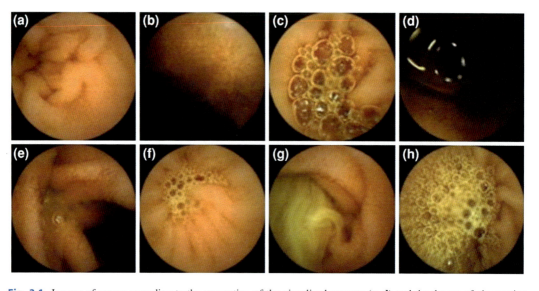

**Fig. 3.1** Images of scores according to the proportion of the visualised mucosa (**a–d**) and the degree of obscuration (**e–h**). **a** Score 3; **b** Score 2; **c** Score 1; **d** Score 0; **e** Score 3; **f** Score 2; **g** Score 1; **h** Score 0

preparation. There are currently 5 commercially available capsules; MiroCam by Intromedic, Pill-Cam by Given Imaging, EndoCapsule by Olympus, OMOM capsule by Jianshan Science and Technology Ltd and CapsoCam by Capsovision.

Most capsule manufacturers advocate a complete fast (no fluid intake at all) for at least 4 h before and 2 h after ingestion of the capsule in addition to oral bowel preparation; these manufacturers rely on radiofrequency transmission. The MiroCam system utilises human body communication for transmission of images from the capsule to the receiver, and the manufacturers do not advocate the need for a water-free fast period, but encourage sipping on water hourly after ingestion as it potentially may enhance image transmission.

### 3.1.5 Practical Issues Related to Delayed Gastric Emptying/Small Bowel Transit

Apart from oral preparation, it is worthwhile considering the characteristic of the patient particularly with regards to preventing an incomplete examination of the small bowel and improving mucosal visualisation. Iron supplementation and loperamide containing medications should be stopped 5–7 days before the procedure; the former obscuring views from unabsorbed iron and the latter having an impact in decreasing intestinal motility.

Gastric and colonic transit times vary greatly in comparison with small bowel transit between individuals. It is known that delayed gastric emptying is mainly responsible for incomplete examinations [23, 24]. Hence, scenarios that may affect gastric transit should be noted by capsule operators. Gastric retention and emptying were studied extensively, even before the advent of small bowel capsule, and it seems that there are numerous factors that can affect gastric emptying [25]. Anecdotally and with reasonable evidence, there are a number of conditions and drugs that are known to effect gastric and possibly small bowel transit. Table 3.2 lists the most common of these. If possible, all contributing drugs should be stopped a few days before the examination.

**Table 3.2** Scenarios affecting capsule transit times

| Conditions | |
|---|---|
| Diabetes (poorly controlled) | [26] |
| Parkinson's | [459] |
| Connective tissue disorders, e.g. scleroderma | [460] |
| *Drugs* | |
| Opiates, e.g. codeine | [461] |
| Anticholinergic effect drugs, e.g. TCAs | [462] |
| Alcohol | [463] |

### 3.1.6 Sample Regimen

The following lists some potential regimens (see post-capsule ingestion preparation in regards to clear water period). All regimens cater for the capsule ingestion occurring in the morning (most practical). Essential medications can be taken as required with sips of water.

1. Breakfast the day before, then clear fluids only from 12:00. Two litres of PEG solution taken between 16:00 and 18:00. Complete fast from midnight.
2. Normal lunch the day before, then clear fluids only from 15:00. Ingestion of 1 L of PEG solution between 30 min and 2 h post-ingestion of capsule

For patients who have had a failed procedure as a consequence of poor cleanliness, consider restricting to a full 24 h of clear liquids only (with possible low residue dietary restriction 48 h before), doubling the volume of prep and adding in 160 mg simethicone at the time of ingestion.

For patients who have had a failed procedure as a consequence of not reaching the caecum in time, consider administration of 10–20 mg metoclopramide 30 min before ingestion or around the time of capsule ingestion if by IM or IV administration.

### 3.1.7 Conclusion

Bowel preparation is essential to provide adequate imaging for small bowel capsule endoscopy. Currently, preparation involves fasting, oral cleanser (usually PEG) and avoiding drugs that

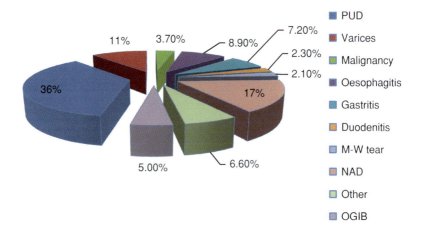

**Fig. 3.2** Causes of gastrointestinal bleeding through the GI tract

would obscure or delay gastrointestinal transit. Promotility drugs are used if required for individual patients. Further research is required with larger studies to devise better tolerated regimens.

## 3.2    Obscure Gastrointestinal Bleeding

**Abstract**  The evaluation of patients with obscure gastrointestinal bleeding (OGIB) has been suboptimal for a long time due to the limited ability to image the small bowel. Over the past 10 years, significant improvements have been made in small bowel imaging techniques. Particularly, since the introduction of capsule endoscopy (CE), the diagnostic approach to OGIB has improved significantly. CE is an extremely well-tolerated examination that allows the evaluation of the entire small bowel mucosa, providing high-quality images and identifying even tiny, flat mucosal changes (i.e. vascular malformations, which represent the most frequent small bowel lesion found in patients with OGIB). Many studies have shown that the diagnostic yield of CE in OGIB patients, which is 50–60 %, is significantly superior to that of most conventional techniques for the study of the small bowel and similar to highly invasive procedures such device-assisted enteroscopy (DAE). Therefore, nowadays, CE is considered the examination of choice in patients with OGIB, after negative gastroscopy and colonoscopy. Its diagnostic yield is especially high in patients with overt bleeding, or when the procedure is performed close to the last episode of acute bleeding, as well as in patients with severe anaemia or with high transfusion requirement. When integrated in a global patient care plan, CE is helpful in achieving effective decision-making concerning subsequent investigations and treatments. Future multicentre prospective studies with standardised surveillance and/or treatment protocol, with long follow-up, are warranted in order to truly estimate the long-term impact of CE in patients with OGIB.

**Keywords**  Obscure gastrointestinal bleeding · Iron-deficiency anaemia · Capsule endoscopy · Device-assisted enteroscopy · Outcomes.

Obscure gastrointestinal bleeding (OGIB) is defined as gastrointestinal (GI) bleeding of unknown origin that persists or recurs following a negative initial endoscopic evaluation (bidirectional gastrointestinal (GI) endoscopy). OGIB is classified as either overt OGIB (which manifests as recurrent melena or haematochezia) or occult OGIB, which presents by recurrent or persistent iron-deficiency anaemia (IDA) [27].

Although OGIB represents only a small proportion (about 5 %) [28] of GI bleeding (Fig. 3.2), it can pose significant diagnostic and management challenges. One of the main reasons is that the small bowel is often the site of bleeding [29, 30]. Indeed, identification and localisation of the bleeding source can be difficult, requiring utilisation of a significant amount of healthcare resources, which leads to reduced cost-effectiveness [31]. Patients with OGIB often require numerous blood transfusions and repeated hospital admissions involving multiple diagnostic procedures. Therefore, the advent of capsule endoscopy (CE) was a major forward leap, leading to a complete redesign of diagnostic algorithms for patients with OGIB [32–36].

The success story of CE lies in its technical characteristics. Hence, its unique ability to provide high-resolution images of the entire (in the majority of cases) [37, 38] small bowel mucosa can account for its superiority over other 'conventional' endoscopic modalities. To date, several studies have shown that, in terms of diagnostic yield (DY), CE is superior, when compared to push enteroscopy (PE) [39–42] (which usually enables the exploration of only 100–150 cm of small intestine), or to DAE [43, 44], if the latter is carried out with a single approach (oral or anal). Conversely, there is a substantial equivalence between CE and DAE when the latter (combining oral and anal approach) assess the entire small bowel [44, 45].

Furthermore, as it was rather expected in patients with OGIB, CE demonstrated better diagnostic performance when compared to classical radiologic modalities, e.g. small bowel follow through. Although most radiological methods provide—just like CE—views of the entire small bowel, they are 'betrayed' by their low spatial resolution in cases of small, superficial lesions such as vascular malformations, erosions or ulcers [46, 47].

### 3.2.1 Findings at Capsule Endoscopy in Patients with OGIB

Essentially, the spectrum of lesions responsible for small bowel bleeding is similar to that seen in other GI tract segments. It includes vascular and inflammatory lesions, as well as polyps/neoplasms. The prevalence of different small

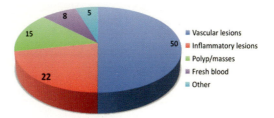

**Fig. 3.3** Patients with OGIB and positive CE: spectrum of findings

bowel findings in patients with OGIB and positive CE is reported in Fig. 3.3.

#### 3.2.1.1 Vascular Lesions

Vascular lesions are the most common causes of bleeding in the small intestine, accounting for about 50–60 % of all small bowel findings [48]. Amongst vascular lesions, angioectasias represent the most frequent small bowel finding in adult patients living in Western countries. Angioectasias (also called arterio-venous malformations–AVM), appear as small, superficial red spots with well-demarcated edges (Fig. 3.4). They are characterised by dilated, distorted blood vessels.

A less common vascular lesion in the small bowel is Dieulafoy's lesion, which consists of an abnormal, submucosal 'calibre-persistent artery' that typically protrudes through a minute 2–5-mm mucosal defect. In most cases, diagnosing a Dieulafoy's lesion is challenging, as by definition, it relies on visualising acute arterial bleeding or a protruding vessel with or without active bleeding during endoscopy. In the absence of these findings, a small mucosal ulceration overlying an artery can be easily overlooked.

Small bowel varices, appearing at CE as tortuous, bluish nodular structures, are seen in the setting of portal hypertension due to chronic liver disease, portal vein thrombosis and/or hepatic vein thrombosis. Ectopic varices are usually located within the proximal small bowel (duodenum and jejunum) and are overall less likely to rupture, compared with oesophageal varices. In portal hypertensive enteropathy (PHE) (Fig. 3.5) small bowel varices may be

**Fig. 3.4** AVMs identified by CE; **a** and **c** are usually classified as P2 lesions whereas **b** as a P1 lesion

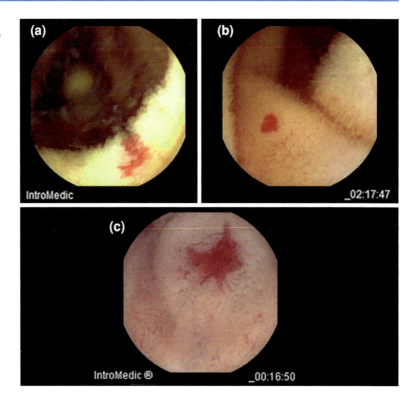

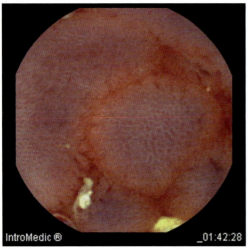

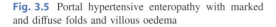

**Fig. 3.5** Portal hypertensive enteropathy with marked and diffuse folds and villous oedema

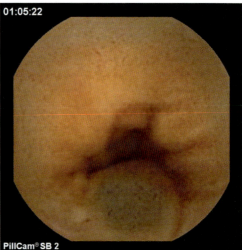

**Fig. 3.6** Phlebectasis

associated with angioectasias, which are usually minute and petechial in appearance [49].

Venous and phlebectasis, (Fig. 3.6) appearing as bluish, flat or slightly elevated spots, are other forms as vascular lesions. This finding is extremely common in the small bowel and usually of no clinical significance; nevertheless, when phlebectasis are multiple, elevated, nodular, large in diameter and/or associated with skin or mucosal venous blebs (cavernous skin haemangioma), can be a manifestation of the blue rubber bleb nevus syndrome or bean syndrome, a

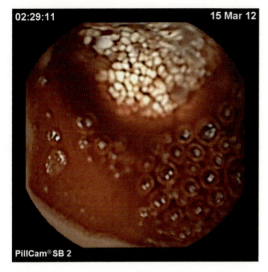

**Fig. 3.7** Giant cavernous haemangioma with active bleeding

rare clinical condition (200 cases are reported in the literature) [50], which is often complicated by profuse GI haemorrhage (which is the main cause of mortality in these patients) [51] (Fig. 3.7).

### 3.2.1.2 Inflammatory Lesions

Although the appearance of inflammatory small bowel lesions is similar to those encountered in other GI segments, they do not appear as depressed at CE, because of the lack of insufflation. Conversely, the fibrin covering the central part of ulcers is often elevated, when compared with the surrounding mucosa (Fig. 3.8).

Small bowel inflammatory changes are seen in several conditions, such as inflammatory bowel disease (IBD), (Fig. 3.9) (previously undiagnosed Crohn's disease is found incidentally in approximately 6 % of patients undergoing CE to evaluate

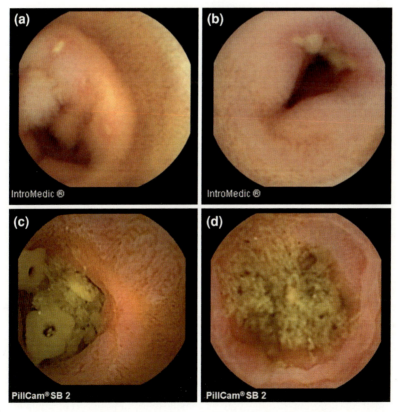

**Fig. 3.8** Inflammatory lesions identified in the small bowel of four patients taking NSAIDs; **a** erosions; **b** small ulcers covered by fibrin; **c, d** circumferential ulcers causing narrowing of the lumen

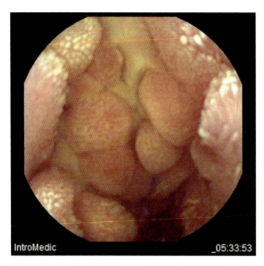

**Fig. 3.9** Cobblestone and linear ulcerations in the terminal ileum of a patient with Crohn's disease

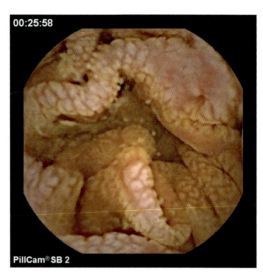

**Fig. 3.11** Proximal small bowel of a patient with refractory coeliac disease; presence of scalloping of folds, mucosal fissures and erosions

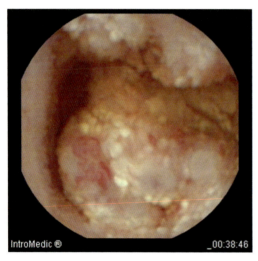

**Fig. 3.10** Small bowel lymphoma appearing at CE as a polypoid lesion by whitish irregular mucosa

OGIB) [48], small bowel lymphomas, (Fig. 3.10) chronic mesenteric ischaemia, complicated coeliac disease, (Fig. 3.11) tuberculosis, Behcet's disease, eosinophilic enteritis, and conditions as chronic non-specific multiple ulcers of the small intestine (CNSU) or cryptogenic multifocal ulcerous stenosing enteritis (CMUSE). Noteworthy, a number of different drugs, such as potassium, chemotherapeutic agents, 6-mercaptopurine, and mainly acetylsalicylic acid and non-

steroidal anti-inflammatory drugs (NSAIDs), can cause small bowel ulcerations and bleeding.

NSAID-induced enteropathy may occur with both cyclooxygenase-1 and cyclooxygenase-2 inhibitors agents [52]. Unfortunately, almost all of the inflammatory lesions in the small bowel have a non-specific appearance; therefore, although CE can be helpful in identifying the source of bleeding, when inflammatory changes are identified a precise diagnosis can seldom be made on the ground of endoscopic findings alone (Fig. 3.8). At present time, this represents one of the main limitations of CE in the setting of the OGIB. Imaging enhancement tools such as virtual chromoendoscopy and/or 3D imaging could potentially have a differential in the classification of such lesions [53, 54].

### 3.2.1.3 Small Bowel Neoplasms/Small Bowel Polyps

Small bowel tumours are discovered in 2–10 % of patients undergoing CE because of OGIB [55, 56], particularly in young patients [57]. Benign and malignant primary tumours, as well as metastatic tumours (i.e. melanoma or breast cancer) [58–60], can be found throughout the small intestine. The endoscopic appearance of

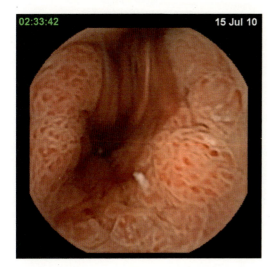

**Fig. 3.12** Small bowel adenocarcinoma actively bleeding

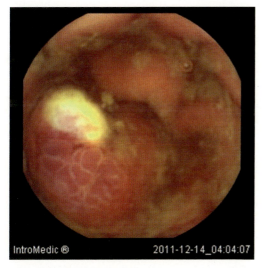

**Fig. 3.13** Large, eroded, small bowel polyp in patient with Peutz–Jeghers syndrome

small bowel tumours varies according to their size, location and site of origin. Tumours originating from the mucosa [i.e. adenocarcinomas (Fig. 3.12)] often appear as ulcerated masses or large polyps (Fig. 3.13), whereas those originating from the submucosal layer [i.e. neuroendocrine tumours (NET) or gastrointestinal stromal tumours (GIST)] often appear as protruding nodules, covered—at the early stages—by normal small bowel mucosa or later in the

course of the disease with superficial erosions or ulcers. The distinction between small bowel submucosal tumours and innocent bulging, due to active peristalsis, is one of the challenging tasks in reviewing CE (Fig. 3.14). A bulge is defined as a round and smooth, large base protrusion in the lumen having an ill-defined edge on the surrounding mucosa; it can be a prominent normal fold or the result of intestinal loop angulation and stiffness, and sometimes, it can be virtually indistinguishable from a small submucosal tumour. Some visual clues may help distinguishing masses from bulges (i.e. changes in mucosal characteristics, presence of bridging folds, of transit abnormalities, of repetitive images, and of synchronous lesions). Some authors [61, 62] have recently proposed, on the ground of these visual clues, a scoring system to distinguish masses from bulges. Unfortunately, none of them has been externally validated yet. Moreover, in everyday clinical practice, the aforementioned indicators are often absent.

Additionally, several studies [63–65] reported patients with negative CE in which further examinations showed small bowel tumours (false negative CE). Lewis et al. [64], analysing data from an industry-maintained trial database, found that CE was negative in about 1.5 % of patients with small bowel tumours. They estimated that the miss rate of CE in neoplastic diseases can reach 18.9 %. Although this percentage is lower than that reported for other diagnostic modalities (63.2 %), it is still alarming, especially considering the clinical relevance of these missing findings. In addition, recent reports showed a relatively low sensitivity of CE, when compared with computed-tomography (CT) enterography in this setting [66]. Therefore, in patients with clinical suspicion of small bowel tumour, CT enterography should precede CE.

### 3.2.1.4 Other Small Bowel Lesions

Small bowel diverticulae are frequently overlooked in CE due to lack of insufflation [67] (Fig. 3.15). The prevalence of small bowel diverticulosis is approximately 0.1–2 % of the

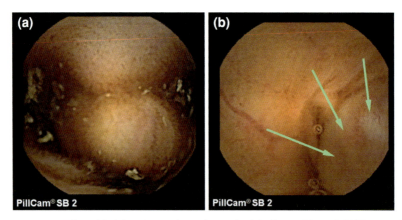

Fig. 3.14  **a** Innocent small bowel bulging due to the active peristalsis; **b** small bowel GIST appearing at CE as a round nodule, covered by slightly congested mucosa (*green arrows*)

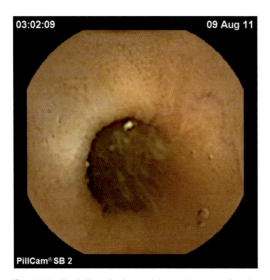

Fig. 3.15  Ileal diverticulum without stigmata of active or recent bleeding

population. Furthermore, Meckel's diverticulum is the commonest cause of small bowel bleeding in patients under the age of 25. It is estimated that fewer than 5 % of subjects with jejunal diverticulae actually bleed from them. Moreover, even when discovered by CE, evidence of active bleeding is necessary to conclude that a diverticulum is the site of blood loss.

Another finding, which is identified in about 8–10 % of OGIB patients with positive CE, is the presence of fresh blood/active bleeding in the lumen (Fig. 3.16). Although by definition not a lesion, it is often considered as a positive finding

when calculating the DY of CE. Indeed, fresh blood in the bowel lumen confirms the bleeding site in the small bowel, provides useful lesion localisation information, and therefore, it can guide further diagnostic/therapeutic procedures, such as DAE [68].

### 3.2.2  Diagnostic Accuracy of Capsule Endoscopy in Patients with OGIB

Large studies identify a definite bleeding source in 50–60 % of patients [37, 38, 69–71]. The DY is usually calculated taking into account only lesion with high bleeding potential; in fact, SB lesions identified at capsule endoscopy are usually divided into three subgroups: (1) *highly relevant lesions* (*P2*) such as angioectasia, large ulcerations, tumours or varices; (2) *uncertain relevance lesions* (*P1*) such as red spots, small isolated erosions; (3) *low relevance lesions* (*P0*) such as visible submucosal veins, non-bleeding diverticula, nodules without mucosal break [72].

In studies concerning CE, the DY is the parameter conventionally used to estimate the diagnostic ability of this examination. That is mostly because, in this setting, it is very difficult to calculate the most common clinical efficacy parameters such as sensitivity, specificity and diagnostic accuracy, as it lacks a true reference standard to which it could be compared with.

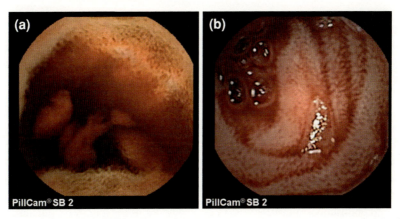

**Fig. 3.16** Red blood in the lumen of the small bowel that covers the mucosa, thus preventing the identification of the actively bleeding lesion

Actually, in the study of the small intestine, a reference standard should allow to explore the entire small bowel, recognising the presence of even small lesions and obtaining histological confirmation, when necessary. These goals, at the present time, can be achieved only through intra-operative enteroscopy (IOE) or bidirectional DAE. The first requires of course surgical intervention (associated with mortality and morbidity), whereas the latter is logistically feasible only in a small proportion of the patients [73].

A recent study that compared CE with IOE found that the sensitivity, specificity, positive and negative predictive values of CE were 95, 75, 95 and 86 %, respectively. In this study, the gold standard, i.e. IOE, had 100 % DY for ongoing bleeding, but only 70.8 % for previous overt OGIB and less so (50 %) for occult OGIB [74]. These data confirmed results from an earlier retrospective study [48] in which CE was compared with a composite reference standard, taking into account both further diagnostic examinations and the follow-up. Moreover, in a more recent paper, Tenembaum et al. [67] compared CE with DAE combining oral and anal approach, according to the type of the lesion identified. These authors found that although CE and DAE yielded similar results, CE had an excellent accuracy profile for masses/tumours (sensitivity and specificity: 100 %), an intermediate performance for vascular and inflammatory lesions (sensitivity: 58 and 50 %

respectively; specificity: 93 and 98 % respectively) and a disappointing accuracy for small bowel diverticulae (sensitivity: 9 %; specificity: 100 %).

On the basis of solid scientific evidence [69, 70, 75], most national and international gastrointestinal scientific societies have issued updated practice guidelines for the diagnosis and management of patients with OGIB, recommending CE as the first-line tool to evaluate the small bowel, after negative bidirectional endoscopy, in the clinical context of OGIB [32–36].

A key factor, which has been demonstrated in several studies, to significantly affect the yield of CE is the timing of the procedure. In fact, several studies [48, 76, 77], mostly focused on patients with overt OGIB, reported a significantly higher DY (75–90 %) in patients undergoing CE in the early stage of their diagnostic work up. Yamada et al. [77] recently showed an inverse linear correlation between the time elapsed from the last episode of overt bleeding and CE.

Unfortunately, less is known about the exact timing for CE in patients with obscure–occult GI bleeding; in these patients, it is often impossible to establish, in a reliable fashion, the length of the clinical history of anaemia; therefore, a more conservative approach can be generally suggested [78]. Recent guidelines [32, 79] suggest first to exclude other causes of persistent/recurrent iron-deficiency anaemia (i.e. malabsorption, menstrual loss) and then an appropriate empiric therapy with iron supplementation (i.e. ferrous sulphate 200 mg twice daily, for 1–3 months) could reasonably precede CE. Another factor, which has been found to have a relevant impact on the yield of CE, is the severity of bleeding. Patients with OGIB and low haemoglobin levels and/or high transfusion requirement are more likely to have small bowel lesions and deserve a small bowel evaluation by means of CE [80, 81].

It should not be underestimated that patients referred for CE can harbour lesions within the reach of standard endoscopes; nevertheless, in a cost-effective analysis as that performed by Vlachogiannakos et al. [30], their incidence is too low [30, 82] to justify a standard policy of second-look endoscopy before CE. Nevertheless, further studies are needed to identify subgroups of patients at increased risk to harbour lesions within the reach of a conventional endoscope in which repeating gastroscopy and/or colonoscopy would be cost-effective. Therefore, at present time, repeating conventional endoscopy before CE has to be decided on an individual basis, taking into account the reason for referral (occult vs. overt OGIB), but also the quality/timing of previous procedures, ongoing/previous therapies and comorbidities.

It is also important to emphasise that, after negative CE, when patients have ongoing or recurrent evidence of bleeding or when clinical suspicion of small bowel pathology is sufficiently high, further investigation with small bowel (total) enteroscopy or cross-sectional imaging is clearly warranted [83].

### 3.2.3 Impact on Long-term Outcomes

Although several [48, 71, 75] studies have assessed the yield of CE in OGIB, the exact significance of the lesions identified and their impact on clinical outcome has not been adequately examined. Unfortunately, the majority of studies on CE in OGIB are focused on potential changes in management, rather than on evaluating long-term outcomes. The studies assessing a change in clinical decision-making after CE showed that about two-thirds of patients with OGIB received specific therapeutic interventions or changes in management based on a finding from CE [84, 85].

Some studies [86, 87] reported that a negative CE in patients with OGIB is associated with a low rate of recurrent bleeding; therefore, it is reasonable to take an expectant approach with these patients, thus avoiding the need for unnecessary additional investigations, but keeping these patients under scheduled surveillance.

As far as the long-term outcome is concerned, the majority of studies evaluating the long-term (2–3 years) outcomes in patients undergoing CE report a favourable outcome in most of patients (about 60 %) managed on the ground of capsule endoscopy results [88, 89]. However, recently published studies [90, 91] are casting some doubts on the real impact on long-term outcome, despite a high diagnostic yield of CE. Several factors can probably explain the differences observed in different studies: there are differences in the population characteristics (i.e. medications, type of bleeding, timing of CE, etc.), there are no standardised approaches for patient management after CE and the different policies adopted at different medical centres can introduce relevant bias.

Therefore, although it is well known that CE has the capability to diagnose small bowel lesions and to drive further management [92–96], in the next few years, large multicentre studies with standardised surveillance and/or treatment protocol, with long follow-up, are warranted in order to truly estimate the long-term impact of CE in patients with OGIB.

**Conflict of interest statement**: Marco Pennazio is a member of the speaker's board of Given Imaging Inc. (Yoqneam, Israel). Anastasios Koulaouzidis has received research Grant from Given® Imaging Ltd., Germany (ESGE-Given® Imaging Research Grant 2011) and material support for capsule endoscopy research from SYNMED©, both unrelated to the present work. Emanuele Rondonotti has no conflict of interest.

## 3.3 The Use of Capsule Endoscopy for Small Bowel Crohn's Disease

**Abstract** The diagnosis of small bowel Crohn's disease (SBCD) can often be a diagnostic challenge due to varied symptomatology, absence of raised inflammatory markers and non-specific radiological and endoscopic findings. Over the past decade, with the introduction of newer therapeutic agents and investigation modalities such as capsule endoscopy, significant progress has been made in the diagnosis of small bowel CD. Capsule endoscopy has gained popularity not only for its use in patients with suspected CD, but also in identifying active small bowel disease in established CD and reclassifying patients with inflammatory bowel disease unclassified (IBDU). In this chapter, we summarise the indications, diagnostic yield and subsequent management change in patients with suspected CD, established CD and IBDU undergoing capsule endoscopy. We also highlight important considerations for its use in these cohorts.

### 3.3.1 Background

Crohn's disease (CD) is a transmural chronic granulomatous inflammatory disorder that can affect any segment of the gastrointestinal tract. Isolated small bowel involvement occurs in up to a third of the patients [97, 98]. Management in these individuals can be challenging due to varying symptoms, absence of raised inflammatory markers and a low sensitivity of small bowel barium study for early mucosal disease [99]. A mean delay in the diagnosis of CD of 1–7 years in published series has been reported [100, 101]. Over the past years, since the introduction of biological therapy for CD, there has been a paradigm shift in the way we manage CD with greater emphasis on mucosal healing rather than symptom control only. Mucosal healing has shown to be associated with improved long-term outcomes for CD and lower rates of hospitalisation and surgery [102]. With the advent of better diagnostic tests and imaging modalities such as capsule endoscopy, early diagnosis of small bowel Crohn's disease (SBCD) has become ever increasingly important.

### 3.3.2 Clinical Features

Small bowel Crohn's disease (SBCD) is often a difficult diagnosis to establish clinically. Patients can present with variable symptoms including abdominal pain, fatigue, diarrhoea, weight loss, with or without evidence of bleeding [103]. Patients can also present with complications of transmural inflammation that include stricturing or fistulating disease.

Apart from GI symptoms, CD can present with extra-intestinal manifestations. These include the following:
- Joint symptoms—Inflammatory arthritis mainly involving large joints
- Eye symptoms—Uveitis, iritis and episcleritis
- Skin manifestations—Erythema nodosum and pyoderma gangrenosum
- Primary Sclerosing Cholangitis

Laboratory markers can be helpful in raising the suspicion of small bowel CD. Patients may present with iron-deficiency anaemia, B12 deficiency and/or raised inflammatory markers. It is unclear that combination of symptoms and/or laboratory markers predicts CD [104]. Faecal calprotectin (fC) has been used as a cost-effective screening tool prior to SBCE in patients with suspected CD and prior normal bidirectional endoscopy [105]. Koulaouzidis et al. [105] showed that an fC > 100 µg/g is a good predictor of positive SBCE findings, whilst fC > 200 µg/g confirmed CD in 50 % of cases. There are published guidelines on the use of SBCE in CD for USA, UK and Europe [106–108].

### 3.3.3 Histology

Typical histological features of CD include the presence of granulomas, areas of chronic inflammatory cell infiltrate (lymphocytes,

known that at least 20 % would require additional surgery for their recurrence [134, 136]. At present, immunosuppressive therapy is recommended in patients who are at high risk of recurrence, i.e. fistulating disease, ileocolonic disease and smokers or those with low risk of recurrence but significant endoscopic changes 6–12 months post-operatively [137, 138].

The use SBCE has been studied in patients with established CD. SBCE was found to have a diagnostic yield of 71 % for active CD compared with 35 and 39 % for small bowel radiology and CT enterography/enteroclysis, respectively [99]. Studies have also compared SBCE and MR enterography (MRE). Both modalities appear complimentary with similar diagnostic yields, yet SBCE is better at identifying mucosal disease whilst MRE is preferred for transmural and extra-intestinal changes [139–142]. There is, however, a small but definite risk of capsule retention, especially in patients with established CD. As a result, the BSG guidelines advocate the use of PillCam Patency$^{TM}$ prior to SBCE if abdominal pain is a significant feature [106]. Although clinical experience with PillCam Patency$^{TM}$ is limited, there are studies in the literature using PillCam Patency$^{TM}$ to detect SB stenosis. It allows an effective assessment of any luminal stenosis amongst established CD and post-operative patients [122, 143–146].

Mehdizadeh et al. [147] published the largest series on symptomatic CD patients ($n = 134$). Although it concluded that SBCE has a higher diagnostic yield, there was no data on long-term outcome. Recently, Long et al. ($n = 86$), Dussault et al. ($n = 71$) and Kalla et al. ($n = 50$) published data on the impact of SBCE on management [122, 148, 149]. All authors concluded that SBCE alters management in the majority of patients with symptomatic IBD, be it surgical resection or intensifying medical therapy.

There is limited published data on the use of SBCE to detect recurrence post-operatively [119, 122, 137]. Bourreille et al. [119] demonstrated that SBCE was inferior to ileocolonoscopy in detecting recurrence of Crohn's disease after surgical resection ($n = 32$ patients), this was not supported by Pons Beltrán et al. [137]. It

has been suggested that this discrepancy could be due to poor views in the distal ileum and irregular propagation of the capsule [119]. In addition, the type of anastomosis in the patient cohorts was different. Whilst one study included patients with end-to-end anastomosis, the other study had patients with side-to-side anastomosis; the latter being more difficult to examine endoscopically [119, 137]. Although these studies have allowed us to appreciate the utility of SBCE in these patients, large prospective trials are lacking.

Studies have shown that patients with established CD seem to have more extensive disease on SBCE than previously seen by ileocolonoscopy [119, 137]. Flamant et al. [150] have suggested that patients with ileal CD are more likely to have jejunal lesions and are at an increased risk of clinical relapse. However, there appears to be no correlation between symptoms and extent of small bowel disease at SBCE [151].

### 3.3.4.6 Inflammatory Bowel Disease Unclassified

Colonic inflammatory bowel disease (IBD) can be classified into either Crohn's disease (CD) or ulcerative colitis (UC). There, however, appears to be a subset of patients that fall short of the endoscopic and histological criteria for CD or UC. These patients are classified as inflammatory bowel disease unclassified (IBDU). This term was first defined by the Montreal World Congress of Gastroenterology working party in 2005 [152]. Population-based studies have shown that up to 20 % of patients with colonic IBD cannot be classified as CD or UC; this prevalence being up to 30 % amongst children [153, 154].

When colitis presentation is severe, it is pertinent to differentiate UC from CD as ileo-anal pouch anastomosis is generally contraindicated in the latter due to high risk of post-op complications such as anastomotic leaks [155]. In addition, pouch salvage surgery is usually unsuccessful in these patients [156]. It is also postulated that the clinical course and outcome could be worse in patients with IBDU [157]. With the introduction of new biological therapies targeted at established CD or UC,

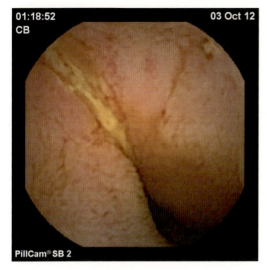

**Fig. 3.17** Linear ulceration on capsule endoscopy

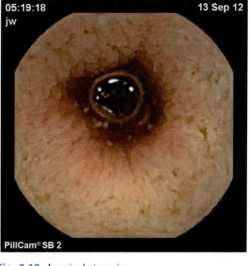

**Fig. 3.19** Luminal stenosis

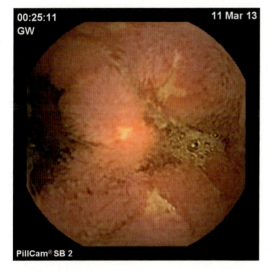

**Fig. 3.18** Multiple erosions in a patient with suspected Crohn's disease

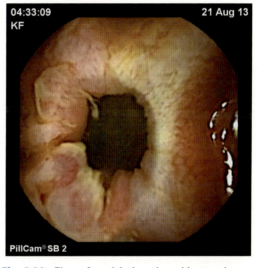

**Fig. 3.20** Circumferential ulceration with stenosis

confirmation of the type of IBD has become increasingly important.

There are a small number of studies, which have looked at the effect of SBCE diagnosis of CD on the management and long-term outcome in patients with IBDU [120, 122, 148, 158, 159]. Lopes et al. felt that the findings on CE did not influence management; however, their study cohort was small with a CD diagnosis of CE in 7 patients. The inclusion criterion for SBCE in their study included asymptomatic individuals with a long-standing diagnosis of IBDU. Hence, on follow-up, although SBCE diagnosed CD in 38 %, management was not altered in any of these patients as they were in clinical remission [158]. In contrast, four other studies felt SBCE was a novel and clinically useful diagnostic tool that altered management in patients with a diagnosis of CD on SBCE [120, 122, 148, 159]. All 4 studies included symptomatic IBDU patients where management was altered as a result of SBCE; this included either step up /step down medical therapy or surgery (Figs. 3.17, 3.18, 3.19, 3.20).

## Summary

| Type of disease | Diagnostic yield (%) | Overall management change (%) | Important considerations |
|---|---|---|---|
| Suspected Crohn's disease [121, 122, 131] | 17–59 (prevalence of 12–13 %) | 62 (Kalla et al.) | Diagnostic yield and prevalence dependant on strict referral and diagnostic criteria at capsule endoscopy |
| Established Crohn's disease [119, 122, 137, 147, 148] | 48–71 | 17–68 | Risk of capsule retention is relatively higher in this cohort, especially if symptoms of abdominal pain are present |
| Inflammatory bowel disease unclassified [120, 122, 148, 158, 159] | 17–43 | 17–73 | Diagnostic yield and post-capsule endoscopy management can vary in asymptomatic versus symptomatic individuals |

## 3.4     Capsule Endoscopy in Coeliac Disease

**Abstract** Coeliac disease is a common auto-immune condition affecting up to 1 % of the adult population. Currently, a duodenal biopsy taken at endoscopy is required to make a conclusive diagnosis. Macroscopic changes of coeliac disease seen at endoscopy and have been shown to have high levels of specificity, especially when combined with coeliac serology. However, standard endoscopy can be poorly tolerated and is contraindicated in a small number of patients. Also changes of coeliac disease may only be apparent more distally in
the small bowel than can be assessed with standard endoscopy. Complications of coeliac disease such as ulcerative jejunitis or small bowel malignancy can also develop throughout the small bowel. This chapter will assess the role of capsule endoscopy for the diagnosis of coeliac disease in routine and equivocal cases. The role of capsule endoscopy in the investigation of non-responsive and refractory coeliac disease and small bowel malignancy will be evaluated. Capsule technology is rapidly evolving and current and potential future developments that may revolutionise capsule endoscopy in coeliac disease will be discussed.

### 3.4.1   Introduction

Coeliac disease is a common autoimmune condition characterised by a heightened immunological response to ingested gluten, with prevalence rates in the USA and European populations estimated to range between 0.2 and 1 % [160, 161]. Furthermore, there is some evidence to suggest that the prevalence of coeliac disease is increasing [162–164]. Finally, clinicians from both China and the Indian subcontinent are now recognising patients with coeliac disease. This had not previously been the case, and one hypothesis is that coeliac disease is emerging due to the introduction of wheat into these ethnic groups (as their diet becomes more westernised). Thus, coeliac disease is a global problem [165, 166]. The current gold standard diagnostic test for coeliac disease is small bowel histology, demonstrating the presence of villous atrophy (VA) (Marsh 3a to 3c) [167]. Corroborative evidence used to support the diagnosis of coeliac disease comes from positive serological tests (tissue transglutaminase (tTG) and endomysial (EMA) antibodies) and a clinical response to a gluten-free diet. Occasionally, when diagnostic uncertainty exists, human leucocyte antigen (HLA) typing is undertaken, which may help to exclude coeliac disease, given the high negative predictive value of this test [168].

Historically, a small bowel biopsy was obtained using a Crosby suction biopsy capsule. With the advent of fiberoptic oesophagogastro-duodenoscopy (EGD), investigators were able to demonstrate that endoscopic duodenal biopsy was comparable to the suction biopsy in terms of its ability to detect VA with three or four endoscopic duodenal biopsies, taken at different levels along the duodenum and jejunum [169–171]. As well as providing a more reliable method of obtaining a small bowel sample, EGD has the advantage over Crosby capsule in that it allows direct visualisation of the duodenal mucosa. Investigators are now able to detect the endoscopic markers of VA—reduction or absence of Kerckring's folds, mosaic mucosal pattern, micronodular pattern, scalloping and possibly duodenal erosions [172–175]. Although these markers can be seen in other conditions that cause VA, they have excellent specificity when combined with positive coeliac serology.

However, there are several potential limitations of EGD as part of this diagnostic pathway. These include its invasive nature and its inability to evaluate small bowel mucosa beyond the duodenum. Changes of coeliac disease are well recognised to be patchy [176], and occasionally, in some patients, the small bowel distal to the reach of a standard gastroscope may be more affected than the proximal bowel where biopsies are taken [177–179]. In addition, duodenal biopsy sampling may be affected by specimen orientation [180]. The distribution of complications of coeliac disease such as ulcerative jejunitis and enteropathy-associated T-cell lymphomas is also particularly important as these appear to be more commonly seen in the distal small bowel [181–183]. For this reason, other endoscopic modalities such as push or double-balloon enteroscopy (DBE) may be employed in order to allow more extensive evaluation of the small bowel and obtain histology [177, 184]. However, these investigations are offered in relatively few centres that are labour intensive and are more invasive than standard EGD.

Capsule endoscopy (CE) could therefore provide a useful alternative for direct visualisation of the small bowel. CE compares favourably with other small bowel imaging techniques such as magnetic resonance imaging (MRI) enteroclysis (Van Weyenberg et al. 2013). CE is a well-tolerated, minimally invasive test, predominantly utilised for the assessment of obscure gastrointestinal bleeding, inflammatory bowel disease and polyposis syndromes. However, there has been increasing interest in the role CE may have in coeliac disease. With an eightfold magnification power comparable to a dissecting microscope, capsule endoscopy has the potential to detect VA and other small bowel complications seen in coeliac disease. In this chapter, we will discuss the potential role of capsule endoscopy in the diagnosis of coeliac disease, its use in complicated cases and the potential for future development.

## 3.4.2 Endoscopic Markers of Coeliac Disease

A number of endoscopic markers for coeliac disease have been identified. The presence of these markers at EGD is sometimes used to determine whether duodenal biopsies are indicated. However, at present, capsule endoscopes are unable to take biopsy samples, so what are the endoscopic markers of coeliac disease? How accurate are they in diagnosis? and Are they applicable to CE? Endoscopic markers of coeliac disease include the following: reduction or absence of Kerckring's duodenal folds; scalloping, which is a notched and nodular appearance of the duodenal folds; increased visualisation of submucosal vasculature; a mosaic pattern, resulting from the cobblestone or micronodular appearance of the mucosal surface; and mucosal fissures and grooves [173]. Endoscopic images of these features are shown in Fig. 3.21. Other endoscopic features such as duodenal erosions have been suggested but are not widely reported and can be seen in multiple other conditions [174]. A wide range of studies have attempted to demonstrate the usefulness of endoscopic markers during EGD with contradictory results. Compared to the gold standard of histology the sensitivity and specificity of all endoscopic

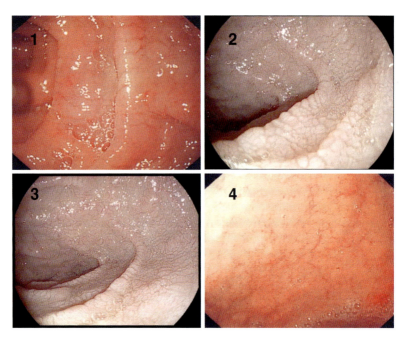

**Fig. 3.21** Endoscopic images showing signs of villous atrophy. *1* Scalloping. *2* Cobblestone appearance. *3* Mosaic pattern and scalloping. *4* Increased visible vessels and loss of duodenal folds

markers combined varies from 37 to 94 % and from 92 to 100 %, respectively [185–188]. There are several possible explanations for the absence of endoscopic markers in patients with coeliac disease. Although histology is the gold standard test, it is known that this does not have 100 % sensitivity particularly if small numbers of biopsies are taken or enteropathy is patchy and if specimens are poorly orientated [176, 180]. Also endoscopic markers might actually be absent for degrees of enteropathy milder than subtotal or total VA [185]. Although coeliac disease is the most common cause of VA, particularly in patients with positive coeliac serology, the specificity of endoscopic markers of coeliac disease is also not 100 % and there are a number of differential diagnoses VA [189]. These include infections such as giardiasis and Whipple's disease or other autoimmune conditions such as Crohn's disease or autoimmune enteropathy. A full list of differential diagnoses is shown in Table 3.3 with capsule images of some of these differentials shown in Fig. 3.22. Particular consideration should be made to these differentials in CE as there is no confirmatory intestinal biopsy.

**Table 3.3** Differential diagnoses for villous atrophy

| Agammaglobulinaemia |
| --- |
| Amyloidosis |
| CMV enteritis |
| Coeliac disease |
| Collagenous sprue |
| Chronic gastroenteritis |
| Crohn's disease |
| Cryptosporidium infection |
| Eosinophilic enteritis |
| Giardiasis |
| Graft-versus-host disease |
| HIV enteropathy |
| Intestinal lymphangiectasia |
| Ischaemia |
| Mastocytosis |
| Radiation enteritis |
| Small bowel bacterial overgrowth |
| Tropical sprue |
| Tuberculosis |
| Whipple's disease |
| Zollinger–Ellison syndrome |

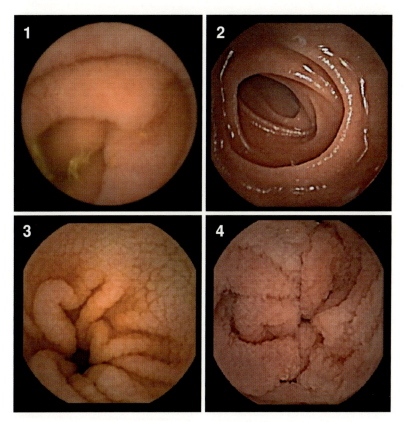

**Fig. 3.22** Capsule images of potential differential diagnoses for villous atrophy. *1* Giardiasis—notching of oedematous duodenal folds. *2* Autoimmune enteropathy—flat mucosa but no other features of coeliac disease. *3* Crohn's disease—mosaic patternation and scalloping seen distally but not proximally. *4* Chronic norovirus infection in an immunosuppressed patient confirmed by PCR in serum and histology—note markedly oedematous folds

**Table 3.4** Indications for capsule endoscopy in coeliac disease

| |
| --- |
| Suspected coeliac disease in patients unwilling to undergo EGD |
| Assessing extent of disease and response to treatment |
| Equivocal cases of possible coeliac disease |
| Investigation of non-responsive coeliac disease |
| Exclusion of enteropathy-associated lymphoma and ulcerative jejunitis in patients with refractory coeliac disease |

The lack of a biopsy is also important when we are considering the wide range of reported sensitivities of endoscopic markers for coeliac disease. The potentially low sensitivity of these markers may lead to a number of missed diagnoses. What is the evidence, therefore, that CE is a suitable tool for diagnosing or assessing coeliac disease? The potential indications for CE in coeliac disease are shown in Table 3.4 and will be discussed in detail below.

### 3.4.3 Suspected Coeliac Disease

Diagnostic EGD with duodenal biopsies has an excellent safety record and is the gold standard test for diagnosing coeliac disease. However, even with adequate sedation, EGD can be poorly tolerated with a small risk of serious complications such as perforation. As a result, some patients are unwilling or unable to undergo the procedure. CE is much better tolerated by patients and as a result may be a potential imaging modality in these patients. CE may also have some other potential advantages over EGD

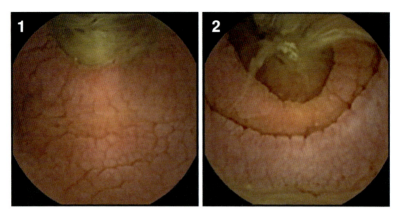

**Fig. 3.23** Capsule images showing **a** mosaic pattern and **b** scalloping

in assessing macroscopic features of coeliac disease. CE is performed without the air insufflation, required for standard endoscopy, which may obscure subtle changes of VA. The optical dome of the capsule is in close contact with the mucosa, which may allow better visualisation of the mucosa. This has a similar effect to water immersion endoscopy, which has been shown to have excellent sensitivity and specificity during standard endoscopy of unselected patients [190]. Characteristic changes of coeliac disease in some patients may only be seen distally, and CE also allows visualisation of the entire length of the small bowel. Capsule images of villous atrophy are shown in Fig. 3.23.

A small study of 10 coeliac patients with VA and 10 controls was the first to assess the utility of CE in diagnosing coeliac disease [191]. All of the images were reviewed by 4 blinded investigators 2 of who had extensive pre-study experience of reporting CE and demonstrated 100 % accuracy in identifying patients with VA. The 100 % accuracy is particularly impressive given that 4 out of the 10 patients with VA had apparently normal looking duodenal mucosa at EGD. However, there was relatively poor inter-observer agreement between some of the investigators with *kappa* coefficients ($\kappa$) as low as 0.26. When results were combined with those of the less experienced clinicians, they achieved a sensitivity, specificity, positive predictive value (PPV) and negative predictive value (NPV) of 70, 100, 100 and 77 %, respectively.

There are several limitations to this study with a small sample size, high degree of ascertainment bias and only one patient included who had partial VA (Marsh 3a). Some of these limitations were addressed in a study of 21 EMA-positive patients and 23 antibody-negative controls [192]. The EMA-positive patients had a range of histology findings from Marsh 1 to 3c including 1 patient with lymphocytic duodenosis (Marsh 1) only and 5 patients with partial VA (Marsh 3a). All of the control patients had normal histology. Seventeen of the 20 patients with VA were correctly identified via CE, and there were no false positives in the control group. A further study of 22 patients with positive serology 8 of whom had normal duodenal histology showed that results were similar when tTG was used for patient selection with sensitivity, specificity, PPV and NPV for CE of 93, 100, 100 and 89 %, respectively [193]. Rondonotti et al. [194] also identified patients with positive serology and showed a sensitivity of 89 % for in 28 patients with confirmed villous atrophy. Finally, in the largest study to date of 37 patients with coeliac disease and 38 gender-matched controls, CE showed a sensitivity of 92 % and specificity of 100 % [178]. Importantly, the disease group included 19 patients with partial VA.

A consistent finding in all of these studies is that the PPV and specificity in the presence of EMA or significantly elevated tTG (usually greater than ten times the upper limit of normal) for the recognition of endoscopic markers of

**Table 3.5** Summary of studies of utility of capsule endoscopy in diagnosing coeliac disease

| Year | Country | Patients | Sensitivity (%) | Specificity (%) | PPV (%) | NPV (%) |
|------|---------|----------|-----------------|-----------------|---------|---------|
| 2005 | Canada | 10 coeliac disease patients and 10 controls | 70 | 10 | 100 | 77 |
| 2007 | USA | 32 coeliac disease patients 11 controls | 87.5 | 90.9 | 96.5 | 71.4 |
| 2007 | UK | 21 EMA-positive patients 20 controls | 85 | 100 | 100 | 88.9 |
| 2006 | Italy | 10 untreated coeliac disease, 10 RCD, 3 treated coeliac disease, 2 EATL, 1 potential coeliac disease, 6 controls | 90.5–95.2 | 63.6 | 100 | 77.8–87.5 |
| 2008 | USA | 38 untreated coeliac disease patients, 38 controls | 92 | 100 | 100 | 93 |
| 2008 | Turkey | 8 untreated coeliac disease patients | 100 | 100 | NA | NA |
| 2011 | Australia | 14 coeliac disease patients and 8 EMA-positive patients with normal duodenal biopsy | 86 | 100 | 100 | 80 |

*PPV* positive predictive value, *NPV* negative predictive value, *EMA* endomysial antibody, *RCD* refractory coeliac disease, *EATL* enteropathy-associated T-cell lymphoma

coeliac disease is 100 %. However, the high pretest probability of coeliac disease in all of these studies may again be a potential limitation, leading to an overestimation of CE performance. However, they accurately reflect real-life clinical practice where patients are likely to be selected for CE of the basis of positive serology and suggest that CE may be an appropriate tool for patients who are unable to undergo EGD. A summary of the studies in suspected coeliac disease is shown in Table 3.5.

### 3.4.4 Assessing Extent of Disease and Response to Treatment

One area where CE may confer an advantage over standard endoscopy is that CE has the potential to image the entire small bowel. The gluten load is highest in the proximal small bowel but the entire length of the small bowel can be affected as demonstrated in a study of terminal ileal biopsies [195]. Patients with newly diagnosed coeliac disease had significantly higher intraepithelial lymphocyte counts when compared to controls. However, not all coeliac disease patients were affected. It would seem intuitive that the more of the bowel that is affected, the more severe symptoms and the

higher the chance of potential complications. However, this has not been proven mainly because it is difficult to assess the extent of disease. Capsule endoscopy may provide a way of doing this.

Also if CE for newly diagnosed coeliac disease patients was common practice, then there is potential for both assessing disease severity response to treatment. This may be pertinent in patients with persistent symptoms as it is known that the villous architecture recovers more quickly in the distal small bowel and proximal duodenal biopsies may show continuing VA. These patients may be labelled as non-adherent. However, the lack of improvement in histology proximally may not represent a significant improvement in the extent of disease. In a recent study of 38 untreated coeliac disease patients and 38 controls, the authors attempted to assess extent of disease by 2 methods [178]. Firstly, the investigator reviewing the images was invited to make a qualitative assessment of severity based on whether disease was patchy or continuous and extent of disease. A second quantitative assessment of severity was also used. The total length of time with changes of VA and time relative to the small bowel transit time were recorded. The authors were unable to show a relationship between either qualitative or quantitative measurements of extent of disease and severity of clinical presentation; however, a positive EMA was associated with more extensive disease. In the 30 coeliac disease patients who agreed to repeat CE after GFD, the mean time with abnormality reduced from 60 to 12 min. A second more recent study of 12 patients with coeliac disease who had repeat CE after 12 months on a GFD has also demonstrated this improvement. The investigators assessed the extent of disease as a percentage of the total small bowel transit time [193]. Although there was no initial correlation between extent of disease and clinical severity, they did demonstrate a significant reduction in the mean time with VA.

These 2 studies have so far failed to demonstrate any relationship between extent of small bowel involvement and clinical severity of disease. However, as experience with CE in coeliac disease increases, this may become possible. The use of CE to assess small bowel healing does appear to be a promising area; however, this will only become relevant as more patients undergo CE at the time of diagnosis. New technologies as discussed later in this chapter may also help to improve the objective measurement of disease severity.

### 3.4.5 Equivocal Cases

Another area where CE may play a role is in the investigation of equivocal cases of coeliac disease. As previously discussed, the changes of coeliac disease can be patchy and a duodenal biopsy in patients with positive serology may not demonstrate VA. Lesser degrees of histology that can be associated with coeliac disease are non-specific and are seen in a variety of other conditions. This can leave some patients without a definitive diagnosis. How therefore should we investigate patients with positive coeliac serology but normal or non-specific duodenal histology? An international consensus conference on the use of capsule and double-balloon enteroscopy advocated the potential use of CE in this situation [196]. There is, however, limited data assessing the role of CE in these equivocal cases.

In a large multicentre study, the investigators identified patients with gastrointestinal symptoms and positive EMA, tTG or antigliadin antibodies (AGA) [194]. Duodenal biopsies and CE were performed at the time of presentation, and 11 patients were found to have normal duodenal histology. Of these, 10 patients also had a normal capsule endoscopy; however, these patients were all positive for AGA only which is non-specific and seen in a variety of other conditions. The one patient that had evidence of VA on capsule endoscopy was also positive for EMA and had biopsy-proven dermatitis herpetiformis making coeliac disease very likely. One patient with Marsh 1 changes and positive EMA had a normal CE; however, the 3 patients with Marsh 2 changes and positive EMA and tTG all had evidence of VA on CE. The authors do not state whether any further confirmatory tests such as HLA genotyping or further small bowel biopsies were taken to confirm coeliac disease but it is likely that these were additional diagnoses that had been missed by conventional EGD and duodenal biopsy.

There is, however, conflicting evidence. In a study of 8 patients with positive serology (EMA or tTG) and a normal duodenal biopsy, CE did not reveal any endoscopic features of coeliac disease [193]. Thus, the investigators concluded that there was no benefit in performing CE for this subgroup of patients. In a further study, 22 irritable bowel syndrome patients with positive AGA, EMA or tTG and normal duodenal histology underwent CE and HLA genotyping [197]. Subtle mucosal abnormalities within in the small bowel, such as mucosal breaks, ulceration or denuded and blunted villi, were seen in 55 % (12/22) of cases. However, the authors felt that none of these features were conclusively characteristic of coeliac disease and these changes were seen in both patients with and without an HLA genotype required for coeliac disease. The majority of the patients only had a positive AGA, which as discussed previously has a low specificity for coeliac disease. The single patient with a positive EMA (the most specific marker for coeliac disease) had a normal CE. Finally, in a study of 30 patients with Marsh 1 or 2 changes, only 6 of whom had positive EMA or tTG, 1 patient was diagnosed with coeliac disease and another with small bowel Crohn's on the basis of CE appearances [198]. It is clear that further work is required to assess the cost-effectiveness of the use of CE in these equivocal cases if the yield is as low as in this final study. CE use may be justified however, in EMA or tTG positive patients with Marsh 1 or 2 changes or gastrointestinal symptoms particularly, if they are unwilling to undergo further EGD and repeat biopsies.

Another diagnostic challenge is antibody-negative VA. As previously discussed, there is a wide range of differential diagnoses for VA. In the study of equivocal cases by Kurien et al. [198], they also included a group of patients with antibody-negative VA to see whether this increased the diagnostic yield. Patients were extensively investigated for coeliac disease including HLA phenotyping, by monitoring response to GFD and, in some cases, repeat duodenal biopsies. On the basis of CE appearances and other ancillary tests, 7 patients could be diagnosed with coeliac disease and 2 further patients were diagnosed with small bowel Crohn's as a cause for VA. Again, this is a single small study and further work needs to be done to clarify the role of CE in antibody-negative VA cases. This is particularly important as CE alone is probably insufficient to confirm a diagnosis of coeliac disease as endoscopic markers are not specific to coeliac disease rather they are predictors of mucosal disease [199].

### 3.4.6 Non-responsive Coeliac Disease, Refractory Coeliac Disease and Enteropathy-Associated T-Cell Lymphoma

Although the majority of patients with diagnosed coeliac disease improve on a gluten-free diet (GFD), up to 30 % patients do not respond as expected. In many of these patients, other causes for their symptoms such as microscopic colitis, small bowel bacterial overgrowth or pancreatic insufficiency are identified [200].

However, many of these patients undergo repeated endoscopy and duodenal biopsy to assess small bowel healing and look for serious complications such as refractory coeliac disease (RCD) or enteropathy-associated T-cell lymphoma (EATL). RCD is defined as persistent malabsorptive symptoms and villous atrophy despite strict adherence to a GFD. It is subdivided into types I and II depending on clonality of intraepithelial lymphocytes. RCD type II carries a worse prognosis and is associated with greater progression to EATL [200]. However, changes may not be confined to the proximal small bowel and may be out of the reach of a standard gastroscope. CE may therefore play a role in the investigation of these patients.

Several studies have attempted to delineate a role for CE in non-responsive patients. In blinded comparison of duodenal biopsy and CE in 18 patients who had failed to respond to a GFD, 67 % of those with histological evidence of coeliac disease had abnormal CE [201]. Six patients with normal histology also had a normal CE. Four patients, however, had evidence of persistent histological changes of coeliac disease but had normal CE appearances. Agreement between histology and CE appearances was therefore fairly modest with a $\kappa$ coefficient of 0.65. Importantly, however, 2 cases of ulcerative jejunitis were identified. Ulcerative jejunitis is usually associated with RCD type II that can result in small bowel stricturing and is associated with a high risk of developing EATL. Early identification of RCD type II may allow effective treatment with immunosuppression and prevent progression to EATL. These findings were replicated in a recent study of 69 patients with coeliac disease and persisting symptoms [198]. Signs of VA were identified in 45 %, and serious complications were identified in 8 patients including 2 cases of EATL, 1 case of ulcerative jejunitis and 4 RCD type 1. However, although the investigators were blinded to the EGD findings, no control groups were included in either of these studies, leading to a high degree of ascertainment bias, which may have overestimated the usefulness of CE. This was addressed in a recent study of 42 non-responsive

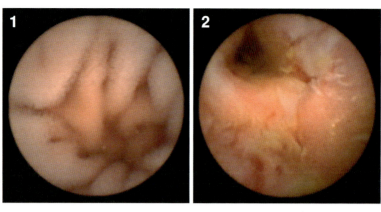

**Fig. 3.24** Ulcerative jejunitis. Capsule appearance from a patient with known coeliac disease and persistent symptoms on a gluten-free diet. *1* shows normal proximal small bowel. *2* shows a complete loss of villi and ulceration consistent with ulcerative jejunitis

patients, 84 controls and 30 patients with uncomplicated coeliac disease who had responded well to a GFD for at least 6 months [182]. Only 9 of 16 patients with villous atrophy on histology had abnormal findings on CE. Four patients with normal histology had apparently abnormal CE appearances. As a result, overall the agreement between histology and CE findings was weak with a $\kappa$ coefficient of 0.44. However, it must be noted that duodenal histology may be a less than perfect gold standard as changes can be patchy. It may be the findings on CE represented VA that was distal to the reach of EGD and standard duodenal biopsy. Also it must be noted that of the 16 patients with VA, 13 had partial VA (Marsh 3a), which may not be seen as clearly as total VA. All 3 of the most severe lesions were correctly identified as abnormal by CE. Again, a case of RCD type II was identified by CE and confirmed by DBE and biopsy. The use of CE to assess the extent and severity of disease in patients with known RCD may also be helpful as shown in a recent study of 29 patients with RCD and 9 patients with symptomatic coeliac disease [202]. Three cases of EATL and 5 cases of ulcerative jejunitis requiring specific treatment in the RCD cohort were identified. The majority of the RCD patients also underwent DBE, and the authors concluded that 17 patients could have avoided this invasive investigation based on CE findings.

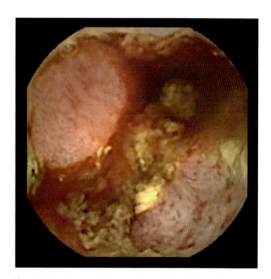

**Fig. 3.25** Enteropathy-associated T-cell Lymphoma

Apart from this final study, where there was an unusually high proportion of patients with RCD, the apparent diagnostic yield for complications such as EATL and ulcerative jejunitis appears low. However, these diagnoses carry significant rates of morbidity and mortality, which may be reduced by prompt diagnosis. The use of capsule in non-responsive patients may therefore be justified. Patients with ulcerative jejunitis and EATL can have a significant risk of small bowel stricturing. CE should therefore be used with caution, and a patency capsule should always be employed to reduce the incidence of capsule retention. Capsule images of ulcerative jejunitis and EATL are shown in Figs. 3.24 and 3.25.

### 3.4.7 New Technology and Future Development

As previously discussed, the main drawback of CE is the inability to perform biopsy. It may, however, be possible to incorporate this function into future incarnations of capsule technology [203]. In the near future, these advances, however, are only likely to allow non-targeted biopsies of the small bowel. As previously discussed, changes of coeliac disease can be patchy and biopsies may miss affected areas. Another method therefore of increasing the diagnostic yield would be to incorporate other image-enhancing techniques. Multiple techniques such as narrow-band imaging or optical-band imaging, amongst others, have been used in conventional endoscopy with limited improvement in diagnostic accuracy [204]. Capsule has already been shown to be more accurate than standard endoscopy for identifying macroscopic features of VA, and as capsule technology and picture resolution improve, these techniques may be incorporated and may prove beneficial in increasing the yield further.

These technologies are, however, not presently available and may never come to fruition. An interesting development that is presently undergoing clinical trials is the use of digital quantitative analysis of CE images. CE interpretation is currently subjective as has been demonstrated by the significant inter-observer variability in some studies. CE can miss lesions as demonstrated by a pooled analysis of 530 examinations where 10.8 % of lesions picked up on conventional endoscopy were missed by CE [64]. There is also a lack of standardisation of severity of CE findings. An objective computerised analysis of CE images would therefore seem advantageous. This has been developed using current CE technology and involves the production of a 3-dimensional representation of 2-dimensional CE images, mucosal protrusions can then be assessed for height, width and number per image. The images are also converted to greyscale and the intensity of each pixel is measured. These techniques were used in 3 recent studies [205–207]. On analysis of these images, patients with villous atrophy showed blunted protrusions with lower height and greater diameter. The mucosal surface also showed greater variability in pixel greyscale intensity in patients with VA, which the authors postulated was due to fissures, scalloping and mosaic pattern seen in patients with VA. Digital enhancement techniques have also been used to estimate small bowel motility, which is known to be impaired in patients with active coeliac disease [208]. With further development, these techniques may prove invaluable in the assessment of patients with suspected or known coeliac disease. Crucially, this objective measurement may also allow for more accurate quantification of severity and improvement in pathology on a GFD.

### 3.4.8 Conclusions

At present, duodenal biopsy remains the gold standard for diagnosing coeliac disease; however, CE may play a role in those patients who are unable or unwilling to undergo standard EGD and biopsy. CE is also proving an important diagnostic tool for investigating patients for possible complications of coeliac disease such as small bowel malignancy, RCD and ulcerative jejunitis. There are potential limitations to CE with high degrees of inter-observer variability, potentially high miss rates for significant lesions and the risk of capsule retention in patients with strictures resulting from complicated coeliac disease. However, technology is evolving and future developments may allow small bowel biopsy or incorporate 'virtual biopsy' technologies that will improve the versatility of CE in coeliac patients.

## 3.5    Polyposis Syndromes

**Abstract** Hereditary gastrointestinal (GI) polyposis syndromes are rare autosomal dominant
disorders that are characterised by the presence
of GI polyps, extra-GI phenotypic manifestations and an increased risk of GI and extra-GI
neoplasia. The histopathology of polyps, nature
of other phenotypic manifestations and degree of
risk of malignancy are governed by the genetic
mutations of the underlying syndrome. Small
bowel (SB) capsule endoscopy (SBCE) has a
role to play in the surveillance and management
of patients with SB polyposis, and this role is
best established for patients with Peutz–Jeghers
syndrome (PJS). Although polyps in PJS have
distinct      hamartomatous      features,      large
(≥1.5 cm) lesions contribute to a major part of
the disease burden in patients with PJS by their
potential to cause SB intussusception and GI
bleeding. Surveillance strategies for the detection of clinically significant PJS SB polyps by
minimally invasive investigations such as SBCE
and magnetic resonance enterography (MRE)
are therefore employed to reduce the risk of
these complications by facilitating pre-emptive
removal of polyps by device-assisted enteroscopy (DAE) or elective surgery. The role of
SBCE in the surveillance of patients with other
polyposis syndromes such as familial adenomatous polyposis (FAP) is less clearly defined.

**Keywords** Small bowel polyposis · Polyps ·
Capsule endoscopy · Peutz–Jeghers syndrome ·
PJS · Familial adenomatous polyposis · FAP ·
Enteroscopy

### 3.5.1    Introduction

Hereditary gastrointestinal (GI) polyposis syndromes are rare autosomal dominant disorders
that are characterised by the presence of GI
polyps, extra-GI phenotypic manifestations and
an increased risk of GI and extra-GI neoplasia.
The histopathology of polyps, nature of other
phenotypic manifestations and degree of risk of
malignancy are governed by the genetic mutations of the underlying syndrome. Small bowel
(SB) capsule endoscopy (SBCE) has a role to
play in the surveillance and management of
patients with SB polyposis. Although this is now
established for patients with Peutz–Jeghers
syndrome (PJS), evidence to support the routine
use of SBCE for the surveillance of patients with
other polyposis syndromes is lacking.

### 3.5.2    Peutz–Jeghers Syndrome

Peutz–Jeghers syndrome (PJS) is a high-pene-
trance autosomal dominant polyposis syndrome,
which is associated with a germline mutation in
the STK11/LKB1 gene (19p13.3) in up to 94 %
of cases [209]. PJS has an incidence of about 1
in 8,500 to 1 in 200,000 live births [210–213]
and is characterised by a phenotype that includes
the presence of distinct mucocutaneous melanin
pigmentation, gastrointestinal (GI) polyposis
[214] and a predisposition to GI and extra-GI
malignant disease [210, 212–218].

   PJS polyps are thought to arise as a result of
GI mucosal prolapse [211, 216] and have a
characteristic    hamartomatous    histopathology
including 'arborisation' of a smooth muscle core
with    'frond-like'    epithelial    lengthening
(Fig. 3.26). Although PJS polyps may occur
anywhere within the GI tract, they occur predominantly within the proximal small bowel
(SB) [214, 218, 219]. PJS SB polyps that are
≥1.5 cm in size are considered to be clinically
significant and contribute to a major part of the
disease burden in patients with this condition,
mainly by resulting in intussusception and SB
obstruction, often requiring emergency surgery
[211–213, 218, 220, 221]. SB complications
arising from large PJS polyps frequently result in
multiple laparotomies throughout a patient's
lifetime [222]. These complications commence
in childhood and early youth [211, 223–225], and
the cumulative risk of SB intussusception may be
as high as 50 % by the age of 20 years [218].

   In view of the high risks associated with
clinically significant SB polyps (≥1.5 cm), current guidelines recommend that patients with PJS

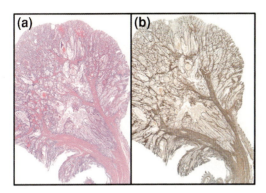

**Fig. 3.26** Scanning view of a PJS polyp(ileum). Haematoxylin and eosin (*H&E*) stain **a** shows a large, pedunculated, lobulated polyp, supported by broad bands of muscularis mucosae smooth muscle. Smooth muscle actin (*SMA*) immuno-stain **b** highlights the tree-like branches of smooth muscle extending from the muscularis mucosae into the periphery of the polyp; the fibrous bands are thicker centrally (images courtesy of Dr TuVinh Luong, Academic Department of Cellular Pathology, The Royal Free Hospital and UCL School of Medicine, London)

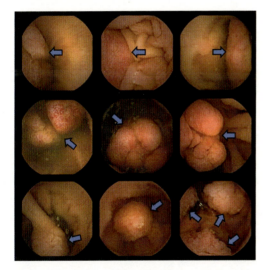

**Fig. 3.27** A variety of PJS SB polyps as seen at video capsule endoscopy (*VCE*) (PillCam™ SB2, Given Imaging, Yokneam, Israel). Polyp tissue is usually darker than the surrounding SB mucosa (*blue arrows*); estimation of polyp size and number can be challenging and often only a small portion of larger polyps can be identified (images courtesy of Ms Aine O'Rourke and Dr Chris Fraser, St Mark's Hospital and Academic Institute, London)

aged ≥8–10 years, should undergo SB surveillance using a minimally invasive modality such as SB capsule endoscopy (SBCE) and/or radiological diagnostic imaging [magnetic resonance enterography/enteroclysis (MRE)] on a biennial to triennial basis [211, 220, 221] in order to facilitate early detection of large PJS polyps and also to investigate for possible occult SB malignancies. SBCE is very well tolerated by patients and is a less invasive option for the surveillance of the SB in patients with PJS [220]. The limitations relating to SBCE include its potential to miss clinically significant polyps, especially if these are located within the proximal SB [220, 221, 226–228] and challenges relating to the estimation of polyp size and location and (Fig. 3.27), possible 'double counting' of polyps [220, 221]. Some of these limitations (such as potential miss rates) may be mitigated by the more advanced technology of newer generation capsules, such as the PillCam SB3® (Given Imaging, Yoqneam, Israel), which also incorporates an 'adaptive frame rate', enabling a higher frequency of frame capture (up to 6 frames per second) during rapid capsule transit.

Before the introduction of SBCE and MRE into clinical practice, SB surveillance in patients with PJS depended on SB follow through (SBFT). However, SBFT is limited by low sensitivity, poor spatial resolution (due to its two-dimensional quality), with poor differentiation of overlapping SB loops and also exposes patients to a significant dose of ionising radiation [220, 229–231]. Radiological imaging of the SB in patients with PJS has therefore been superseded by MRE [220, 221]. A recent prospective comparative study of MRE versus SBCE for this indication showed that although patients tolerated SBCE better and preferred it to MRE [220], the 2 modalities were comparable for the detection of clinically significant (≥1.5 cm) PJS SB polyps. Currently, MRE may also allow for more accurate estimation of PJS polyp size and respective polyp location (Fig. 3.28) [220, 221, 232] and therefore appears to be a useful, alternative modality to SBCE for surveillance or for further evaluation of polyps detected by SBCE [220, 221].

Minimally invasive SB surveillance for clinically significant (≥1.5 cm) polyps allows pre-emptive removal, before an episode of

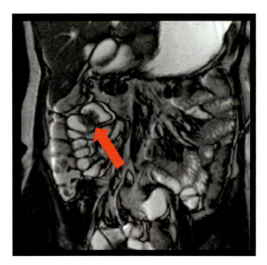

**Fig. 3.28** A large (2.5 cm) PJS ileal polyp (*red arrow*) as seen at magnetic resonance enterography (*MRE*) (image courtesy of Dr Arun Gupta, St Mark's Hospital, London)

intussusception occurs, potentially avoiding the need for emergency surgery and possible SB resection [211, 222]. This minimally invasive approach to the management of PJS SB polyposis has been enhanced by the introduction of device-assisted enteroscopy (DAE). DAE facilitates endoscopic excision of PJS polyps located deep within the SB (Fig. 3.29) [233–243] and therefore has the potential to obviate the need for laparotomy with intra-operative enteroscopy (IOE), which until recently was the sole option available for removal of PJS polyps deep within the SB [244, 245]. Laparotomy with IOE, however, exposes patients to major abdominal surgery and its potential complications such as

post-operative intra-abdominal adhesions and short-bowel syndrome [246–248]. Data on DAE for this indication mainly relate to the double-balloon enteroscopy (DBE)and suggest that this endotherapeutic modality may offer a minimally invasive alternative to laparotomy and IOE for selected patients with PJS [216, 219, 236–238, 240]. The introduction of a DAE-based therapeutic strategy in childhood (before the patient's first laparotomy has been required) may enhance its success, since DAE may be hindered by the presence of post-surgical intra-abdominal adhesions [249, 250]. In patients who have already developed post-surgical adhesive disease, division of adhesions by mini-port laparoscopic assistance during DAE may still provide a less invasive alternative to laparotomy with IOE for SB polypectomy [251]. However, in certain patients, laparotomy with IOE shall continue to have a major role to play in the management of SB polyps and the overall strategy should be tailored to the requirements of the individual patient. The current recommendations for the surveillance and management of PJS SB polyposis using minimally invasive strategies are presented as an algorithm (Fig. 3.30).

### 3.5.3 Other Polyposis Syndromes

Familial adenomatous polyposis (FAP) is an important autosomal dominant polyposis syndrome with an incidence of about 1 in 10,000 live births [252–254]. FAP is associated with a germline mutation in the APC gene (5q21)

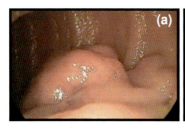
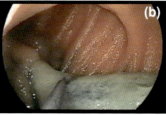
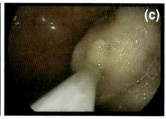

**Fig. 3.29** Large (2 cm) semi-pedunculated PJS jejunal polyp (**a**) as seen at double-balloon enteroscopy (*DBE*) (Fujifilm, Saitama, Japan). Prior to polypectomy, the submucosal of the polyp base/stalk is injected with a dilute solution of adrenaline (1 in 100,000) in normal saline and 2 drops of 0.005 % methylene blue, in order to reduce the risk of perforation and bleeding at polypectomy (**b**). After polypectomy, the polyp is then retrieved using a Roth Net (US Endoscopy, USA) (**c**)

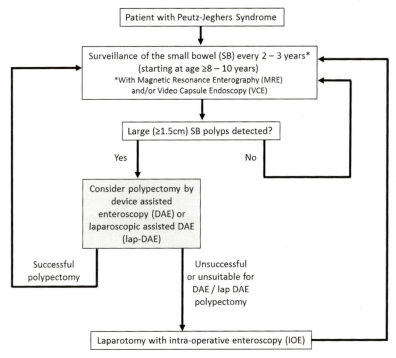

**Fig. 3.30** A proposed algorithm for the surveillance and management of small bowel (*SB*) polyps in patients with Peutz–Jeghers syndrome (*PJS* based on current recommendations [211])

[252–254] and is characterised mainly by the development of tens to thousands of adenomatous polyps in the colon and rectum and other parts of the gastrointestinal (GI) tract with a hazard of colorectal cancer (CRC) of up to 100 % [253]. Patients with FAP may also develop extra-GI neoplasia and mesenteric fibromatosis (desmoid tumours) [255]. The second most commonly affected GI site in FAP is the duodenum, and the lifetime risk of developing duodenal adenomas has been reported to be as high as 100 %. It has also been estimated that about 5 % of duodenal (specifically peri-ampullary) adenomas progress to cancer within 10 years, and although rare in the general population, the risk of duodenal or peri-ampullary cancer is increased several hundred fold in FAP patients and remains the most common cause of death in FAP patients who have had a prophylactic colectomy [253, 256–259]. Duodenal polyposis has been shown to progress in an orderly fashion depending on the severity of the disease as described in the staging system by

**Table 3.6** Modified classification of the severity of duodenal polyposis (according to Spigelman et al. [259–262])

| | No of points | | |
|---|---|---|---|
| | 1 | 2 | 3 |
| No of polyps | 1–4 | 5–20 | >20 |
| Polyp size (mm) | 1–4 | 5–10 | >10 |
| Histology | Tubulous | Tubulovillous | Villous |
| Dysplasia | Low-grade | | High-grade |

*Stage 0* 0 points; *stage I* 1–4 points; *stage II* 5–6 points; *stage III* 7–8 points; *stage IV* 9–12 points

Spigelman et al. [259], Caspari et al. [260], Saurin et al. [261], Schlemper et al. [262] (Table 3.6). This is used to guide duodenal surveillance of patients with FAP who undertake upper GI endoscopies with a side-viewing duodenoscope at 1–5-year intervals in order to determine the need for endotherapy or surgery [253, 259, 260, 262]. Although several studies of SBCE in FAP patients have also shown that a higher Spigelman stage may also correlate with an increased presence of jejunal and ileal polyposis [254, 260, 263, 264], the clinical relevance of these lesions is unclear and likely to be small, given the low incidence of extra-duodenal SB cancers in patients with FAP [265]. Furthermore, it is also important to note that SBCE provides poor visualisation of the duodenal ampulla and peri-ampullary duodenal mucosa and cannot replace surveillance with a forward and side-viewing duodenoscope in its current form [254, 266]. The evidence to support a role of SBCE in patients with FAP is lacking, and its use for routine surveillance in this condition cannot be recommended at present.

Although the use of SBCE has also been described in case reports and small case series of patients with juvenile polyposis syndrome (JPS) [267] and Cowden's syndrome [268, 269], there is currently no evidence to support the routine use of SBCE in these rarer forms of GI polyposis.

### 3.5.4 Summary

In summary, SBCE has been shown to be useful for the detection of clinically significant ($\geq 1.5$ cm) SB polyps in patients with PJS, and its use as a surveillance instrument at 2–3-year intervals is recommended. SB surveillance in PJS should be commenced in childhood (before patients become symptomatic) in order to attempt pre-emptive endotherapy of clinically significant PJS polyps and reduce the need for surgery. The routine use of SBCE in other GI polyposis syndromes (such as FAP) appears to be of limited value at present.

## 3.6     Less Common Indications for Small Bowel Capsule Endoscopy

**Abstract** Typical indications for small bowel capsule endoscopy (SBCE) are mid-gastrointestinal (GI) bleeding, iron-deficiency anaemia, suspected and established Crohn's disease, complicated coeliac disease and polyposis syndromes. However, SBCE may be useful in any case in which endoscopically visible mucosal abnormalities affect patient management. Patients with advanced melanoma or with anaemia have a high risk of small bowel metastasis. Even a small primary neuroendocrine tumour causing hepatic metastasis may be found by SBCE.

Diagnostic yield of SBCE in abdominal pain alone is low, but may increase in the presence of additional symptoms. SBCE can be used in isolated cases of malabsorption syndromes if standard tests are inconclusive. Infections that cause intestinal lymphangiectasia are Whipple's disease, atypical mycobacteriosis or HIV enteropathy. Small bowel ulcers can be seen in cytomegalovirus infection and in tuberculosis. Intraluminal helminths have also been diagnosed by SBCE.

SBCE has been used successfully in the diagnosis of iatrogenic small bowel injury due to radiation enteritis, acute graft-versus-host disease and enteropathy due to non-steroidal anti-inflammatory drugs. Pharmacological studies have used SBCE to investigate the harmful as well as protective effects of drugs on the small bowel mucosa.

Video capsule endoscopy has been used in the emergency room for patients with upper GI bleeding, especially to identify those who require urgent endoscopic haemostasis. Portal hypertensive enteropathy is occasionally seen in patients with liver cirrhosis and GI bleeding. IgA vasculitis frequently affects the small bowel, unlike other systemic diseases.

Although some case series and a few prospective studies exist for these less common indications, SBCE is considered on an individual patient basis.

Established indications for small bowel capsule endoscopy (SBCE) are mid-GI bleeding, iron-deficiency anaemia not otherwise explained, suspected Crohn's disease, established non-stricturing Crohn's disease in case of potential therapeutic consequences, complicated coeliac

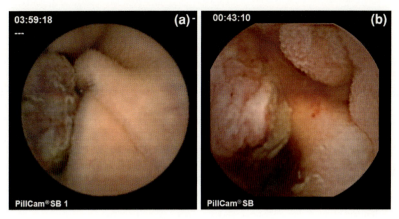

Fig. 3.31 **a** Melanotic melanoma of the small bowel. **b** Amelanotic melanoma

sprue and polyposis syndrome. Many other indications exist, as the number of small bowel diseases is high. However, before applying SBCE for any indication, it should be clear that the suspected disease is associated with endoscopically visible lesions. In this chapter, some rather unusual indications for SBCE are discussed.

### 3.6.1 Tumours

Examination of the small bowel by small bowel capsule endoscopy (SBCE) is useful in detecting small bowel tumours. These tumours usually present with mid-GI bleeding or anaemia. However, there are some scenarios in which metastases of certain primary tumours may be suitable for further therapy.

Patients suffering from a malignant melanoma have a high risk of small bowel metastasis. Depending on the tumour stage, the probability ranges from 5 to 17 %. In these patients, the resection of all detected neoplastic lesions is a known positive prognostic marker [270]. A study including 390 melanoma patients by Albert et al. came to the conclusion that a small bowel examination via SBCE is useful in patients with a positive faecal occult blood test (FOBT) and in every patient with a stage IV melanoma (AJCC). Obviously, this applies to all patients in whom detection of a small bowel metastasis would change the therapeutic course [271] (Fig. 3.31).

Gastrointestinal **follicular lymphoma** is predominantly located in the duodenum (81–96 %; [272, 273]). In most of these cases, additional lesions across the entire small bowel are present. Since the optimal treatment depends on the initial extent of the disease, a complete small bowel examination is recommended if a follicular lymphoma is detected by upper or lower GI endoscopy. Due to the small size of the lesions, radiologic diagnostic alone is not sufficient. Nakamura et al. showed in a single centre study that SBCE has a similar detection rate compared to double-balloon enteroscopy. However, if a small bowel examination is required after treatment, SBCE is not recommended as only histological specimens can reliably differentiate between lymphoid hyperplasia and residual lymphoma [272].

For primary **gastric marginal zone B-cell lymphoma** (MBZCL) of mucosa-associated lymphoid tissue (MALT), a few cases have been reported with additional lesions found by VCE in the small bowel. However, in a retrospective study of 40 patients with MBZCL who underwent conventional upper and lower endoscopy, SBCE did not reveal additional intestinal lesions [274]. Hence, screening of the small bowel via SBCE as a routine work up does not seem necessary.

**Neuroendocrine tumours** (NET) occur predominantly in the gastrointestinal tract and bronchi. Lymph nodes and liver are the most

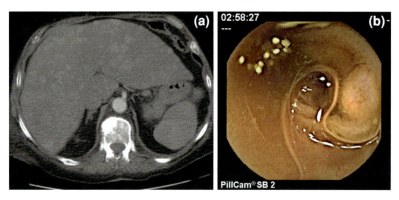

**Fig. 3.32** **a** Female patient with liver metastasis, histology showed a neuroendocrine carcinoma. **b** SBCE identified the small primary tumour in the ileum

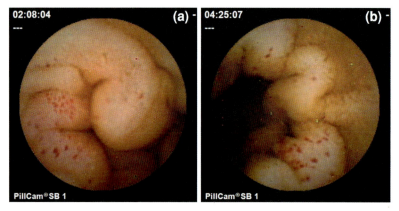

**Fig. 3.33** **a**, **b** NET located in the small bowel mesentery. Erythema and multiple red spots are the intraluminal findings with SBCE

common sites of metastatic lesions. Patients presenting with hepatic metastasis of neuroendocrine origin and unknown primary tumour should undergo gastrointestinal examination in addition to biochemical assays and advanced imaging techniques [275] (Fig. 3.32). A small study implicated that SBCE is superior to CT scan and enteroclysis in the search of a primary small bowel NET. Nuclear imaging presented a similar detection rate but failed to provide a sufficient localisation [276]. Another small study showed similar diagnostic yields for SBCE and CT enteroclysis, whilst CT enteroclysis had more false-positive findings [277]. Although SBCE is capable of detecting even small intestinal lesions, it may be limited in detecting those neuroendocrine tumours located predominately in the mesentery. Non-specific mucosal alterations may

be the only endoscopic sign in these cases (Fig. 3.33). Hence, a combination of SBCE with imaging technique may be appropriate.

Patients with **acromegaly** have been studied with SBCE in the search of small bowel tumours [278]. Amongst 18 patients with acromegaly, 3 polyps of the small bowel were detected, in the control group, only one in 36 patients suggesting a relative risk for SB polyps of 2.50 (95 % CI: 1.23–5.07). Incidence of tumours (relative risk 1.69) was not significantly higher than in the control group. Hence, larger studies are necessary.

### 3.6.2 Abdominal Pain

Abdominal pain is a common symptom associated with a heterogeneous group of underlying

**Fig. 3.34** **a, b** Female patient with abdominal pain and anaemia, EGD and colonoscopy were inconclusive. SBCE showed aphthous lesions of the proximal and distal small bowel consistent with Crohn's disease [shown in image **b** with flexible image colour enhancement (*FICE1*)]. Clinical condition improved following therapy

diseases and conditions. In 20 patients with chronic abdominal pain and negative upper and lower endoscopy, abdominal ultrasound and unremarkable laboratory tests, capsule endoscopy presented no findings that could be correlated to the symptoms [279]. Additional small studies from single centres came to a similar conclusion, resulting in the recommendation that capsule endoscopy should not be performed in patients with the sole symptom of abdominal pain [280, 281].

A prospective multicentre study of 50 patients undergoing SBCE for chronic abdominal pain as the dominant complaint and additional symptoms ('plus' signs) reported a higher diagnostic yield (Fig. 3.34). These signs were weight loss >10 % in 3 months, suspected gastrointestinal bleeding and/or elevated laboratory markers of inflammation. Relevant pathological findings were reported in up to 40 % of these cases. Laboratory signs of inflammation had the highest prognostic value [282].

In a study of 110 patients with abdominal pain, chances of positive SBCE findings were significantly increased if accompanied by weight loss (OR, 18.6; 95 % CI (1.6, 222.4), $p = 0.02$). A positive correlation was also suggested in patients with elevated erythrocyte sedimentation rate, elevated C-reactive protein and hypalbuminaemia [283].

In 23 patients with abdominal pain and suspected Crohn's disease, the diagnostic yield of SBCE was raised from 12.5 to 57 % ($p = 0.04$) if anaemia and an elevated platelet count as an inflammatory marker was present as well [284]. In another study, 112 patients with abdominal pain, iron-deficiency anaemia and/or diarrhoea underwent SBCE in search of Crohn's disease. SBCE showed signs of inflammation in only 6 %. The diagnostic yield was raised to 33 % if patients had the combination of abdominal pain and diarrhoea [285].

Patients with abdominal pain and (recurring) signs of **intestinal obstruction** may profit from SBCE. Although SBCE is generally contraindicated in suspected bowel obstruction, a small retrospective analysis of 19 patients with signs of obstruction, with inconclusive conventional diagnostics reports a definite diagnosis by SBCE in 5 of these cases. However, a surgical resection was performed in 4 of these cases due to a retained capsule [286].

In conclusion, SBCE should not be performed with the sole indication of abdominal pain. Yet, with additional symptoms like weight loss, suspected bleeding and/or signs of inflammation SBCE seem to be a valuable diagnostic tool. Suspected obstruction as a cause of abdominal pain can be an indication within the right setting.

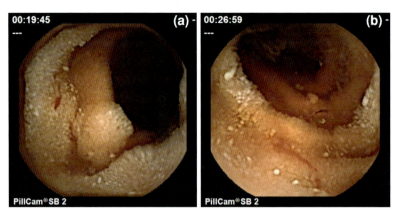

**Fig. 3.35** **a**, **b** Radiation enteropathy with bleeding

### 3.6.3 Acute Gastrointestinal Graft-Versus-Host Disease

Patients developing diarrhoea, nausea, vomiting, abdominal pain, anorexia or hematochezia after allogenic stem cell transplantation may suffer from acute gastrointestinal graft-versus-host disease (aGI GvHD). As a common complication, it is associated with an increased morbidity and mortality rate [287]. Differential diagnosis includes viral and bacterial infections such as cytomegalovirus, Epstein-barr virus or Clostridium difficile. Additionally, chemotherapeutic toxicity presents with similar symptoms [288]. An exact and early diagnosis is important to initiate a specific treatment or adapt the ongoing immunomodulating therapy.

In several small series, patients with suspected aGI GvHD underwent SBCE without complications in any stage of the disease with the procedure being well tolerated [287, 289, 290]. Endoscopic findings correlated with the histopathologic staging. One series reported that aGI GvHD was only visible at SBCE in 2/14 patients [291]. In two series, 7/9 and 3/7 patients, respectively, with lesions detected by upper and lower endoscopy had more severe lesions detected by SBCE in the small bowel, which were not accessible by conventional endoscopy. In these cases, SBCE made the overall assessment more accurate [287, 289]. A normal SBCE study essentially ruled out aGI

GvHD effectively changing the therapeutic course [291]. However, patients suffering from a chronic gastrointestinal GvHD may have a normal SBCE study [290].

In conclusion, SBCE appears to be at least equal to conventional endoscopy in identifying and staging aGI GVHD. The visualisation of the small bowel led to a change in therapeutic approach in numerous cases.

### 3.6.4 Radiation Enteritis

Abdominopelvic radiotherapy can lead to radiation enteritis of the small bowel, presenting itself with anaemia, abdominal pain, chronic diarrhoea, melena or hematochezia. Fifteen patients who had at least one of these signs after radiochemotherapy for pancreatic cancer were examined by SBCE. Nine patients showed mild to severe small bowel lesions, especially in patients who received therapy within the last 6 months. Capsule retention did not occur in the small bowel in this study early after radiotherapy. Other case reports showed a higher risk in patients with a distant history of radiotherapy [292]. Endoscopic findings are neo-vascularisation, red spots, bleeding, lymphangiectasia, fibrosis and stenosis (Fig. 3.35). If possible, SBCE should be performed within the first months after radiotherapy; otherwise, a patency capsule should be considered to exclude relevant stenosis (Fig. 3.34).

### 3.6.5 Intestinal Dysmotility

Patients presenting with recurring abdominal distension, bloating, abdominal pain, nausea and constipation might suffer from chronic intestinal dysmotility (CID) [293] or an underlying disease with a secondary intestinal motility disorder like coeliac disease or food allergy [294].

In 86 patients, SBCE with computerised evaluation of contractile patterns, intestinal content and endoluminal motion was tested against conventional intestinal manometry. The assessment based on the SBCE was reliable and accurate in identifying intestinal dysmotility as well as less time consuming [295].

A prospective study of 18 patients with known CID (neuropathic, myopathic or indeterminate) who underwent SBCE showed erosions and ulcers in 16/18 patients and an overall increased small bowel transit time (346 to 241 min of the control group, $p = 0.061$). Capsule retention with the need of a surgical or endoscopic intervention did not occur in any of these cases. A differentiation between myopathic and neuropathic CID was not possible by means of SBCE. Furthermore, the relevance of the detected mucosal alterations remains unclear. For now, SBCE seems feasible in patients with CID but with an unknown diagnostic relevance [296].

In general, abnormal intestinal motility can be detected by SBCE. Yet, as a sole finding, it cannot be linked to a specific underlying disease [294].

### 3.6.6 Non-steroidal Anti-inflammatory Drug Enteropathy

Enteropathy due to non-steroidal anti-inflammatory drugs (NSAIDs) including low-dose aspirin (LDA) may cause intestinal bleeding, iron-deficiency anaemia, protein loss, small bowel obstruction or even perforation. Symptoms and mucosal damage can persist for months even if the NSAID medication is stopped [297]. Although an elevated level of faecal calprotectin correlates with the presence of a mucosal injury, it does not seem to be a viable predictor to assess the extent of the mucosal damage [298].

Recent analysis using SBCE revealed that NSAID-induced lesions occur more often in the small bowel than it does in the stomach, especially when combined with proton pump inhibitors [299, 300]. Maiden et al. [301] discovered mucosal lesions (Fig. 3.36) in the small bowel in 60 % of patients taking 150 mg diclofenac daily. The severity ranged from reddened spots to bleeding ulcers with the possibility of small bowel perforation. Furthermore, long-term alterations may lead to diaphragm-like strictures with partial or total obstruction [299]

As a consequence, numerous single centre trials reported promising results in reducing NSAID or LDA induced lesions, for example with Lactobacillus casei [302], misoprostol [303], polaprezinc [304], rebamipide [305] or mesalazine [306]. In all of these pharmaceutical

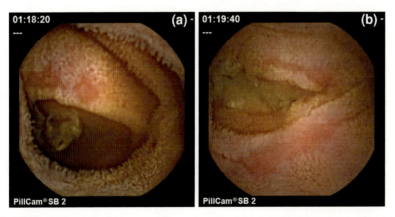

**Fig. 3.36** **a**, **b** SBCE shows small erosions, patchy erythema and patchy villous atrophy (*mucosal breaks*) due to NSAID

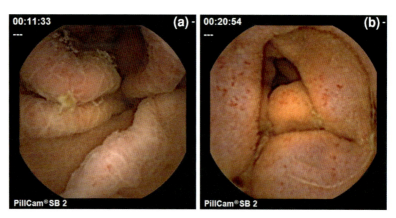

**Fig. 3.37** **a**, **b** Portal hypertensive gastropathy (**a**) and portal hypertensive enteropathy (**b**) in a patient with liver cirrhosis

trials, SBCE was successfully used at baseline to identify NSAID-induced small bowel enteropathy and at the end of treatment to evaluate the protective effects of the agent.

### 3.6.7 Capsule Endoscopy in the Emergency Department

In a pilot study, 25 patients presenting acute upper gastrointestinal haemorrhage immediately underwent SBCE in the emergency department. The procedure was performed to identify fresh blood or coffee ground in the stomach. It was well tolerated and by patients choice preferable to a nasogastric tube. Data were analysed in real time via a portable monitor. Compared to information acquired by conventional upper gastrointestinal endoscopy, SBCE had a sensitivity of 88 % and specificity of 64 % in the detection of blood. Advanced knowledge of SBCE was not necessary to identify a haemorrhage, making it a feasible procedure for emergency physicians. Yet, further studies are necessary to determine the diagnostic value of SBCE in the emergency department [307].

### 3.6.8 Compensated Liver Cirrhosis and Anaemia

Aoyama et al. examined 60 patients with liver cirrhosis Child-Pugh Class A or B and an associated anaemia (haemoglobin <12 g/dl) who showed no clinical signs of an active gastrointestinal bleeding and had an non-diagnostic upper and lower gastrointestinal endoscopy in this regard. Small bowel abnormalities were found in 67 % including erythema, erosions, angioectasias and varices. Small bowel lesions were significantly more prevalent in patients with Child-Pugh Class B, ascites, and portal hypertensive gastropathy (Fig. 3.37). Although the value of the additional information needs to be further explored, SBCE should be considered in patients who meet these criteria and have an unexplained anaemia [308].

### 3.6.9 Small Bowel Capsule Endoscopy in Systemic Diseases

Systemic diseases are generally rare with a wide etiological spectrum. Involvement of the small bowel may occur in many systemic diseases, with a high variation in frequency, severity and extent. Small bowel ulcers can be detected by SBCE in patients suffering from iron-deficiency anaemia, gastrointestinal bleeding or malabsorption with or without abdominal pain. Differentiation from ulcers in Crohn's disease can be challenging and requires additional clinical and laboratory tests as well as biopsies. In patients with an established diagnosis, capsule endoscopy may document extent and severity with which the small bowel is involved.

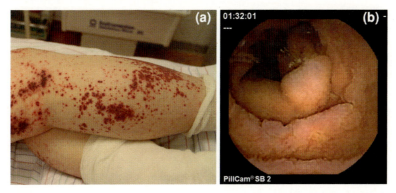

**Fig. 3.38** IgA-Vasculitis. **a** Male adult patient with Henoch-Schoenlein Purpura, typical purpura of the skin. **b** Ulcers, erosions and oedema documented by SBCE

### 3.6.9.1 Sarcoidosis

Sarcoidosis may be asymptomatic, especially in chronic disease. Clinical symptoms are often non-specific like fatigue or weight loss. Gastrointestinal involvement in systemic sarcoidosis is rare and often silent. Cases of gastric sarcoidosis have been reported [309, 310], whilst involvement of the small bowel is extremely rare. Patients may be asymptomatic or present with iron-deficiency anaemia or even haemorrhage [311, 312]. SBCE can reveal nodular and ulcerated lesions of the mucosa. Diagnosis can be established by clinical presentation and histology.

### 3.6.9.2 IgA-vasculitis (Henoch-Schoenlein Purpura)

Henoch-Schoenlein purpura (HSP) is an immune complex vasculitis characterised by deposition of IgA-immune complexes. Whilst common in children, the disease is rare in adults and may be hard to diagnose. HSP often manifests with acute abdominal pain and bloody diarrhoea [313], whilst typical palpable purpura of the skin may develop later and delay correct diagnosis (Fig. 3.38a). SBCE can facilitate correct diagnosis when being performed in patients with acute onset of abdominal pain and haemorrhage of uncertain cause. It is useful to document extent and severity of small bowel disease. SBCE usually shows haemorrhagic ulcerating enteritis with a wide range of additional lesions. In-between areas with normal mucosa can be

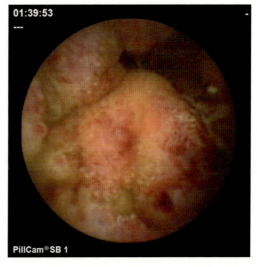

**Fig. 3.39** IgA-Vasculitis with severe inflammation and stenosis of the small bowel

found (Fig. 3.38b), and the severity of the lesions may decrease towards the distal small bowel. Inflammatory stenosis has been observed [314, 315] (Fig. 3.39)

### 3.6.9.3 Behçet's Syndrome

Behçet's syndrome is a recurrent systemic disease predominately affecting young adults between 20 and 40 years. It is characterised by vasculitis of arteries and veins of all sizes. Clinically, patients often present with the triple-symptom complex of uveitis, oral aphthous ulcers and genital ulcers. Involvement of the intestine occurs amongst other manifestations.

Association with HLA B51 has been described. In the presence of gastrointestinal symptoms, case series have shown frequent involvement of the small bowel with ulcers as the main findings [316, 317].

### 3.6.9.4 Rheumatoid Arthritis

In patients with rheumatoid arthritis, changes of the small bowel mucosa are often induced by medication including NSAIDs, corticosteroids or disease-modifying anti-rheumatic drugs (DMARDS), leading to typical SBCE findings such as mucosal breaks with erosions, ulcers or webs [318]. In patients with rheumatic arthritis, SBCE can be helpful to monitor complications of therapy.

### 3.6.9.5 Systemic Lupus Erythematosus

Systemic lupus erythematosus (SLE) may imitate multiple other diseases, and therefore, diagnosis may be challenging. Intestinal involvement, especially of the small bowel, is rare but may occur, e. g. due to secondary vasculitis [319]. Endoscopy may show aphthous lesions or ulcers, even perforation or pseudo-obstruction has been described [320].

### 3.6.9.6 Amyloidosis

Amyloidosis is a clinical disorder characterised by extracellular or intracellular deposition of insoluble abnormal fibrillar protein (amyloid). The most common systemic type is lambda light-chain amyloidosis (AL) associated with multiple myeloma or monoclonal gammopathy. AA-amyloidosis may occur in chronic inflammatory diseases (e.g. Crohn's disease, rheumatoid arthritis), chronic local or systemic infections (e.g. tuberculosis) or occasionally in neoplasms (e.g. Hodgkin disease). In patients undergoing dialysis, amyloidosis (A$\beta$2M-amyloidosis) may occur. Affection of the gastrointestinal tract may cause non-specific symptoms like abdominal pain, constipation, diarrhoea or gastrointestinal bleeding. In these patients, SBCE can be used to detect involvement of the small bowel. Endoscopic changes vary from ulcers and erosions to submucosal haematomas and pseudo-obstruction [321]. Biopsy samples

are warranted to establish the diagnosis. Involvement of the gastrointestinal tract has been shown to have a negative impact on survival and quality of life [322–324].

## 3.6.10 Infections of the Small Bowel

Most infectious diseases of the small bowel are self-limiting. Often stool cultures are used as the first-line diagnostic tool, sometimes complemented by toxin or antigen detection. Further investigation is warranted in cases with persistent, severe or extra-intestinal symptoms such as fever or weight loss or pathological findings of anaemia or elevated inflammatory markers. Although indication for SBCE is rarely given in infectious diseases, it may occasionally reveal even small lesions of the small bowel and guide further diagnostic and therapy.

### 3.6.10.1 Tuberculosis and Infection with Atypical Mycobacteria

Gastrointestinal tuberculosis may be due to a primary infection with Mycobacterium bovis or secondary to pulmonary infection with Mycobacterium tuberculosis. It affects the small bowel and the ileocaecal region in the majority of cases [325]. Intestinal tuberculosis may mimic other diseases as symptoms are often non-specific including abdominal pain, weight loss, diarrhoea and anaemia. Even intestinal obstruction and perforation with subsequent peritonitis have been described [326]. Therefore, SBCE may be indicated in patients with tuberculosis and gastrointestinal symptoms, especially in regions with a high prevalence of tuberculosis. Gastrointestinal infection may occur in asymptomatic patients with pulmonary tuberculosis [327]. Findings are often non-specific. Affected mucosa may present with swelling or patchy redness. Ileocaecal ulcers are the commonest finding, sometimes leading to strictures or obstruction [328]. Differentiation from other diseases such as Crohn's or NSAID-related lesions might be challenging [329, 330] because of the morphologic resemblance biopsy sampling is crucial.

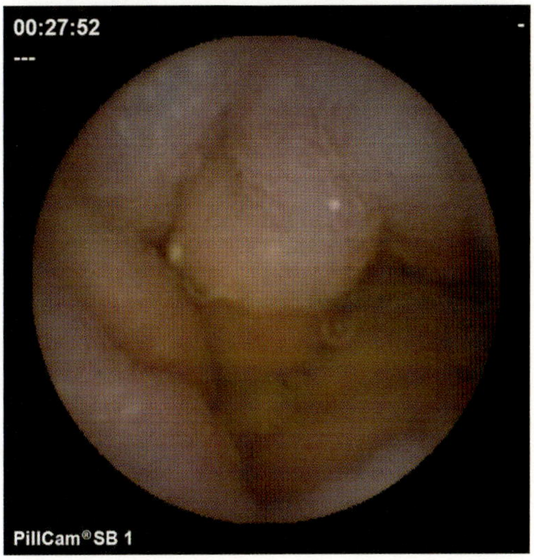

Fig. 3.40 Atypical mycobacteriosis causing oedema and lymphangiectasia

Atypical mycobacteria do not cause tuberculosis or leprosy but have been described as occurring in patients with immunodeficiency and gastrointestinal symptoms such as abdominal pain or diarrhoea [331]. SBCE may reveal oedema, diffuse haemorrhage, lymphangiectasia, erosions and ulcers. The endoscopic resemblance to Whipple's diseases led to the term 'pseudo-Whipple' (Fig. 3.40).

### 3.6.10.2  Whipple's Disease
Whipple's disease is caused by the organism Tropheryma whipplei and characterised by diarrhoea, malabsorption, arthritis, neurological symptoms and psychiatric abnormalities. Affected patients may suffer from a cellular immune defect [332]. Although small bowel involvement is very rare, it may be the cause of chronic diarrhoea and should be considered, especially in the presence of immunosuppression [333]. Endoscopic findings are oedema, ulcers, erosions and lymphangiectasia, sometimes with diffuse haemorrhage [334]. These findings have been shown to decrease during therapy, with SBCE being used to monitor these changes [335].

### 3.6.10.3  Cytomegalovirus Enteritis
Cytomegalovirus (CMV) is a DNA virus belonging to the group of herpes viruses. After primary infection and persistence, it may be reactivated. Infection often remains asymptomatic but severe disease may occur in immunosuppression, e. g. in malignant diseases, pharmacological treatment or Acquired Immunodeficiency Syndrome (AIDS) [336, 337]. It may affect all portions of the gastrointestinal tract, sometimes causing mid-gastrointestinal bleeding, obstruction or perforation [338, 339]. Indication for SBCE is mid-gastrointestinal bleeding in most patients. CMV ulcers appear punched out without inflammatory reaction.

### 3.6.10.4  Acquired Immunodeficiency Syndrome
Patients with Acquired Immunodeficiency Syndrome (AIDS) may suffer from enteritis due to a variety of causes including mycobacteriosis, cryptosporidiosis, histoplasmosis or CMV infections [340, 341]. Besides, these infectious reasons HIV enteropathy may occur, often presenting with non-specific lymphangiectasia [342]. It is diagnosed by exclusion of other underlying reasons. Pathological findings by SBCE were more common in patients with gastrointestinal symptoms and low CD4 cell count [331]. Capsule endoscopy might be beneficial because of its single use and the possibility of visualisation of oesophagus, stomach, small bowel and parts of the colon. However, microbiological testing is essential in patients with AIDS and enteritis. Although it is limited by the inability to obtain biopsies, SBCE can be indicated in case of persistent symptoms in patients with AIDS.

### 3.6.10.5  Helminthiases
Helminths are more prevalent in the tropics and subtropics [343]. Infestation may remain asymptomatic, whereas severe cases may cause diarrhoea, anaemia, pruritus, abdominal pain and even obstruction. Indication for SBCE is mid-gastrointestinal bleeding or anaemia in most cases. Ascarids are often found incidentally but SBCE may be helpful for early detection in regions with high prevalence [344]. In patients with hookworm infections besides anaemia or diarrhoea, eosinophilia may guide the diagnosis [345, 346]. Enterobius is normally prevalent in

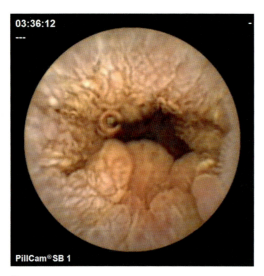

**Fig. 3.41** Idiopathic non-granulomatous ulcerative jejuno-ileitis in an elderly patient with severe malabsorption

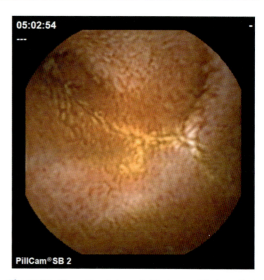

**Fig. 3.42** Ulcerative jejuno-ileitis in an elderly patient with malabsorption and previously undiagnosed coeliac disease

the caecum. Due to rectal–oral autoinfection, perianal itching is the main symptom. However, sometimes, SBCE may identify enterobius in the colon [347]. Tapeworms present as large parasites with multiple proglottids, sometimes reaching a length of several metres and often leading to anaemia or abdominal pain. Tapeworms can be found incidentally. SBCE may be helpful to monitor therapy [348, 349].

### 3.6.11 Gastrointestinal Food Allergy

SBCE has been applied in 15 patients with documented food allergy: 12 had small bowel findings. In 4 cases, erosions, aphthae, and petechiae were seen, whilst in 8 oedema, erythema or lymphoid hyperplasia could be detected [350]. Anaemia in these patients improved after anti-allergic treatment.

### 3.6.12 Malabsorption Syndromes

In unexplained malabsorption syndrome, SBCE can be useful in selected cases to detect mucosal alterations of the small bowel. Diffuse lymphangiectasia may be due to either idiopathic

Waldman's disease [351] or may be secondary to radiation, medication (NSAIDs) or infection (Whipple's disease, atypical mycobacteriosis or HIV). Diffuse ulceration or villous atrophy can be detected in a large variety of diseases. Rare causes of malabsorption like chronic idiopathic non-granulomatous ulcerative jejuno-ileitis (Fig. 3.41) [352, 353], ulcerative jejuno-ileitis in previously undiagnosed coeliac disease (Fig. 3.42) eosinophilic enteritis [354] or amyloidosis [355] have been reported.

Two-nine of 42 patients with cystic fibrosis had pancreatic insufficiency. In this group, faecal calprotectin was markedly elevated and most of these patients had small bowel lesions as erythema, oedema, mucosal breaks and ulcers detected at SBCE [356].

Malabsorption as an indication for SBCE seems to be more frequent in children than in adults. In an early paediatric study [357], suspected Crohn's disease was the most common indication. However, 5 of 37 children underwent SBCE for protein loss or malabsorption. [358] studied 83 children under the age of 8 years with SBCE. Four of 9 children with intestinal protein loss had diffuse lymphangiectasia and in 6 of 12 with malabsorption, SBCE-diagnosed enteropathy, and in one case, ascariasis.

**Table 3.7** Contraindications to capsule endoscopy

| Contraindications | Relative contraindications |
| --- | --- |
| Gastrointestinal obstruction, strictures or fistulae, unless patency has been confirmed by patency testing or surgery is planned | Swallowing disorders |
| Pseudo-obstruction | Zenker's diverticulum |
| Pregnancy | Cardiac pacemaker/defibrillator |
| Planned magnetic resonance imaging | |

## 3.7  Optimising Safety in Small Bowel Capsule Endoscopy

As a non-invasive procedure, capsule endoscopy (CE) has an excellent safety profile with an overall complication rate of 1–3 % [359, 360]. Whilst there are few limitations to its use, contraindications do exist and there are some special situations that require careful management to minimise the risk of complications.

### 3.7.1  Contraindications

The number of contraindications to CE is small, and some of these are relative (Table 3.7). Contraindications include suspected or known obstruction (unless patency has been previously confirmed or surgical intervention is warranted), pseudo-obstruction, pregnancy and impending magnetic resonance imaging [361]. The safety of CE in pregnancy has not been established, with specific concerns relating to the effect of radiofrequency emissions on the foetus, as well as the risk of capsule retention with clinical obstruction. Two case reports have documented the use of CE in pregnant patients without any immediate complication, the first within the third trimester at 28 weeks [362], and the second within the first trimester [363]. However, as safety outcomes have not been addressed, and in

the absence of robust data, CE in pregnancy remains contraindicated.

Patients requiring magnetic resonance imaging (MRI) should defer CE until completion of the MRI procedure, or where MRI is required after CE, capsule excretion should be verified by patient-reported passage of the capsule or by performing a plain abdominal radiograph. With ongoing CE manufacturer warnings against exposure to strong magnetic fields with a capsule inside the body, there is concern for the potential danger of capsule migration, causing injury to the intestinal tract or abdominal cavity [364]. Although two episodes of inadvertent magnetic resonance scanning with a retained capsule in the colon, resulting in no harm to the patients, have been reported [365, 366], retained capsules are considered a danger and remain a contraindication to MRI [364, 367].

Historically, the use of CE in patients with swallowing disorders and pacemakers or implanted cardiac defibrillators (ICDs) has also been contraindicated. With the exception of obstructive dysphagia, these factors can now be effectively managed to reduce clinical risk, and no longer present a barrier for these patients who require capsule imaging.

### 3.7.2  Risks of Capsule Endoscopy

Risk factors associated with CE can be broadly categorised into three main areas for discussion of risk assessment, preventative strategies and management of complications: (i) capsule retention, (ii) risk associated with swallowing the capsule (non-obstructive dysphagia and diverticula), (iii) additional factors that may impact on patient safety, including pacemakers and implantable defibrillators and altered gastrointestinal anatomy.

### 3.7.3  Capsule Retention

Capsule retention in the small intestine is the main complication associated with capsule endoscopy. The capsule is normally excreted

**Table 3.8** Stratified risk of small bowel capsule retention according to indication

| | |
|---|---|
| Healthy controls (%) [370] | 0 |
| Overall retention rate (%) [359] | 1.4 |
| Obscure GI bleeding (%) [359] | 1.2 |
| Suspected small bowel Crohn's disease (%) [371, 464–466] | 1.48 |
| Established small bowel Crohn's disease [359, 371, 392, 467] | Up to 13 % (pooled rate 2.6 %) |
| Suspected small bowel obstruction (%) [286] | 21 |

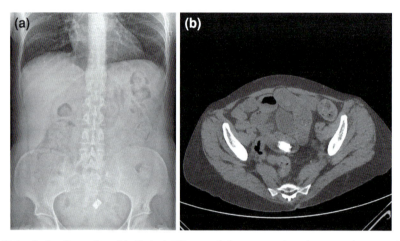

**Fig. 3.43** **a** Abdominal radiograph and **b** limited CT scan of the same patient demonstrating retention of patency capsule secondary to small bowel stricture

after an average time of 72 h [368]. Retention is defined as the presence of the capsule within the digestive tract for more than 2 weeks after ingestion, or when the capsule is retained indefinitely in the bowel lumen unless a targeted medical, endoscopic or surgical intervention is initiated [369].

The overall rate of capsule retention is 1.4 % [359]. The level of retention risk can be stratified according to the clinical indication for the examination (Table 3.8), with obscure gastrointestinal bleeding presenting the lowest risk, 1.2 % [359]. It is important to note that the risk of capsule retention in healthy individuals is 0 % [370]. Retention is usually due to previously undiagnosed small bowel strictures (Fig. 3.43a–b) or tumours, with the three most common causes being Crohn's disease, NSAID-induced strictures and tumours [359, 371–375]. Rarely, capsules have been reported to be retained in a Zenker diverticulum [376], Meckel's diverticulum [377–379] and umbilical hernia [380].

As well as suspected or known Crohn's disease, other factors that are known to significantly increase retention risk include previous major abdominal surgery or small bowel resection [381], previous abdominopelvic radiotherapy [359] and prolonged non-steroidal anti-inflammatory drug use [373].

Retention of the capsule is detected primarily during the process of video image review. Images may show an obstructive lesion, repetitive views with no clear progress and/or excessive luminal contents; all of which may be indicative of small bowel retention. In the absence of patient confirmed passage, failure of the capsule to reach the colon should prompt investigation (at 2 weeks post-ingestion unless the patient reports symptoms sooner) with an abdominal radiograph or CT to detect the presence of the radio-opaque foreign body, thus confirming the diagnosis.

Up to 85 % of retained capsules are asymptomatic and, in some cases, may be retained for several years with minimal clinical sequelae

**Table 3.9** Informed consent: key elements to be discussed

| |
|---|
| Preparation requirements |
| How the procedure is performed |
| Purpose, benefits and alternatives to the procedure |
| Risks and potential complications: |
| – Retention of capsule with potential consequence of surgical intervention |
| – Option of patency test to evaluate gut patency |
| – Complications relating to swallowing (aspiration) |
| – Study incompletion (capsule does not reach the colon within the recording period), requiring repetition |
| – Potential risk of electromagnetic interference |
| – MRI contraindication until verification of capsule excretion is verified |

Verbal information should be supplemented with printed information/leaflets

[359, 375, 382]. Although less common, capsule retention can cause partial or complete small bowel obstruction [359, 383, 384] and, very rarely, can result in small bowel perforation. At the time of writing, only 6 reports of capsule-induced perforation have been published [385–390].

### 3.7.3.1 Minimising the Risk of Retention

To identify potential risk factors and minimise the occurrence of complications, patients should be appropriately selected and carefully assessed. With a thorough knowledge of the patient's medical and surgical background, the assessing clinician should identify any co-morbidities, drug history and special considerations that may present or increase risk. An informed consent process should be undertaken prior to the procedure being performed. This should include information regarding the procedure, the intended benefits, as well as the nature and level of risk associated with the procedure. A summary of the key elements to be discussed with the patient during the consent process is outlined in Table 3.9.

For high-risk patient groups, further small bowel imaging to evaluate small bowel patency should be considered in advance of the procedure [373]. Conventional radiological imaging methods such as barium contrast radiography

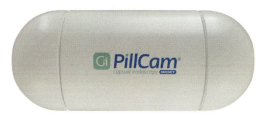

**Fig. 3.44** Pillcam Patency Capsule (Courtesy of Given Imaging Ltd)

and CT or magnetic resonance enterography (using oral contrast) may be used. Whilst negative studies suggest that the capsule will most likely pass without incident [391], significant stenoses can be missed [286, 369, 374, 392–395]. Enteroclysis techniques using nasojejunal intubation to distend the small bowel have been shown to more accurately detect intestinal strictures in patients with Crohn's disease [396]; however, they may miss diaphragmatic webs associated with NSAID enteropathy [373]. In addition, this test is time consuming, uncomfortable for the patient and thus less commonly available [391]. An alternative and increasingly used approach to establish patency of the small bowel in patients with a high risk of retention is the use of the Pillcam Patency test (Given Imaging Ltd).

### 3.7.3.2 Pillcam Patency Test

The Pillcam Patency test (Given Imaging Ltd) is a system designed to non-invasively verify sufficient patency of the small bowel in order to enable the safe passage of a video capsule. It provides a direct indication of functional patency even in cases where radiological imaging indicates a small bowel stricture. When the patency capsule is excreted intact, the video capsule will pass naturally, when performed without undue delay. Retention of the patency capsule is indicative of pathology.

The system comprises a non-video, dissolvable patency capsule (Fig. 3.44) identical in size to the Given Pillcam video capsule (11 mm × 26 mm). The capsule body contains barium sulphate to make it radio-opaque, lactose to enable the capsule to dissolve quickly in gastrointestinal fluids, and a small

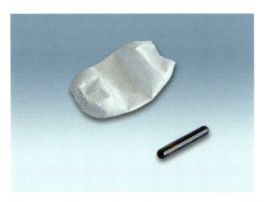

**Fig. 3.45** Disintegrated capsule remnants: empty shell and RFID tag

radiofrequency identification tag (RFID) to assist with capsule detection. Two timer plugs at each end of the capsule allow controlled disintegration, beginning approximately 30 h after ingestion. The remnants of the capsule (Fig. 3.45), including the RFID tag, can be passed through even small orifices [397].

Assessment of capsule excretion may be done in one of three ways:

- Patient-reported passage
- Patency scan test
- Abdominal radiograph (if scanner not available or contraindicated)

The patency scan test requires a hand-held, battery-operated patency scanner to transmit a radiofrequency signal to the capsule RFID, which in turn emits a signal that is detected by the scanner. The scanner is operated 30 h post-ingestion to determine whether the capsule has been excreted. A positive scan indicates the presence of the capsule within the gastrointestinal tract. Where a scanner is not available, a plain abdominal radiograph may be used to determine excretion.

Approximately half the number of patients undergoing a patency test will screen positive [398–400]. Whilst a positive scan indicates that the capsule remains inside the gastrointestinal tract, it is not possible to verify successful transverse of the small bowel with passage through the ileocaecal valve using the scanner alone. In the majority of cases, the capsule will be in the colon [399], but occasionally may be

held up in the stomach. In order to accurately localise the capsule position, further imaging is necessary. Some centres utilise abdominal radiograph as the first-line approach; however, this requires access to radiologists who are experienced and competent in the assessment of post-patency capsule imaging [398]. Even experienced radiologists are not always accurate in determining capsule position on abdominal radiograph [399, 400]. Where there is uncertainty, a limited low-dose CT (unprepared, without contrast) should be performed the same day to confirm position.

Some centres have opted to replace abdominal radiograph with a CT scout film and subsequent targeted limited CT, reporting an accuracy rate of 99.5 % in capsule localisation ([400]).

Whichever imaging protocol is used, it is essential that radiological imaging is undertaken within a few hours of the patency scan (maximum of 36 h post-capsule ingestion) before dissolution of the capsule begins. A prolonged time lapse between ingestion and imaging increases the risk of a false negative, rendering the test non-diagnostic.

### 3.7.3.3 Patency Procedure

Minimal preparation is required for the patency procedure. Informed consent should be undertaken, with the patient informed of the very rare risk of temporary intestinal occlusion caused by the disintegrating capsule and the potential need for surgery [401]. Any drugs that affect gut motility, including narcotics should be reviewed and, if possible, withheld for at least 48 h before the procedure. A 12-h fasting period is recommended by the manufacturer. Prior to ingestion, the capsule should be tested with the patency scanner to ensure whether the signal is detected. The capsule is swallowed with a glass of water at 08.00 a.m. Normal activities including eating and drinking may then be resumed. Where patients have swallowing or gastric motility disorders, or anatomical abnormalities, the patency capsule may be placed endoscopically into the duodenum using a specialised capsule delivery device. Endoscopic placement is

**Table 3.10** Standard patency capsule procedure protocol

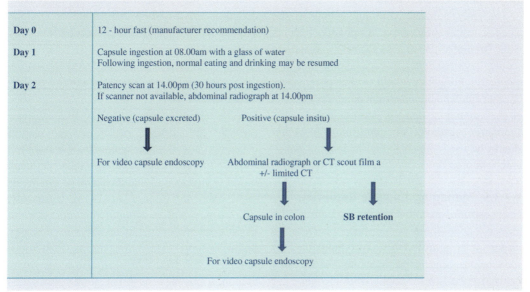

| Day 0 | 12 - hour fast (manufacturer recommendation) |
| --- | --- |
| Day 1 | Capsule ingestion at 08.00am with a glass of water |
| | Following ingestion, normal eating and drinking may be resumed |
| Day 2 | Patency scan at 14.00pm (30 hours post ingestion). |
| | If scanner not available, abdominal radiograph at 14.00pm |

Negative (capsule excreted) → For video capsule endoscopy

Positive (capsule insitu) → Abdominal radiograph or CT scout film a +/- limited CT → Capsule in colon → For video capsule endoscopy / SB retention

a Depending on clinically agreed protocol and resource availability

discussed further below in *Dysphagia and diverticula*. At 30 h post-ingestion, the patient should attend for the patency scan (or abdominal radiograph), unless excretion has already been confirmed. A summary of the standard patency capsule procedure and scanning protocol is outlined in Table 3.10. Once safe small bowel passage of the patency capsule has been verified, the patient may proceed to video capsule endoscopy.

### 3.7.3.4 Application of the Patency Test in Clinical Practice

A number of studies have demonstrated that the patency capsule is safe to use within routine clinical practice and is more sensitive than radiological imaging as a screening test for retention [397, 399, 402–406]. The test is indicated for patient groups who are deemed to be at high risk of small bowel retention:

- Established (or suspected + abdominal pain) Crohn's disease
- Long-term (>1 year) use of non-steroidal anti-inflammatory medications (NSAIDS)
- Previous abdominopelvic radiotherapy
- Previous small bowel resection
- Previous abdominal surgery with suspected adhesions
- Suspected or confirmed small bowel strictures based on symptoms or radiological imaging
- Patients with significant co-morbidities who are considered high surgical risk

Minimal complications of the patency test have been reported; the most common of which is transient abdominal pain in approximately 20 % cases [403], usually resolving when the capsule is excreted. Although temporary intestinal occlusion has previously been reported (Gay et al. 2004), this case involved the use of a 'first-generation' patency capsule, and subsequent design modifications to the capsule have significantly reduced the risk of this very rare adverse event. Delayed transit of the patency capsule without true small bowel retention has been documented as a failed test or study incompletion [407]. Risk factors for study incompletion include type II diabetes mellitus, gastroparesis, hypothyroidism and constipating drugs. A careful assessment of medical and drug history with consideration of endoscopic placement for those at risk of delayed transit can help to minimise such risks.

The only absolute contraindication to the patency test is obstructive dysphagia. Patients with non-obstructive swallowing disorders should have the patency capsule placed endoscopically. For patients with cardiac pacemakers or other implantable electromedical devices, use of the patency scanner is contraindicated, and alternative methods of confirming excretion should be used (for example, abdominal radiograph, fluoroscopy).

### 3.7.3.5 Managing Capsule Retention

Once capsule retention has been confirmed, it may be appropriate to consider conservative management in those who are asymptomatic, as spontaneous capsule passage may occur, especially if there is a medically treatable cause for the retention [359, 372, 375, 408]. This may be medical treatment of Crohn's disease and tuberculous enterocolitis, or stopping NSAID use in NSAID-associated small bowel strictures [372]. The majority are, however, likely to require further intervention. Current literature suggests 15 % pass with conservative management, 12 % are removed endoscopically and 58 % undergo surgery for the removal of the capsule [359].

Various endoscopic retrieval methods have been used including gastroscopy and colonoscopy if the retained capsule is within reach, and also push and pull enteroscopy [409]. Increasingly, double-balloon enteroscopy has been used in multiple cases of capsule retention [410–413]. In the largest study, this was shown to be safe and effective, with all using the antegrade route for successful proximal small bowel retrieval. Most of these subsequently underwent surgery to treat the underlying cause of retention [413]. Establishing the site of the capsule retention without knowing small bowel transit time is difficult. Conventional CE methods of estimating pathology location rely on transit time with the small bowel broadly divided into tertiles; however, this technique requires completion of small bowel transit with confirmed entry of the capsule into the colon. In the absence of these

localisation methods, using a combination of the clinical history, capsule imaging and likely diagnosis can assist in estimating the position and thus determine which endoscopic modality is appropriate.

Although capsule retention is a complication of capsule endoscopy, it is not always considered to be an adverse event. With the premise that the retained capsule leads to surgical treatment of the diseased bowel and removal of capsule to alleviate the symptoms, CE has been used in the setting of recurrent subacute small bowel obstruction to find the cause of symptoms and localise the disease [414, 415]. Ultimately, surgical intervention is required in most cases of capsule retention due to underlying pathology requiring surgical resection such as small bowel tumours [359, 372, 373], and also to deal with complications such as small bowel obstruction or perforation. Although surgery is traditionally performed via open approaches, there are cases of laparoscopic capsule retrieval [416].

Whilst capsule endoscopy is overall a safe procedure, patients should be adequately counselled about the retention risk and likelihood of subsequent surgery. They can, however, be reassured that capsule retention is not always considered a bad thing and, in some cases, has been shown to have clear benefit in identifying and treating the underlying aetiology of symptoms [414].

### 3.7.4 Dysphagia and Diverticula

During assessment, it is important to identify potential difficulties that the patient may encounter when swallowing the capsule endoscope. Even though the history may not reveal dysphagia, occult oropharyngeal dysfunction should be considered in patients who are elderly or with a history of cerebrovascular disease. In patients with oropharyngeal dysfunction, the capsule may be aspirated into the upper and, more rarely, lower respiratory tract [417, 418]. The management of patients with dysphagia is dependent on a number of factors including patient comorbidity, the extent of the dysphagia,

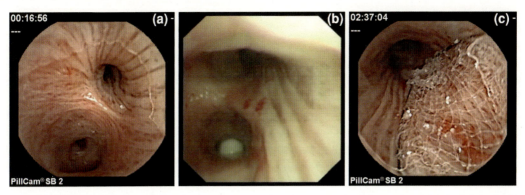

**Fig. 3.46** Capsule aspiration into the respiratory tract: **a** real-time viewing shows the capsule positioned within the left main bronchus **b** position confirmed at bronchoscopy **c** bronchoscopic retrieval of the capsule using Roth Net™ (US Endoscopy)

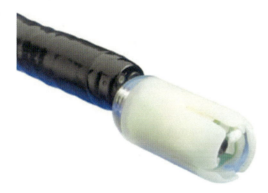

**Fig. 3.47** AdvanCE™ accessory device (US endoscopy) for endoscopic capsule placement. The capsule is held at the tip of the endoscope during intubation and released directly into the duodenum

and whether it is functional or structural. Patients with functional dysphagia may reasonably be able to swallow the capsule if they are provided with a clear explanation to minimise misperceptions or fears.

In rare situations, the capsule can be held up by diverticula in the retro-pharynx or oesophagus. Accordingly, capsule endoscopy is relatively contraindicated in patients with known Zenker's diverticulum, and for these patients, the capsule is best delivered endoscopically [419, 420].

Endoscopic placement of the capsule directly into the duodenum should be considered in cases where the patient is unable to swallow the capsule, or where a risk factor exists that may decrease the chances of the capsule reaching the small intestine. This procedure requires the use of either a proprietary device, AdvanCE™ (US endoscopy) designed to hold the capsule at the tip of the endoscope (Fig. 3.47) [421], or the use of other endoscopic accessories (snare or basket) with or without the use of an overtube or banding cap [420, 422]. A 'scouting' endoscopy is performed to review the anatomy before the AdvanCE™ device is used. Passage of the scope through the pylorus during the 'scouting' endoscopy aids passage of the capsule once it is loaded in the placement device. The capsule is held within the placement device in front of the endoscope tip during intubation, such that the capsule is facing away from the tip. Often endoscopic placement of the capsule is performed with the combination of local anaesthetic throat spray and conscious sedation to minimise the additional discomfort that might be associated with the procedure. In addition, it is best to try to utilise all features associated with optimal endoscopic intubations of the oesophagus, e.g. flexing the neck to mitigate the loss of angle deflection at the tip of the endoscope when an accessory is placed in front of the endoscope tip. Intubation of the oesophagus with direct visualisation is not possible once the capsule is loaded in the AdvanCE™ device; however, once the oesophagus is intubated, the device can be advanced through the scope 1–2 cm to improve endoscopic views.

### 3.7.4.1 Detection and Management of Aspiration

Capsule aspiration into the respiratory tract is a rare occurrence, with a recent case series citing a risk level of 1 in 800–1,000 capsule ingestions [417]. Patients may be symptomatic [423] or asymptomatic [424, 425]. Indeed, a capsule has been retained in the airway for up to 6 days without causing pneumonitis or airway compromise [424]. In the absence of symptoms, inadvertent aspiration may only be detected during review of the CE video [426].

Within the published literature to date, a number of features have been documented [417, 427]:

(i) capsule aspirations occur with a greater than 90 % predominance in elderly (older than 65) male patients
(ii) most patients who aspirated did not have history of dysphagia
(iii) most patients had some coughing post-capsule ingestion

Although the reported cases suggest that age may be an independent risk factor for aspiration, a study involving 195 patients over the age of 80 demonstrated no increased risk compared with a control group under the age of 80 years [428].

If aspiration is suspected, it is important to verify urgently. This can be achieved by real-time viewing, by aborting the study and downloading and reviewing capsule images, or by radiographic imaging [429, 430]. Although no direct fatalities have been reported to date, a putative connection has been made between the cough caused by capsule aspiration and the development of an intra-cerebral haemorrhage [431]. As airway compromise and pneumonitis are the primary concern, the capsule should be removed.

The mechanism by which the capsule is removed depends on several factors: how deeply and firmly the capsule is lodged, the strength of the patient cough reflex and the facilities available. Certainly, the intra-thoracic pressures generated by a strong cough reflex can be very helpful and, in most cases, the patient expectorates the capsule naturally [42]. If this proves unsuccessful,

possible invasive methods include rigid or flexible bronchoscopy using a retrieval device [432]. There have been a number of reports of capsules being aspirated into the main bronchi and subsequently removed (Fig. 3.46a–c). Although removal has been achieved with several methods, including 'crocodile' forceps, Roth Net™ (US Endoscopy USA), flexible bronchoscopy with a Roth Net [433], rigid bronchoscopy [430] and via esophagogastroduodenoscopy [434], the optimal method depends on local resource availability and expertise as well as degree of patient compromise, if any [432].

Whilst taking a careful history to look for clues suggesting an increased risk of aspiration may help to predict which patients should be monitored more carefully, the experience to date has shown that neither the history nor the post-ingestion symptoms are sensitive enough to detect the majority of capsule aspirations. Accordingly, the routine use of real-time viewing is recommended post-ingestion to confirm that the capsule is within the gastrointestinal tract [435, 436]. Every study should include real-time viewing 30–45 min after ingestion to confirm that the capsule has reached the duodenum; however, for those patients deemed to be at risk of aspiration or who develop symptoms, real-time viewing should be done immediately after the capsule has been swallowed to confirm gastric entry.

### 3.7.5 Impaired Luminal Motility

Motility disorders of the oesophagus and stomach may impair movement of the capsule to the small intestine. Whilst oesophageal motility disorders are less likely to cause problems due to the effect of gravity (assuming the patient is not in a prone or supine position), gastroparesis can lead to significant delays in the capsule reaching the small intestine. Gastric transit time (GTT) longer than 45 min has been suggested as an independent risk factor for incomplete CE studies [437]. Prolonged GTT can now be quickly identified with real-time viewing, thus providing an opportunity to instigate timely interventions to induce capsule passage through the pylorus. Possible interventions include lateral positioning and/or asking the patient to take a walk, use of pharmacologic agents (prokinetics) and endoscopic capture and advancement of the capsule. The use of prokinetics to decrease gastric transit time and increase the completion rate of capsule endoscopy has been advocated by some with mixed results [438–440]. Whilst studies indicate that these agents reduce gastric transit time, there is insufficient evidence that they improve small bowel completion rates [440–446].

In cases where there is established or suspected gastric dysmotility, real-time viewing should be used to monitor capsule progression [447]. Where this technology is not available, direct endoscopic placement of the capsule can be performed safely and effectively [421, 422, 448].

### 3.7.6 Pacemakers and Implantable Defibrillators

There has always been a theoretical concern that the signals between capsule endoscopy and cardiac pacemakers/implanted cardioverters (ICDs) might interfere with each other. The theoretical outcome of such interference would be possible malfunction of the pacemakers/implanted cardioverters on one hand and image degradation/non-capture on the other. Some manufacturers of capsules have listed the presence of cardiac pacemakers/implanted cardioverters (ICDs) as a contraindication for the use of capsule endoscopy, placing product label warnings to advise that use of capsule endoscopy in patients with electromechanical devices is not recommended.

Over the last 13 years, this theoretical risk has to a great extent, been unsubstantiated. To date, there have been approximately 500 published cases of capsule use with pacemakers and over 100 with ICD, and none of the data have shown any significant adverse effect on pacemaker/ICD function [449–452]. Although there are a few reports of image degradation or non-

capture [453, 454], the main concern with this capsule/cardiac device interaction has focused on possible cardiac sequelae.

Although the problem may appear easy to resolve, it is complicated due to the numerous types of pacemakers currently in use, thus making it difficult to issue all-inclusive statements about capsule/pacemaker interaction with any certainty. To partially address this issue, several studies have been performed in vitro where capsules were tested with different cardiac pacemakers, demonstrating no adverse interference with any device [455, 456].

Despite multiple small clinical in vivo and in vitro studies reporting no adverse interaction, and favourable recommendations of scientific societies [106, 457], capsule manufacturers have maintained a warning on their product inserts alluding to potential interactions. In the face of this product warning and in ideal circumstances, a decision to use the capsule must be reached using a multidisciplinary consensus approach involving a cardiology, ethical, medico-legal perspective, and administrative perspective to protect patient and provider interests. Knowledge of the indication for the pacemaker and whether the patient is 'pacemaker dependent' can assist in the decision-making process. In practice, many centres have adopted a risk reduction approach and perform capsule endoscopy in patients with pacemakers/ICDs in a cardiac monitored setting, with testing of capsule/pacemaker compatibility prior to ingestion. This can be done by holding the activated capsule adjacent to the pacemaker, and monitoring for any rhythm disturbance before the patient swallows the capsule.

### 3.7.7 Altered Gastrointestinal Anatomy

Capsule passage to the duodenum may be more difficult in patients who have altered gastrointestinal anatomy as a consequence of surgery. This may be because the normal anatomy of the connection of the stomach to the duodenum is altered, e.g. dual intestinal loop anatomy such as a Billroth-II procedure, Whipple surgery, Roux-en-Y gastric bypass, or due to other forms of surgery (esophagectomy or Nissen fundoplication). In most cases, the best option is to place the capsule endoscopically using the techniques described above [422, 448, 458].

# References

1. Neale JR, James S, Callaghan J, Patel P. Premedication with N-acetylcysteine and simethicone improves mucosal visualization during gastroscopy: a randomized, controlled, endoscopist-blinded study. Eur J Gastroenterol Hepatol. 2013;25(7):778–83.
2. Mathus-Vliegen E, Pellisier M, Heresbach D, Fischbach W, Dixon T, Belsey J, Parente F, Rio-Tinto R, Brown A, Toth E, Crosta C, Layer P, Epstein O, Boustiere C. Consensus guidelines for the use of bowel preparation prior to colonic diagnostic procedures: colonoscopy and small bowel video capsule endoscopy. Curr Med Res Opin. 2013;29(8):931–45.
3. Rex DK, Imperiale TF, Latinovich DR, Bratcher LL. Impact of bowel preparation on efficiency and cost of colonoscopy. Am J Gastroenterol. 2002;97:1696–700.
4. Belsey J, Crosta C, Epstein O, Fischbach W, Layer P, Parente F, Halphen M. Meta-analysis: efficacy of small bowel preparation for small bowel video capsule endoscopy. Curr Med Res Opin. 2012;28:1883–90.
5. Rokkas T, Papaxoinis K, Triantafyllou K, Pistiolas D, Ladas SD. Does purgative preparation influence the diagnostic yield of small bowel video capsule endoscopy? A meta-analysis. Am J Gastroenterol. 2009;104(1):219–27.
6. Niv Y. Efficiency of bowel preparation for capsule endoscopy examination: a meta-analysis. World J Gastroenterol. 2008;14(9):1313–7.
7. Onlusen G, Akgun H, Ertan A, Olivero J, Truong LD. Renal failure and nephrocalcinosis associated with oral sodium phosphate bowel cleansing: clinical patterns and renal biopsy findings. Arch Pathol Lab Med. 2006;130(1):101–6.
8. Singal AK, Rosman AS, Post JB, Bauman WA, Spungen AM, Korsten MA. The renal safety of bowel preparations for colonoscopy: a comparative study of oral sodium phosphate solution and polyethylene glycol. Aliment Pharmacol Ther. 2008;27(1):41–7.
9. Park SC, Keum B, Seo YS, Kim YS, Jeen YT, Chun HJ, Um SH, Kim CD, Ryu HS. Effect of bowel preparation with polyethylene glycol on quality of capsule endoscopy. Dig Dis Sci. 2011;56:1769–75.
10. Ito T, Ohata K, Ono A, Chiba H, Tsuji Y, Sato H, Matsuhashi N. Prospective controlled study on the effects of polyethylene glycol in capsule endoscopy. World J Gastroenterol. 2012;18(15):1789–92.
11. Endo H, Kondo Y, Inamori M, Ohya TR, Yanagawa T, Asayama M, Hisatomi K, Teratani T, Yoneda M, Nakajima A, Matsuhashi N. Ingesting 500 ml of polyethylene glycol solution during capsule endoscopy improves the image quality and completion rate to the cecum. Dig Dis Sci. 2008;53(12):3201–5.
12. Osono K, Endo H, Sakai E, Sekino Y, Uchiyama T, Watanabe S, Iida H, Sakamoto Y, Koide T, Takahashi H, Yoneda M, Tokoro C, Abe Y, Inamori M, Kobayashi N, Kubota K, Nakajima A. Optimal approach for small bowel capsule endoscopy using polyethylene glycol and metoclopramide with the assistance of a real-time viewer. Digestion. 2011;84(2):119–25.
13. Basit AW, Newton JM, Short MD, Waddington WA, Ell PJ, Lacey LF. The effect of polyethylene glycol 400 on gastrointestinal transit: implications for the formulation of poorly-water soluble drugs. Pharm Res. 2001;18(8):1146–50.
14. Fang YH, Chen CX, Zhang BL. Effect of small bowel preparation with simethicone on capsule endoscopy. J Zhejiang Univ Sci B. 2009;10:46–51.
15. Ge ZZ, Chen HY, Gao YJ, Hu YB, Xiao SD. The role of simeticone in small-bowel preparation for capsule endoscopy. Endoscopy. 2006;38:836–40.
16. Albert J, Göbel CM, Lesske J, Lotterer E, Nietsch H, Fleig WE. Simethicone for small bowel preparation for capsule endoscopy: a systematic, single-blinded, controlled study. Gastrointest Endosc. 2004;59:487–91.
17. Wei W, Ge ZZ, Lu H, Gao YJ, Hu YB, Xiao SD. Purgative bowel cleansing combined with simethicone improves capsule endoscopy imaging. Am J Gastroenterol. 2008;103:77–82.
18. Spada C, Riccioni ME, Familiari P, et al. Polyethylene glycol plus simethicone in small-bowel preparation for capsule endoscopy. Dig Liver Dis. 2010;42:365–70.
19. Koulaouzidis A, Giannakou A, Yung DE, Dabos KJ, Plevris JN. Do prokinetics influence the completion rate in small-bowel capsule endoscopy? A systematic review and meta-analysis. Curr Med Res Opin. 2013.
20. Taylor WB, Proctor SJ, Bateman DN. Pharmacokinetics and efficacy of high-dose metoclopramide given by continuous infusion for the control of cytotoxic drug-induced vomiting. Br J Clin Pharmacol. 1984;18(5):679–84.
21. Niv E, Ovadia B, Ron Y, Santo E, Mahajna E, Halpern Z, Fireman Z. Ensure preparation and capsule endoscopy: a two-center prospective study. World J Gastroenterol. 2013;19(8):1264–70.
22. Park SC, Keum B, Hyun JJ, Seo YS, Kim YS, Jeen YT, Chun HJ, Um SH, Kim CD, Ryu HS. A novel cleansing score system for capsule endoscopy. World J Gastroenterol. 2010;16(7):875–80.

23. Westerhof J, Weersma RK, Koornstra JJ. Risk factors for incomplete small-bowel capsule endoscopy. Gastrointest Endosc. 2009;69(1):74–80.
24. Höög CM, Bark LÅ, Arkani J, Gorsetman J, Broström O, Sjöqvist U. Capsule retentions and incomplete capsule endoscopy examinations: an analysis of 2300 examinations. Gastroenterol Res Pract. 2012;2012:518718.
25. Olsson C, Holmgren S. The control of gut motility. Comp Biochem Physiol A: Mol Integr Physiol. 2001;128(3):481–503.
26. Laway BA, Malik TS, Khan SH, Rather TA. Prevalence of abnormal gastric emptying in asymptomatic women with newly detected diabetes and its reversibility after glycemic control-a prospective case control study. J Diabetes Complications. 2013;27(1):78–81.
27. Raju GS, Gerson L, Das A, Lewis B. American Gastroenterological Association (AGA) Institute technical review on obscure gastrointestinal bleeding. Gastroenterology. 2007;133:1697–717.
28. Lewis BS. Small intestinal bleeding. Gastroenterol Clin North Am. 1994;23:67–91.
29. Lara LF, Bloomfeld RS, Pineau BC. The rate of lesions found within reach of esophagogastroduodenoscopy during push enteroscopy depends on the type of obscure gastrointestinal bleeding. Endoscopy. 2005;37:745–50.
30. Vlachogiannakos J, Papaxoinis K, Viazis N, Kegioglou A, Binas I, Karamanolis D, Ladas SD. Bleeding lesions within reach of conventional endoscopy in capsule endoscopy examinations for obscure gastrointestinal bleeding: is repeating endoscopy economically feasible? Dig Dis Sci. 2011;56:1763–8.
31. Gerson LB. Small bowel endoscopy: cost-effectiveness of the different approaches. Best Pract Res Clin Gastroenterol. 2012;26:325–35.
32. ASGE Standards of Practice Committee, Fisher L, Lee Krinsky M, Anderson MA, Appalaneni V, Banerjee S, Ben-Menachem T, Cash BD, Decker GA, Fanelli RD, Friis C, Fukami N, Harrison ME, Ikenberry SO, Jain R, Jue T, Khan K, Maple JT, Strohmeyer L, Sharaf R, Dominitz JA. The role of endoscopy in the management of obscure gastrointestinal bleeding. Gastrointest Endosc. 2010;72:471–9.
33. Ladas SD, Triantafyllou K, Spada C, Riccioni ME, Rey JF, Niv Y, Delvaux M, de Franchis R, Costamagna G, ESGE Clinical Guidelines Committee. European Society Gastrointestinal Endoscopy (ESGE): recommendations (2009) on clinical use of video capsule endoscopy to investigate small-bowel, esophageal and colonic diseases. Endoscopy. 2010;42:220–7.
34. Pérez-Cuadrado E, Pons V, Bordas JM, Gonzalez B, Llach J, Menchén P, Pellicer F, Rodriguez S. Small bowel endoscopic exploration Spanish GI endoscopy society recommendations. Endoscopy. 2012;44:979–87.
35. Sidhu R, Sanders DS, Morris AJ, McAlindon ME. Guidelines on small bowel enteroscopy and capsule endoscopy in adults. Gut. 2008;57:125–36.
36. Shim KN, Moon JS, Chang DK, Do JH, Kim JH, Min BH, Jeon SR, Kim JO, Choi MG, Korean Gut Image Study Group. Guideline for capsule endoscopy: obscure gastrointestinal bleeding. Clin Endosc. 2013;46:45–53.
37. Liao Z, Gao R, Xu C, Li ZS. Indications and detection, completion, and retention rates of small-bowel capsule endoscopy: a systematic review. Gastrointest Endosc. 2010;71:280–6.
38. Rondonotti E, Soncini M, Girelli C, Ballardini G, Bianchi G, Brunati S, Centenara L, Cesari P, Cortelezzi C, Curioni S, Gozzini C, Gullotta R, Lazzaroni M, Maino M, Mandelli G, Mantovani N, Morandi E, Pansoni C, Piubello W, Putignano R, Schalling R, Tatarella M, Villa F, Vitagliano P, Russo A, Conte D, Masci E, de Franchis R. Small bowel capsule endoscopy in clinical practice: a multicenter 7-year survey. EurJ Gastroenterol Hepatol. 2010;22:1380–6.
39. Peterson WL. Capsule endoscopy was superior to push enteroscopy for identifying sources of obscure gastrointestinal bleeding. ACP J Club. 2007;147:39.
40. de Leusse A, Vahedi K, Edery J, Tiah D, Fery-Lemonnier E, Cellier C, Bouhnik Y, Jian R. Capsule endoscopy or push enteroscopy for first-line exploration of obscure gastrointestinal bleeding? Gastroenterology. 2007;132:855–62.
41. Sidhu R, McAlindon ME, Kapur K, Sanders DS. Should push enteroscopy be reserved for therapeutic intervention after capsule endoscopy? Experience from a tertiary centre in the United Kingdom. Gastroenterology. 2007;133:729.
42. Koulaouzidis A, Rondonotti E, Karargyris A. Small-bowel capsule endoscopy: a ten-point contemporary review. World J Gastroenterol. 2013;19(24):3726–46.
43. Keum B, Chun HJ. Capsule endoscopy and double balloon enteroscopy for obscure gastrointestinal bleeding: which is better? Gastroenterol Hepatol. 2011;26:794–5.
44. Pasha SF, Leighton JA, Das A, Harrison ME, Decker GA, Fleischer DE, Sharma VK. Double-balloon enteroscopy and capsule endoscopy have comparable diagnostic yield in small-bowel disease: a meta-analysis. Clin Gastroenterol Hepatol. 2008;6:671–6.
45. Shishido T, Oka S, Tanaka S, Aoyama T, Watari I, Imagawa H, Yoshida S, Chayama K. Diagnostic yield of capsule endoscopy vs. double-balloon endoscopy for patients who have undergone total enteroscopy with obscure gastrointestinal bleeding. Hepatogastroenterology. 2012;59:955–9.
46. Heo HM, Park CH, Lim JS, Lee JH, Kim BK, Cheon JH, Kim TI, Kim WH, Hong SP. The role of capsule endoscopy after negative CT enterography in patients with obscure gastrointestinal bleeding. Eur Radiol. 2012;22:1159–66.

47. Wang Z, Chen JQ, Liu JL, Qin XG, Huang Y. CT enterography in obscure gastrointestinal bleeding: a systematic review and meta-analysis. J Med Imaging Radiat Oncol. 2013;57:263–73.

48. Pennazio M, Santucci R, Rondonotti E, Abbiati C, Beccari G, Rossini FP, De Franchis R. Outcome of patients with obscure gastrointestinal bleeding after capsule endoscopy: report of 100 consecutive cases. Gastroenterology. 2004;126:643–53.

49. Higaki N, Matsui H, Imaoka H, Ikeda Y, Murakami H, Hiasa Y, Matsuura B, Onji M. Characteristic endoscopic features of portal hypertensive enteropathy. J Gastroenterol. 2008;43(5):327–31.

50. Agnese M, Cipolletta L, Bianco MA, Quitadamo P, Miele E, Staiano A. Blue rubber bleb nevus syndrome. Acta Paediatr. 2010;99(4):632–5.

51. Yuksekkaya H, Ozbek O, Keser M, Toy H. Blue rubber bleb nevus syndrome: successful treatment with sirolimus. Pediatrics. 2012;129(4):e1080–4.

52. Brady RR, Fineron P, Potter MA. Analgesics block more than pain. Gastroenterology. 2011;141(5):e9–10.

53. Spada C, Hassan C, Costamagna G. Virtual chromoendoscopy: will it play a role in capsule endoscopy? Dig Liver Dis. 2011;43(12):927–8.

54. Koulaouzidis A, Karargyris A, Rondonotti E, Noble CL, Douglas S, Alexandridis E, Zahid AM, Bathgate AJ, Trimble KC, Plevris JN. Three-dimensional representation software as image enhancement tool in small-bowel capsule endoscopy: a feasibility study. Dig Liver Dis. 2013 (Epub ahead of print).

55. Rondonotti E, Pennazio M, Toth E, Menchen P, Riccioni ME, De Palma GD, Scotto F, De Looze D, Pachofsky T, Tacheci I, Havelund T, Couto G, Trifan A, Kofokotsio A, Cannizzaro R, Perez-Quadrado E, de Franchis R, European Capsule Endoscopy Group, Italian Club for Capsule Endoscopy (CICE), Iberian Group for Capsule Endoscopy. Small-bowel neoplasms in patients undergoing video capsule endoscopy: a multicenter European study. Endoscopy. 2008;40:488–95.

56. Lewis BS, Kornbluth A, Waye JD. Small bowel tumours: yield of enteroscopy. Gut. 1991;32:763–5.

57. Koulaouzidis A, Yung DE, Lam JH, Smirnidis A, Douglas S, Plevris JN. The use of small-bowel capsule endoscopy in iron-deficiency anemia alone; be aware of the young anemic patient. Scand J Gastroenterol. 2012;47(8–9):1094–100.

58. Kruger S, Noack F, Blachle C, Feller AC. Primary malignant melanoma of the small bowel: a case report and review of the literature. Tumori. 2005;91:73–6.

59. Prakoso E, Fulham M, Thompson JF, Selby WS. Capsule endoscopy versus positron emission tomography for detection of small-bowel metastatic melanoma: a pilot study. Gastrointest Endosc. 2011;73(4):750–6.

60. Prakoso E, Selby WS. Capsule endoscopy in patients with malignant melanoma. Am J Gastroenterol. 2007;102(6):1204–8.

61. Shyung LR, Lin SC, Shih SC, Chang WH, Chu CH, Wang TE. Proposed scoring system to determine small bowel mass lesions using capsule endoscopy. J Formos Med Assoc. 2009;108(7):533–8.

62. Girelli CM, Porta P, Colombo E, Lesinigo E, Bernasconi G. Development of a novel index to discriminate bulge from mass on small-bowel capsule endoscopy. Gastrointest Endosc. 2011;74(5):1067–74.

63. Mehdizadeh S, Ross A, Gerson L, Leighton J, Chen A, Schembre D, Chen G, Semrad C, Kamal A, Harrison EM, Binmoeller K, Waxman I, Kozarek R, Lo SK. What is the learning curve associated with double-balloon enteroscopy? Technical details and early experience in 6 U.S. tertiary care centers. Gastrointest Endosc. 2006;64:740–50.

64. Lewis BS, Eisen GM, Friedman S. A pooled analysis to evaluate results of capsule endoscopy trials. Endoscopy. 2005;37:960–5.

65. Chong AK, Chin BW, Meredith CG. Clinically significant small-bowel pathology identified by double-balloon enteroscopy but missed by capsule endoscopy. Gastrointest Endosc. 2006;64:445–9.

66. Hakim F, Alexander J, Huprich J, Alexander G, Enders F, Schreiber J. CT-enterography is more sensitive than capsule endoscopy in the diagnosis of endoscopy-negative small bowel tumors. The Mayo Clinic Rochester experience. Am J Gastroenterol. 2009;104:S100.

67. Tenembaum D, Sison C, Rubin M. Accuracy of community based video capsule endoscopy in patients undergoing follow up double balloon enteroscopy. World J Gastrointest Endosc. 2013;5:154–9.

68. Marmo R, Rotondano G, Casetti T, Manes G, Chilovi F, Sprujevnik T, Bianco MA, Brancaccio ML, Imbesi V, Benvenuti S, Pennazio M. Degree of concordance between double-balloon enteroscopy and capsule endoscopy in obscure gastrointestinal bleeding: a multicenter study. Endoscopy. 2009;41:587–92.

69. Marmo R, Rotondano G, Piscopo R, Bianco MA, Cipolletta L. Meta-analysis: capsule enteroscopy vs. conventional modalities in diagnosis of small bowel diseases. Aliment Pharmacol Ther 1. 2005;22(7):595–604.

70. Leighton JA, Triester SL, Sharma VK. Capsule endoscopy: a meta-analysis for use with obscure gastrointestinal bleeding and Crohn's disease. Gastrointest Endosc Clin N Am. 2006;16:229–50.

71. Koulaouzidis A, Rondonotti E, Giannakou A, Plevris JN. Diagnostic yield of small-bowel capsule endoscopy in patients with iron-deficiency anemia: a systematic review. Gastrointest Endosc. 2012;76(5):983–92.

72. Saurin JC, Delvaux M, Gaudin JL, Fassler I, Villarejo J, Vahedi K, Bitoun A, Canard JM,

Souquet JC, Ponchon T, Florent C, Gay G. Diagnostic value of endoscopic capsule in patients with obscure digestive bleeding: blinded comparison with video push-enteroscopy. Endoscopy. 2003;35(7):576–84.

73. Rondonotti E, Sunada K, Yano T, Paggi S, Yamamoto H. Double-balloon endoscopy in clinical practice: where are we now? Dig Endosc. 2012;24:209–19.

74. Hartmann D, Schmidt H, Bolz G, Schilling D, Kinzel F, Eickhoff A, Huschner W, Muller K, Jakobs R, Reitzig P, Weickert U, Gellert K, Schultz H, Guenther K, Hollerbuhl H, Schoenleben K, Schulz HJ, Riemann J. A prospective two-center study comparing wireless capsule endoscopy with intraoperative enteroscopy in patients with obscure GI bleeding. Gastrointest Endosc. 2005;61:826–32.

75. Triester SL, Leighton JA, Leontiadis GI, Fleischer DE, Hara AK, Heigh RI, Shiff AD, Sharma VK. A meta-analysis of the yield of capsule endoscopy compared to other diagnostic modalities in patients with obscure gastrointestinal bleeding. Am J Gastroenterol. 2000;100(11):2407–18.

76. Singh A, Marshall C, Chaudhuri B, Okoli C, Foley A, Person SD, Bhattacharya K, Cave DR. Timing of video capsule endoscopy relative to overt obscure GI bleeding: implications from a retrospective study. Gastrointest Endosc. 2013;77:761–6.

77. Yamada A, Watabe H, Kobayashi Y, Yamaji Y, Yoshida H, Koike K. Timing of capsule endoscopy influences the diagnosis and outcome in obscure-overt gastrointestinal bleeding. Hepatogastroenterology. 2012;59:676–9.

78. Riccioni ME, Urgesi R, Cianci R, Rizzo G, D'Angelo L, Marmo R, Costamagna G. Negative capsule endoscopy in patients with obscure gastrointestinal bleeding reliable: recurrence of bleeding on long-term follow-up. World J Gastroenterol. 2013;19(28):4520–5.

79. Goddard AF, James MW, McIntyre AS, Scott BB, British Society of Gastroenterology. Guidelines for the management of iron deficiency anaemia. Gut. 2011;60:1309–16.

80. May A, Wardak A, Nachbar L, Remke S, Ell C. Influence of patient selection on the out come of capsule endoscopy in patients with chronic gastrointestinal bleeding. J Clin Gastroenterol. 2005;39:684–8.

81. Estevez E, Gonzalez-Conde B, Vazquez-Iglesias JL, de Los Angeles Vázquez-Millán M, Pértega S, Alonso PA, Clofent J, Santos E, Ulla JL, Sánchez E. Diagnostic yield and clinical outcomes after capsule endoscopy in 100 consecutive patients with obscure gastrointestinal bleeding. Eur J Gastroenterol Hepatol. 2006;18:881–8.

82. Gilbert D, O'Malley S, Selby W. Are repeat upper gastrointestinal endoscopy and colonoscopy necessary within six months of capsule endoscopy in patients with obscure gastrointestinal bleeding. J Gastroenterol Hepatol. 2008;23:1806–9.

83. Rondonotti E, Marmo R, Petracchini M, de Franchis R, Pennazio M. The American Society for Gastrointestinal Endoscopy (ASGE) diagnostic algorithm for obscure gastrointestinal bleeding: eight burning questions from everyday clinical practice. Dig Liver Dis. 2013;45(3):179–85.

84. Albert JG, Schulbe R, Hahn L, Heinig D, Schoppmeyer K, Porst H, Lorenz R, Plauth M, Dollinger MM, Massner J, Caca K, Fleig WE. Impact of capsule endoscopy on outcome in mid-intestinal bleeding: a multicentre cohort study in 285 patients. Eur J Gastroenterol Hepatol. 2008;20(10):971–7.

85. Baichi MM, Arifuddin RM, Mantry PS. Capsule endoscopy for obscure GI bleeding: therapeutic yield of follow-up procedures. Dig Dis Sci. 2007;52(5):1370–5.

86. Lai LH, Wong GL, Chow DK, Lau JY, Sung JJ, Leung WK. Long-term follow-up of patients with obscure gastrointestinal bleeding after negative capsule endoscopy. Am J Gastroenterol. 2006;101:1224–8.

87. Koh SJ, Im JP, Kim JW, Kim BG, Lee KL, Kim SG, Kim JS, Jung HC. Long-term outcome in patients with obscure gastrointestinal bleeding after negative capsule endoscopy. World J Gastroenterol. 2013;19(10):1632–8.

88. Hindryckx P, Botelberge T, De Vos M, De Looze D. Clinical impact of capsule endoscopy on further strategy and long-term clinical outcome in patients with obscure bleeding. Gastrointest Endosc. 2008;68(1):98–104.

89. Delvaux M, Fassler I, Gay G. Clinical usefulness of the endoscopic video capsule as the initial intestinal investigation in patients with obscure digestive bleeding: validation of a diagnostic strategy based on the patient outcome after 12 months. Endoscopy. 2004;36(12):1067–73.

90. Holleran GE, Barry SA, Thornton OJ, Dobson MJ, McNamara DA. The use of small bowel capsule endoscopy in iron deficiency anaemia: low impact on outcome in the medium term despite high diagnostic yield. Eur J Gastroenterol Hepatol. 2013;25(3):327–32.

91. Laine L, Sahota A, Shah A. Does capsule endoscopy improve outcomes in obscure gastrointestinal bleeding? Randomized trial versus dedicated small bowel radiography. Gastroenterology. 2010;138(5):1673–80.

92. Ahmad NA, Iqbal N, Joyce A. Clinical impact of capsule endoscopy on management of gastrointestinal disorders. Clin Gastroenterol Hepatol. 2008;6(4):433–7.

93. Toy E, Rojany M, Sheikh R, Mann S, Prindiville T. Capsule endoscopy's impact on clinical management and outcomes: a single-center experience with 145 patients. Am J Gastroenterol. 2008;103(12):3022–8.

94. Sidhu R, Sanders DS, Kapur K, Hurlstone DP, McAlindon ME. Capsule endoscopy changes

patient management in routine clinical practice. Dig Dis Sci. 2007;52(5):1382–6.

95. Garcıa-Compean D, Armenta JA, Marrufo C, Gonales JA, Maldonado H. Impact of therapeutic interventions induced by capsule endoscopy on long term outcome in chronic obscure GI bleeding. Gastroenterol Clin Biol. 2007;31(10):806–11.

96. Redondo-Cerezo E, Perez-Vigara G, Perez-Sola A, Gomez-Ruiz CJ, Chicano MV, Sanchez-Manjavacas N, Morillas J, Perez-Garcia JI, Garcia-Cano JD. Diagnostic yield and impact of capsule endoscopy on management of patients with gastrointestinal bleeding of obscure origin. Dig Dis Sci. 2007;52(5):1376–81.

97. Lashner B. Clinical features, laboratory findings, and course of Crohn's disease. In: Kirsner JV, editor. Inflammatory bowel disease. 5th ed. Philadelphia: Saunders; 2000. p. 305–14.

98. Molinié F, Gower-Rousseau C, Yzet T, Merle V, Grandbastien B, Marti R, Lerebours E, Dupas J-L, Colombel J-F, Salomez J-L, Cortot A. Opposite evolution in incidence of Crohn's disease and ulcerative colitis in Northern France (1988–1999). Gut. 2004;53(6):843–8.

99. Dionisio PM, Gurudu SR, Leighton JA, Leontiadis GI, Fleischer DE, Hara AK, Heigh RI, Shiff AD, Sharma VK. Capsule endoscopy has a significantly higher diagnostic yield in patients with suspected and established small-bowel Crohn's disease: a meta-analysis. Am J Gastroenterol. 2010;105(6):1240–8; quiz 1249.

100. Pimentel M, Chang M, Chow EJ, Tabizadeh S, Kirit-Kiriak V, Targan SR, Lin HC. Identification of a prodromal period in Crohn's disease but not ulcerative colitis. Am J Gastroenterol. 2000;95(12):3458–62.

101. Timmer A, Breuer-Katschinski B, Goebell H. Time trends in the incidence and disease location of Crohn's disease 1980–1995: a prospective analysis in an urban population in Germany. Inflamm Bowel Dis. 1999;5(2):79–84.

102. Schnitzler F, Fidder H, Ferrante M, Noman M, Arijs I, Van Assche G, Hoffman I, Van Steen K, Vermeire S, Rutgeerts P. Mucosal healing predicts long-term outcome of maintenance therapy with infliximab in Crohn's disease. Inflamm Bowel Dis. 2009;15(9):1295–301.

103. Mekhjian HS, Switz DM, Melnyk CS, Rankin GB, Brooks RK. Clinical features and natural history of Crohn's disease. Gastroenterology. 1979;77(4 Pt 2): 898–906.

104. Kornbluth A, Colombel JF, Leighton JA, Loftus E. ICCE consensus for inflammatory bowel disease. Endoscopy. 2005;37(10):1051–4.

105. Koulaouzidis A, Douglas S, Rogers MA, Arnott ID, Plevris JN. Fecal calprotectin: a selection tool for small bowel capsule endoscopy in suspected IBD with prior negative bi-directional endoscopy. Scand J Gastroenterol. 2011;46(5):561–6.

106. Sidhu R, Sanders DS, Morris AJ, McAlindon ME. Guidelines on small bowel enteroscopy and capsule endoscopy in adults. Gut. 2008;57(1):125–36.

107. Bourreille A, Ignjatovic A, Aabakken L, Loftus EV, Eliakim R, Pennazio M, Bouhnik Y, Seidman E, Keuchel M, Albert JG, Ardizzone S, Bar-Meir S, Bisschops R, Despott EJ, Fortun PF, Heuschkel R, Kammermeier J, Leighton JA, Mantzaris GJ, et al. Role of small-bowel endoscopy in the management of patients with inflammatory bowel disease: an international OMED-ECCO consensus. Endoscopy. 2009;41(7):618–37.

108. Leighton JA, Shen B, Baron TH, Adler DG, Davila R, Egan JV, Faigel DO, Gan S-I, Hirota WK, Lichtenstein D, Qureshi WA, Rajan E, Zuckerman MJ, VanGuilder T, Fanelli RD. ASGE guideline: endoscopy in the diagnosis and treatment of inflammatory bowel disease. Gastrointest Endosc. 2006;63(4):558–65.

109. Morson BC. Histopathology of Crohn's disease. Scand J Gastroenterol. 1971;6(7):573–5.

110. Yantiss RK, Odze RD. Diagnostic difficulties in inflammatory bowel disease pathology. Histopathology. 2006;48(2):116–32.

111. Costamagna G, Shah SK, Riccioni ME, Foschia F, Mutignani M, Perri V, Vecchioli A, Brizi MG, Picciocchi A, Marano P. A prospective trial comparing small bowel radiographs and video capsule endoscopy for suspected small bowel disease. Gastroenterology. 2002;123(4):999–1005.

112. Hara AK, Leighton JA, Heigh RI, Sharma VK, Silva AC, De Petris G, Hentz JG, Fleischer DE. Crohn disease of the small bowel: preliminary comparison among CT enterography, capsule endoscopy, small-bowel follow-through, and Ileoscopy. Radiology. 2006;238(1):128–34.

113. Leighton JA, Gralnek IM, Richner RE, Lacey MJ, Papatheofanis FJ. Capsule endoscopy in suspected small bowel Crohn's disease: economic impact of disease diagnosis and treatment. World J Gastroenterol. 2009;15(45):5685–92.

114. Marmo R, Rotondano G, Piscopo R, Bianco MA, Cipolletta L. Meta-analysis: capsule enteroscopy vs. conventional modalities in diagnosis of small bowel diseases. Aliment Pharmacol Ther. 2005;22(7):595–604.

115. Farmer RG, Hawk WA, Turnbull RB. Clinical patterns in Crohn's disease: a statistical study of 615 cases. Gastroenterology. 1975;68(4 Pt 1): 627–35.

116. Burgmann T, Clara I, Graff L, Walker J, Lix L, Rawsthorne P, McPhail C, Rogala L, Miller N, Bernstein CN. The Manitoba Inflammatory Bowel Disease Cohort Study: prolonged symptoms before diagnosis–how much is irritable bowel syndrome? Clin Gastroenterol Hepatol. 2006;4(5):614–20.

117. Solem CA, Loftus EV, Fletcher JG, Baron TH, Gostout CJ, Petersen BT, Tremaine WJ, Egan LJ, Faubion WA, Schroeder KW, Pardi DS, Hanson

KA, Jewell DA, Barlow JM, Fidler JL, Huprich JE, Johnson CD, Harmsen WS, Zinsmeister AR, et al. Small-bowel imaging in Crohn's disease: a prospective, blinded, 4-way comparison trial. Gastrointest Endosc. 2008;68(2):255–66.

118. Siddiki HA, Fidler JL, Fletcher JG, Burton SS, Huprich JE, Hough DM, Johnson CD, Bruining DH, Loftus EV, Sandborn WJ, Pardi DS, Mandrekar JN. Prospective comparison of state-of-the-art MR enterography and CT enterography in small-bowel Crohn's disease. AJR Am J Roentgenol. 2009;193(1):113–21.

119. Bourreille A, Jarry M, D'Halluin PN, Ben-Soussan E, Maunoury V, Bulois P, Sacher-Huvelin S, Vahedy K, Lerebours E, Heresbach D, Bretagne JF, Colombel JF, Galmiche JP. Wireless capsule endoscopy versus ileocolonoscopy for the diagnosis of postoperative recurrence of Crohn's disease: a prospective study. Gut. 2006;55(7):978–83.

120. Mow WS, Lo SK, Targan SR, Dubinsky MC, Treyzon L, Abreu-Martin MT, Papadakis KA, Vasiliauskas EA. Initial experience with wireless capsule enteroscopy in the diagnosis and management of inflammatory bowel disease. Clin Gastroenterol Hepatol. 2004;2(1):31–40.

121. Tukey M, Pleskow D, Legnani P, Cheifetz AS, Moss AC. The utility of capsule endoscopy in patients with suspected Crohn's disease. Am J Gastroenterol. 2009;104(11):2734–9.

122. Kalla R, McAlindon ME, Drew K, Sidhu R. Clinical utility of capsule endoscopy in patients with Crohn's disease and inflammatory bowel disease unclassified. Eur J Gastroenterol Hepatol. 2013;25(6):706–13.

123. Rosa B, Moreira MJ, Rebelo A, Cotter J. Lewis Score: a useful clinical tool for patients with suspected Crohn's disease submitted to capsule endoscopy. J Crohn's Colitis. 2012;6(6):692–7.

124. Gal E, Geller A, Fraser G, Levi Z, Niv Y. Assessment and validation of the new capsule endoscopy Crohn's disease activity index (CECDAI). Dig Dis Sci. 2008;53(7):1933–7.

125. Goldstein JL, Eisen GM, Lewis B, Gralnek IM, Zlotnick S, Fort JG. Video capsule endoscopy to prospectively assess small bowel injury with celecoxib, naproxen plus omeprazole, and placebo. Clin Gastroenterol Hepatol. 2005;3(2):133–41.

126. Yang L, Ge Z-Z, Gao Y-J, Li X-B, Dai J, Zhang Y, Xue H-B, Zhao Y-J. Assessment of capsule endoscopy scoring index, clinical disease activity and C-reactive protein in small bowel Crohn's disease. J Gastroenterol Hepatol. 2013.

127. Lashner BA. Sensitivity-specificity trade-off for capsule endoscopy in IBD: is it worth it? Am J Gastroenterol. 2006;101(5):965–6.

128. Maiden L, Thjodleifsson B, Theodors A, Gonzalez J, Bjarnason I. A quantitative analysis of NSAID-induced small bowel pathology by capsule enteroscopy. Gastroenterology. 2005;128(5):1172–8.

129. Maiden L. Capsule endoscopic diagnosis of nonsteroidal antiinflammatory drug-induced enteropathy. J Gastroenterol. 2009;44(Suppl 1):64–71.

130. Goldstein JL, Eisen GM, Lewis B, Gralnek IM, Aisenberg J, Bhadra P, Berger MF. Small bowel mucosal injury is reduced in healthy subjects treated with celecoxib compared with ibuprofen plus omeprazole, as assessed by video capsule endoscopy. Aliment Pharmacol Ther. 2007;25(10):1211–22.

131. Girelli CM, Porta P, Malacrida V, Barzaghi F, Rocca F. Clinical outcome of patients examined by capsule endoscopy for suspected small bowel Crohn's disease. Dig Liver Dis. 2007;39(2):148–54.

132. Goldfarb NI, Pizzi LT, Fuhr JP, Salvador C, Sikirica V, Kornbluth A, Lewis B. Diagnosing Crohn's disease: an economic analysis comparing wireless capsule endoscopy with traditional diagnostic procedures. Dis Manage: DM. 2004;7(4):292–304.

133. Hoffmann JC, Preiss JC, Autschbach F, Buhr HJ, Häuser W, Herrlinger K, Höhne W, Koletzko S, Krieglstein CF, Kruis W, Matthes H, Moser G, Reinshagen M, Rogler G, Schreiber S, Schreyer AG, Sido B, Siegmund B, Stallmach A, et al. Clinical practice guideline on diagnosis and treatment of Crohn's disease. Zeitschrift für Gastroenterologie. 2008;46(9):1094–146.

134. Jess T, Riis L, Vind I, Winther KV, Borg S, Binder V, Langholz E, Thomsen OØ, Munkholm P. Changes in clinical characteristics, course, and prognosis of inflammatory bowel disease during the last 5 decades: a population-based study from Copenhagen, Denmark. Inflamm Bowel Dis. 2007;13(4):481–9.

135. Rutgeerts P. Protagonist: Crohn's disease recurrence can be prevented after ileal resection. Gut. 2002;51(2):152–3.

136. Binder V, Hendriksen C, Kreiner S. Prognosis in Crohn's disease–based on results from a regional patient group from the county of Copenhagen. Gut. 1985;26(2):146–50.

137. Pons Beltrán V, Nos P, Bastida G, Beltrán B, Argüello L, Aguas M, Rubín A, Pertejo V, Sala T. Evaluation of postsurgical recurrence in Crohn's disease: a new indication for capsule endoscopy? Gastrointest Endosc. 2007;66(3):533–40.

138. D'Haens G, Rutgeerts P. Postoperative recurrence of Crohn's disease: pathophysiology and prevention. Inflamm Bowel Dis. 1999;5(4): 295–303.

139. Gölder SK, Schreyer AG, Endlicher E, Feuerbach S, Schölmerich J, Kullmann F, Seitz J, Rogler G, Herfarth H. Comparison of capsule endoscopy and magnetic resonance (MR) enteroclysis in suspected small bowel disease. Int J Colorectal Dis. 2006;21(2):97–104.

140. Albert JG, Martiny F, Krummenerl A, Stock K, Lesske J, Göbel CM, Lotterer E, Nietsch HH, Behrmann C, Fleig WE. Diagnosis of small bowel Crohn's disease: a prospective comparison of capsule endoscopy with magnetic resonance imaging and fluoroscopic enteroclysis. Gut. 2005;54(12):1721–7.

141. Crook DW, Knuesel PR, Froehlich JM, Eigenmann F, Unterweger M, Beer H-J, Kubik-Huch RA. Comparison of magnetic resonance enterography and video capsule endoscopy in evaluating small bowel disease. Eur J Gastroenterol Hepatol. 2009;21(1):54–65.

142. Tillack C, Seiderer J, Brand S, Göke B, Reiser MF, Schaefer C, Diepolder H, Ochsenkühn T, Herrmann KA. Correlation of magnetic resonance enteroclysis (MRE) and wireless capsule endoscopy (CE) in the diagnosis of small bowel lesions in Crohn's disease. Inflamm Bowel Dis. 2008;14(9):1219–28.

143. Spada C, Spera G, Riccioni M, Biancone L, Petruzziello L, Tringali A, Familiari P, Marchese M, Onder G, Mutignani M, Perri V, Petruzziello C, Pallone F, Costamagna G. A novel diagnostic tool for detecting functional patency of the small bowel: the Given patency capsule. Endoscopy. 2005;37(9):793–800.

144. Boivin ML, Lochs H, Voderholzer WA. Does passage of a patency capsule indicate small-bowel patency? A prospective clinical trial? Endoscopy. 2005;37(9):808–15.

145. Delvaux M, Ben Soussan E, Laurent V, Lerebours E, Gay G. Clinical evaluation of the use of the M2A patency capsule system before a capsule endoscopy procedure, in patients with known or suspected intestinal stenosis. Endoscopy. 2005;37(9):801–7.

146. Signorelli C, Rondonotti E, Villa F, Abbiati C, Beccari G, Avesani EC, Vecchi M, de Franchis R. Use of the Given Patency System for the screening of patients at high risk for capsule retention. Dig Liver Dis. 2006;38(5):326–30.

147. Mehdizadeh S, Chen GC, Barkodar L, Enayati PJ, Pirouz S, Yadegari M, Ippoliti A, Vasiliauskas EA, Lo SK, Papadakis KA. Capsule endoscopy in patients with Crohn's disease: diagnostic yield and safety. Gastrointest Endosc. 2010;71(1):121–7.

148. Long MD, Barnes E, Isaacs K, Morgan D, Herfarth HH. Impact of capsule endoscopy on management of inflammatory bowel disease: a single tertiary care center experience. Inflamm Bowel Dis. 2011;17(9):1855–62.

149. Dussault C, Gower-Rousseau C, Salleron J, Vernier-Massouille G, Branche J, Colombel J-F, Maunoury V. Small bowel capsule endoscopy for management of Crohn's disease: a retrospective tertiary care centre experience. Dig Liver Dis. 2012;45(7):558–61.

150. Flamant M, Trang C, Maillard O, Sacher-Huvelin S, Le Rhun M, Galmiche J-P, Bourreille A. The prevalence and outcome of jejunal lesions visualized by small bowel capsule endoscopy in Crohn's disease. Inflamm Bowel Dis. 2013;19(7):1390–6.

151. Petruzziello C, Onali S, Calabrese E, Zorzi F, Ascolani M, Condino G, Lolli E, Naccarato P, Pallone F, Biancone L. Wireless capsule endoscopy and proximal small bowel lesions in Crohn's disease. World J Gastroenterol. 2010;16(26):3299–304.

152. Silverberg MS, Satsangi J, Ahmad T, Arnott ID, Bernstein CN, Brant SR, Caprilli R, Colombel J-F, Gasche C, Geboes K, Jewell DP, Karban A, Loftus Jr EV, Peña AS, Riddell RH, Sachar DB, Schreiber S, Steinhart AH, Targan SR, et al. Toward an integrated clinical, molecular and serological classification of inflammatory bowel disease: report of a working party of the 2005 Montreal world congress of gastroenterology. Can J Gastroenterol. 2005;19(Suppl A):5–36.

153. Stewénius J, Adnerhill I, Ekelund G, Florén CH, Fork FT, Janzon L, Lindström C, Mars I, Nyman M, Rosengren JE. Ulcerative colitis and indeterminate colitis in the city of Malmö, Sweden. A 25-year incidence study. Scand J Gastroenterol. 1995;30(1):38–43.

154. Vind I, Riis L, Jess T, Knudsen E, Pedersen N, Elkjaer M, Bak Andersen I, Wewer V, Nørregaard P, Moesgaard F, Bendtsen F, Munkholm P. Increasing incidences of inflammatory bowel disease and decreasing surgery rates in Copenhagen City and County, 2003–2005: a population-based study from the Danish Crohn colitis database. Am J Gastroenterol. 2006;101(6):1274–82.

155. Tekkis PP, Heriot AG, Smith O, Smith JJ, Windsor ACJ, Nicholls RJ. Long-term outcomes of restorative proctocolectomy for Crohn's disease and indeterminate colitis. Colorectal Dis. 2005;7(3):218–23.

156. Tekkis PP, Heriot AG, Smith JJ, Das P, Canero A, Nicholls RJ. Long-term results of abdominal salvage surgery following restorative proctocolectomy. Br J Surg. 2006;93(2):231–7.

157. Stewénius J, Adnerhill I, Ekelund GR, Florén CH, Fork FT, Janzon L, Lindström C, Ogren M. Risk of relapse in new cases of ulcerative colitis and indeterminate colitis. Dis Colon Rectum. 1996;39(9):1019–25.

158. Lopes S, Figueiredo P, Portela F, Freire P, Almeida N, Lérias C, Gouveia H, Leitão MC. Capsule endoscopy in inflammatory bowel disease type unclassified and indeterminate colitis serologically negative. Inflamm Bowel Dis. 2010;16(10):1663–8.

159. Maunoury V, Savoye G, Bourreille A, Bouhnik Y, Jarry M, Sacher-Huvelin S, Ben Soussan E, Lerebours E, Galmiche J-P, Colombel J-F. Value of wireless capsule endoscopy in patients with

indeterminate colitis (inflammatory bowel disease type unclassified). Inflamm Bowel Dis. 2007;13(2):152–5.

160. Ludvigsson JF, Rubio-Tapia A, van Dyke CT, Melton 3rd LJ, Zinsmeister AR, Lahr BD, Murray JA. Increasing incidence of celiac disease in a North American population. Am J Gastroenterol. 2013;108:818–24.

161. Mustalahti K, Catassi C, Reunanen A, Fabiani E, Heier M, Mcmillan S, Murray L, Metzger MH, Gasparin M, Bravi E, Maki M, Coeliac EU Cluster PE. The prevalence of celiac disease in Europe: results of a centralized, international mass screening project. Ann Med. 2010;42:587–95.

162. Catassi C, Kryszak D, Bhatti B, Sturgeon C, Helzlsouer K, Clipp SL, Gelfond D, Puppa E, Sferruzza A, Fasano A. Natural history of celiac disease autoimmunity in a USA cohort followed since 1974. Ann Med. 2010;42:530–8.

163. Lohi S, Mustalahti K, Kaukinen K, Laurila K, Collin P, Rissanen H, Lohi O, Bravi E, Gasparin M, Reunanen A, Maki M. Increasing prevalence of coeliac disease over time. Aliment Pharmacol Ther. 2007;26:1217–25.

164. Rubio-Tapia A, Kyle RA, Kaplan EL, Johnson DR, Page W, Erdtmann F, Brantner TL, Kim WR, Phelps TK, Lahr BD, Zinsmeister AR, Melton 3rd LJ, Murray JA. Increased prevalence and mortality in undiagnosed celiac disease. Gastroenterology. 2009;137:88–93.

165. Kochhar R, Sachdev S, Kochhar R, Aggarwal A, Sharma V, Prasad KK, Singh G, Nain CK, Singh K, Marwaha N. Prevalence of coeliac disease in healthy blood donors: a study from north India. Dig Liver Dis. 2012;44:530–2.

166. Wang XQ, Liu W, Xu CD, Mei H, Gao Y, Peng HM, Yuan L, Xu JJ. Celiac disease in children with diarrhea in 4 cities in China. J Pediatr Gastroenterol Nutr. 2011;53:368–70.

167. Jones HJ, Warner JT. NICE clinical guideline 86. Coeliac disease: recognition and assessment of coeliac disease. Arch Dis Child. 2010;95:312–3.

168. Cassinotti A, Birindelli S, Clerici M, Trabattoni D, Lazzaroni M, Ardizzone S, Colombo R, Rossi E, Porro GB. HLA and autoimmune digestive disease: a clinically oriented review for gastroenterologists. Am J Gastroenterol. 2009;104, 195–217; quiz 194, 218.

169. Achkar E, Carey WD, Petras R, Sivak MV, Revta R. Comparison of suction capsule and endoscopic biopsy of small bowel mucosa. Gastrointest Endosc. 1986;32:278–81.

170. Gillberg R, Ahren C. Coeliac disease diagnosed by means of duodenoscopy and endoscopic duodenal biopsy. Scand J Gastroenterol. 1977;12:911–6.

171. Mee AS, Burke M, Vallon AG, Newman J, Cotton PB. Small bowel biopsy for malabsorption: comparison of the diagnostic adequacy of endoscopic forceps and capsule biopsy specimens. Br Med J (Clin Res Ed). 1985;291:769–72.

172. Brocchi E, Corazza GR, Brusco G, Mangia L, Gasbarrini G. Unsuspected celiac disease diagnosed by endoscopic visualization of duodenal bulb micronodules. Gastrointest Endosc. 1996;44:610–1.

173. Brocchi E, Tomassetti P, Misitano B, Epifanio G, Corinaldesi R, Bonvicini F, Gasbarrini G, Corazza G. Endoscopic markers in adult coeliac disease. Dig Liver Dis. 2002;34:177–82.

174. Dickey W, Hughes D. Erosions in the second part of the duodenum in patients with villous atrophy. Gastrointest Endosc. 2004;59:116–8.

175. Stevens FM, McCarthy CF. The endoscopic demonstration of coeliac disease. Endoscopy. 1976;8:177–80.

176. Hopper AD, Cross SS, Sanders DS. Patchy villous atrophy in adult patients with suspected gluten-sensitive enteropathy: is a multiple duodenal biopsy strategy appropriate? Endoscopy. 2008;40:219–24.

177. Horoldt BS, McAlindon ME, Stephenson TJ, Hadjivassiliou M, Sanders DS. Making the diagnosis of coeliac disease: is there a role for push enteroscopy? Eur J Gastroenterol Hepatol. 2004;16:1143–6.

178. Murray JA, Rubio-Tapia A, van Dyke CT, Brogan DL, Knipschield MA, Lahr B, Rumalla A, Zinsmeister AR, Gostout CJ. Mucosal atrophy in celiac disease: extent of involvement, correlation with clinical presentation, and response to treatment. Clin Gastroenterol Hepatol. 2008;6:186–93; quiz 125.

179. Ravelli A, Bolognini S, Gambarotti M, Villanacci V. Variability of histologic lesions in relation to biopsy site in gluten-sensitive enteropathy. Am J Gastroenterol. 2005;100:177–85.

180. Ravelli A, Villanacci V. Tricks of the trade: how to avoid histological pitfalls in celiac disease. Pathol Res Pract. 2012;208:197–202.

181. Apostolopoulos P, Alexandrakis G, Giannakoulopoulou E, Kalantzis C, Papanikolaou IS, Markoglou C, Kalantzis N. M2A wireless capsule endoscopy for diagnosing ulcerative jejunoileitis complicating celiac disease. Endoscopy. 2004;36:247.

182. Atlas DS, Rubio-Tapia A, van Dyke CT, Lahr BD, Murray JA. Capsule endoscopy in nonresponsive celiac disease. Gastrointest Endosc. 2011;74:1315–22.

183. Joyce AM, Burns DL, Marcello PW, Tronic B, Scholz FJ. Capsule endoscopy findings in celiac disease associated enteropathy-type intestinal T-cell lymphoma. Endoscopy. 2005;37:594–6.

184. Hadithi M, Al-Toma A, Oudejans J, van Bodegraven AA, Mulder CJ, Jacobs M. The value of double-balloon enteroscopy in patients with refractory celiac disease. Am J Gastroenterol. 2007;102:987–96.

185. Dickey W, Hughes D. Prevalence of celiac disease and its endoscopic markers among patients having routine upper gastrointestinal endoscopy. Am J Gastroenterol. 1999;94:2182–6.

186. Lo A, Guelrud M, Essenfeld H, Bonis P. Classification of villous atrophy with enhanced magnification endoscopy in patients with celiac disease and tropical sprue. Gastrointest Endosc. 2007;66:377–82.

187. Maurino E, Capizzano H, Niveloni S, Kogan Z, Valero J, Boerr L, Bai JC. Value of endoscopic markers in celiac disease. Dig Dis Sci. 1993;38:2028–33.

188. Oxentenko AS, Grisolano SW, Murray JA, Burgart LJ, Dierkhising RA, Alexander JA. The insensitivity of endoscopic markers in celiac disease. Am J Gastroenterol. 2002;97:933–8.

189. Shah VH, Rotterdam H, Kotler DP, Fasano A, Green PH. All that scallops is not celiac disease. Gastrointest Endosc. 2000;51:717–20.

190. Cammarota G, Pirozzi GA, Martino A, Zuccala G, Cianci R, Cuoco L, Ojetti V, Landriscina M, Montalto M, Vecchio FM, Gasbarrini G, Gasbarrini A. Reliability of the "immersion technique" during routine upper endoscopy for detection of abnormalities of duodenal villi in patients with dyspepsia. Gastrointest Endosc. 2004;60:223–8.

191. Petroniene R, Dubcenco E, Baker JP, Ottaway CA, Tang SJ, Zanati SA, Streutker CJ, Gardiner GW, Warren RE, Jeejeebhoy KN. Given capsule endoscopy in celiac disease: evaluation of diagnostic accuracy and interobserver agreement. Am J Gastroenterol. 2005;100:685–94.

192. Hopper AD, Sidhu R, Hurlstone DP, McAlindon ME, Sanders DS. Capsule endoscopy: an alternative to duodenal biopsy for the recognition of villous atrophy in coeliac disease? Dig Liver Dis. 2007;39:140–5.

193. Lidums I, Cummins AG, Teo E. The role of capsule endoscopy in suspected celiac disease patients with positive celiac serology. Dig Dis Sci. 2011;56:499–505.

194. Rondonotti E, Spada C, Cave D, Pennazio M, Riccioni ME, de Vitis I, Schneider D, Sprujevnik T, Villa F, Langelier J, Arrigoni A, Costamagna G, de Franchis R. Video capsule enteroscopy in the diagnosis of celiac disease: a multicenter study. Am J Gastroenterol. 2007;102:1624–31.

195. Hopper AD, Hurlstone DP, Leeds JS, McAlindon ME, Dube AK, Stephenson TJ, Sanders DS. The occurrence of terminal ileal histological abnormalities in patients with coeliac disease. Dig Liver Dis. 2006;38:815–9.

196. Delvaux M, Gay G. International conference on capsule and double-balloon endoscopy (ICCD), Paris, 27–28 August 2010. Endoscopy. 2011;43:533–9.

197. Adler SN, Jacob H, Lijovetzky G, Mulder CJ, Zwiers A. Positive coeliac serology in irritable bowel syndrome patients with normal duodenal biopsies: video capsule endoscopy findings and HLA-DQ typing may affect clinical management. J Gastrointestin Liver Dis. 2006;15:221–5.

198. Kurien M, Evans KE, Aziz I, Sidhu R, Drew K, Rogers TL, McAlindon ME, Sanders DS. Capsule endoscopy in adult celiac disease: a potential role in equivocal cases of celiac disease? Gastrointest Endosc. 2013;77:227–32.

199. Tursi A. Endoscopic diagnosis of celiac disease: what is the role of capsule endoscopy? Gastrointest Endosc. 2013;78:381.

200. Mooney PD, Evans KE, Singh S, Sanders DS. Treatment failure in coeliac disease: a practical guide to investigation and treatment of non-responsive and refractory coeliac disease. J Gastrointestin Liver Dis. 2012;21:197–203.

201. Maiden L, Elliott T, McLaughlin SD, Ciclitira P. A blinded pilot comparison of capsule endoscopy and small bowel histology in unresponsive celiac disease. Dig Dis Sci. 2009;54:1280–3.

202. Barret M, Malamut G, Rahmi G, Samaha E, Edery J, Verkarre V, Macintyre E, Lenain E, Chatellier G, Cerf-Bensussan N, Cellier C. Diagnostic yield of capsule endoscopy in refractory celiac disease. Am J Gastroenterol. 2012;107:1546–53.

203. Swain P. The future of wireless capsule endoscopy. World J Gastroenterol. 2008;14:4142–5.

204. Cammarota G, Fedeli P, Gasbarrini A. Emerging technologies in upper gastrointestinal endoscopy and celiac disease. Nat Clin Pract Gastroenterol Hepatol. 2009;6:47–56.

205. Ciaccio EJ, Bhagat G, Tennyson CA, Lewis SK, Hernandez L, Green PH. Quantitative assessment of endoscopic images for degree of villous atrophy in celiac disease. Dig Dis Sci. 2011;56:805–11.

206. Ciaccio EJ, Tennyson CA, Bhagat G, Lewis SK, Green PH. Robust spectral analysis of videocapsule images acquired from celiac disease patients. Biomed Eng Online. 2011;10:78.

207. Ciaccio EJ, Tennyson CA, Bhagat G, Lewis SK, Green PH. Transformation of videocapsule images to detect small bowel mucosal differences in celiac versus control patients. Comput Methods Programs Biomed. 2012;108:28–37.

208. Ciaccio EJ, Tennyson CA, Bhagat G, Lewis SK, Green PH. Quantitative estimates of motility from videocapsule endoscopy are useful to discern celiac patients from controls. Dig Dis Sci. 2012;57:2936–43.

209. Aretz S, Stienen D, Uhlhaas S, Loff S, Back W, Pagenstecher C, et al. High proportion of large genomic STK11 deletions in Peutz-Jeghers syndrome. Hum Mutat. 2005;26(6):513–9.

210. Riegert-Johnson D, Gleeson FC, Westra W, Hefferon T, Wong Kee Song LM, Spurck L, et al. Peutz-Jeghers Syndrome. 2009.

211. Beggs AD, Latchford AR, Vasen HF, Moslein G, Alonso A, Aretz S, et al. Peutz-Jeghers syndrome: a systematic review and recommendations for management. Gut. 2010;59(7):975–86.
212. Giardiello FM, Welsh SB, Hamilton SR, Offerhaus GJ, Gittelsohn AM, Booker SV, et al. Increased risk of cancer in the Peutz-Jeghers syndrome. N Engl J Med. 1987;316(24):1511–4.
213. Giardiello FM, Trimbath JD. Peutz-Jeghers syndrome and management recommendations. Clin Gastroenterol Hepatol. 2006;4(4):408–15.
214. Utsunomiya J, Gocho H, Miyanaga T, Hamaguchi E, Kashimure A. Peutz-Jeghers syndrome: its natural course and management. Johns Hopkins Med J. 1975;136(2):71–82.
215. Latchford AR, Phillips RK. Gastrointestinal polyps and cancer in Peutz-Jeghers syndrome: clinical aspects. Fam Cancer. 19 Apr 2011.
216. Latchford AR, Neale K, Phillips RK, Clark SK. Peutz-Jeghers syndrome: intriguing suggestion of gastrointestinal cancer prevention from surveillance. Dis Colon Rectum. 2011;54(12):1547–51.
217. van Lier MG, Westerman AM, Wagner A, Looman CW, Wilson JH, de Rooij FW, et al. High cancer risk and increased mortality in patients with Peutz-Jeghers syndrome. Gut. 2011;60(2):141–7.
218. van Lier MG, Mathus-Vliegen EM, Wagner A, van Leerdam ME, Kuipers EJ. High cumulative risk of intussusception in patients with Peutz-Jeghers syndrome: time to update surveillance guidelines? Am J Gastroenterol. 2011;106(5):940–5.
219. Gao H, van Lier MG, Poley JW, Kuipers EJ, van Leerdam ME, Mensink PB. Endoscopic therapy of small-bowel polyps by double-balloon enteroscopy in patients with Peutz-Jeghers syndrome. Gastrointest Endosc. 2010;71(4):768–73.
220. Gupta A, Postgate AJ, Burling D, Ilangovan R, Marshall M, Phillips RK, et al. A prospective study of MR enterography versus capsule endoscopy for the surveillance of adult patients with Peutz-Jeghers syndrome. AJR Am J Roentgenol. 2010;195(1):108–16.
221. Korsse SE, Dewint P, Kuipers EJ, van Leerdam ME. Small bowel endoscopy and Peutz-Jeghers syndrome. Best Pract Res Clin Gastroenterol. 2012;26(3):263–78.
222. Hinds R, Philp C, Hyer W, Fell JM. Complications of childhood Peutz-Jeghers syndrome: implications for pediatric screening. J Pediatr Gastroenterol Nutr. 2004;39(2):219–20.
223. Hyer W. Polyposis syndromes: pediatric implications. Gastrointest Endosc Clin N Am. 2001;11(4):659-vii.
224. Hyer W. Implications of Peutz-Jeghers syndrome in children and adolescents. 2009.
225. Will OC, Phillips RK, Hyer W, Clark SK. Symptomatic polyposis in a 4-year-old: the exception proves the rule. J Paediatr Child Health. 2009;45(5):320–1.
226. Postgate A, Despott E, Burling D, Gupta A, Phillips R, O'Beirne J, et al. Significant small-bowel lesions detected by alternative diagnostic modalities after negative capsule endoscopy. Gastrointest Endosc. 2008;68(6):1209–14.
227. Ross A, Mehdizadeh S, Tokar J, Leighton JA, Kamal A, Chen A, et al. Double balloon enteroscopy detects small bowel mass lesions missed by capsule endoscopy. Dig Dis Sci. 2008;53(8):2140–3.
228. Soares J, Lopes L, Vilas BG, Pinho C. Wireless capsule endoscopy for evaluation of phenotypic expression of small-bowel polyps in patients with Peutz-Jeghers syndrome and in symptomatic first-degree relatives. Endoscopy. 2004;36(12):1060–6.
229. de Berrington GA, Darby S. Risk of cancer from diagnostic X-rays: estimates for the UK and 14 other countries. Lancet. 2004;363(9406):345–51.
230. Bessette JR, Maglinte DD, Kelvin FM, Chernish SM. Primary malignant tumors in the small bowel: a comparison of the small-bowel enema and conventional follow-through examination. AJR Am J Roentgenol. 1989;153(4):741–4.
231. Maglinte DD, Kelvin FM, O'Connor K, Lappas JC, Chernish SM. Current status of small bowel radiography. Abdom Imaging. 1996;21(3):247–57.
232. Maccioni F, Al AN, Mazzamurro F, Barchetti F, Marini M. Surveillance of patients affected by Peutz-Jeghers syndrome: diagnostic value of MR enterography in prone and supine position. Abdom Imaging. 2012;37(2):279–87.
233. Akarsu M, Ugur KF, Akpinar H. Double-balloon endoscopy in patients with Peutz-Jeghers syndrome. Turk J Gastroenterol. 2012;23(5):496–502.
234. Akerman PA, Agrawal D, Cantero D, Pangtay J. Spiral enteroscopy with the new DSB overtube: a novel technique for deep peroral small-bowel intubation. Endoscopy. 2008;40(12):974–8.
235. Akerman PA, Cantero D. Spiral enteroscopy and push enteroscopy. Gastrointest Endosc Clin N Am. 2009;19(3):357–69.
236. Kopacova M, Tacheci I, Rejchrt S, Bures J. Peutz-Jeghers syndrome: diagnostic and therapeutic approach. World J Gastroenterol. 2009;15(43):5397–408.
237. Ohmiya N, Taguchi A, Shirai K, Mabuchi N, Arakawa D, Kanazawa H, et al. Endoscopic resection of Peutz-Jeghers polyps throughout the small intestine at double-balloon enteroscopy without laparotomy. Gastrointest Endosc. 2005;61(1):140–7.
238. Ohmiya N, Nakamura M, Takenaka H, Morishima K, Yamamura T, Ishihara M, et al. Management of small-bowel polyps in Peutz-Jeghers syndrome by using enteroclysis, double-balloon enteroscopy, and

videocapsule endoscopy. Gastrointest Endosc. 2010;72(6):1209–16.

239. Riccioni ME, Urgesi R, Cianci R, Spada C, Nista EC, Costamagna G. Single-balloon push-and-pull enteroscopy system: does it work? A single-center, 3-year experience. Surg Endosc. 2011;25(9):3050–6.

240. Sakamoto H, Yamamoto H, Hayashi Y, Yano T, Miyata T, Nishimura N, et al. Nonsurgical management of small-bowel polyps in Peutz-Jeghers syndrome with extensive polypectomy by using double-balloon endoscopy. Gastrointest Endosc. 2011;74(2):328–33.

241. Thomson M, Venkatesh K, Elmalik K, van der Veer W, Jaacobs M. Double balloon enteroscopy in children: diagnosis, treatment, and safety. World J Gastroenterol. 2010;16(1):56–62.

242. Yamamoto H, Sekine Y, Sato Y, Higashizawa T, Miyata T, Iino S, et al. Total enteroscopy with a nonsurgical steerable double-balloon method. Gastrointest Endosc. 2001;53(2):216–20.

243. Yamamoto H, Yano T, Kita H, Sunada K, Ido K, Sugano K. New system of double-balloon enteroscopy for diagnosis and treatment of small intestinal disorders. Gastroenterology. 2003;125(5):1556–7.

244. Oncel M, Remzi FH, Church JM, Connor JT, Fazio VW. Benefits of 'clean sweep' in Peutz-Jeghers patients. Colorectal Dis. 2004;6(5):332–5.

245. Spigelman AD, Thomson JP, Phillips RK. Towards decreasing the relaparotomy rate in the Peutz-Jeghers syndrome: the role of peroperative small bowel endoscopy. Br J Surg. 1990;77(3):301–2.

246. Parker MC, Ellis H, Moran BJ, Thompson JN, Wilson MS, Menzies D, et al. Postoperative adhesions: ten-year follow-up of 12,584 patients undergoing lower abdominal surgery. Dis Colon Rectum. 2001;44(6):822–9.

247. Parker MC, Wilson MS, Menzies D, Sunderland G, Clark DN, Knight AD, et al. The SCAR-3 study: 5-year adhesion-related readmission risk following lower abdominal surgical procedures. Colorectal Dis. 2005;7(6):551–8.

248. You YN, Wolff BG, Boardman LA, Riegert-Johnson DL, Qin R. Peutz-Jeghers syndrome: a study of long-term surgical morbidity and causes of mortality. Fam Cancer. 23 Jan 2010.

249. Despott EJ, Murino A, Fraser C. Management of deep looping when failing to progress at double-balloon enteroscopy. Endoscopy 2011;43(Suppl 2 UCTN):E275–6.

250. Gerson LB, Flodin JT, Miyabayashi K. Balloon-assisted enteroscopy: technology and troubleshooting. Gastrointest Endosc. 2008;68(6):1158–67.

251. Ross AS, Dye C, Prachand VN. Laparoscopic-assisted double-balloon enteroscopy for small-bowel polyp surveillance and treatment in patients with Peutz-Jeghers syndrome. Gastrointest Endosc. 2006;64(6):984–8.

252. Bodmer WF, Bailey CJ, Bodmer J, Bussey HJ, Ellis A, Gorman P, et al. Localization of the gene for familial adenomatous polyposis on chromosome 5. Nature. 1987;328(6131):614–6.

253. Half E, Bercovich D, Rozen P. Familial adenomatous polyposis. Orphanet J Rare Dis. 2009;4:22.

254. Katsinelos P, Kountouras J, Chatzimavroudis G, Zavos C, Pilpilidis I, Fasoulas K, et al. Wireless capsule endoscopy in detecting small-intestinal polyps in familial adenomatous polyposis. World J Gastroenterol. 2009;15(48):6075–9.

255. Gurbuz AK, Giardiello FM, Petersen GM, Krush AJ, Offerhaus GJ, Booker SV, et al. Desmoid tumours in familial adenomatous polyposis. Gut. 1994;35(3):377–81.

256. Bjork J, Akerbrant H, Iselius L, Bergman A, Engwall Y, Wahlstrom J, et al. Periampullary adenomas and adenocarcinomas in familial adenomatous polyposis: cumulative risks and APC gene mutations. Gastroenterology. 2001;121(5):1127–35.

257. Burke CA, Beck GJ, Church JM, van Stolk RU. The natural history of untreated duodenal and ampullary adenomas in patients with familial adenomatous polyposis followed in an endoscopic surveillance program. Gastrointest Endosc. 1999;49(3 Pt 1):358–64.

258. Schulmann K, Hollerbach S, Kraus K, Willert J, Vogel T, Moslein G, et al. Feasibility and diagnostic utility of video capsule endoscopy for the detection of small bowel polyps in patients with hereditary polyposis syndromes. Am J Gastroenterol. 2005;100(1):27–37.

259. Spigelman AD, Williams CB, Talbot IC, Domizio P, Phillips RK. Upper gastrointestinal cancer in patients with familial adenomatous polyposis. Lancet. 1989;2(8666):783–5.

260. Caspari R, von FM, Krautmacher C, Schild H, Heller J, Sauerbruch T. Comparison of capsule endoscopy and magnetic resonance imaging for the detection of polyps of the small intestine in patients with familial adenomatous polyposis or with Peutz-Jeghers' syndrome. Endoscopy. 2004;36(12):1054–9.

261. Saurin JC, Gutknecht C, Napoleon B, Chavaillon A, Ecochard R, Scoazec JY, et al. Surveillance of duodenal adenomas in familial adenomatous polyposis reveals high cumulative risk of advanced disease. J Clin Oncol. 2004;22(3):493–8.

262. Schlemper RJ, Riddell RH, Kato Y, Borchard F, Cooper HS, Dawsey SM, et al. The Vienna classification of gastrointestinal epithelial neoplasia. Gut. 2000;47(2):251–5.

263. Burke CA, Santisi J, Church J, Levinthal G. The utility of capsule endoscopy small bowel

surveillance in patients with polyposis. Am J Gastroenterol. 2005;100(7):1498–502.

264. Wong RF, Tuteja AK, Haslem DS, Pappas L, Szabo A, Ogara MM, et al. Video capsule endoscopy compared with standard endoscopy for the evaluation of small-bowel polyps in persons with familial adenomatous polyposis (with video). Gastrointest Endosc. 2006;64(4):530–7.

265. Ruys AT, Alderlieste YA, Gouma DJ, Dekker E, Mathus-Vliegen EM. Jejunal cancer in patients with familial adenomatous polyposis. Clin Gastroenterol Hepatol. 2010;8(8):731–3.

266. Koornstra JJ. Small bowel endoscopy in familial adenomatous polyposis and Lynch syndrome. Best Pract Res Clin Gastroenterol. 2012;26(3):359–68.

267. Postgate AJ, Will OC, Fraser CH, Fitzpatrick A, Phillips RK, Clark SK. Capsule endoscopy for the small bowel in juvenile polyposis syndrome: a case series. Endoscopy. 2009;41(11):1001–4.

268. Hatogai K, Hosoe N, Imaeda H, Rey JF, Okada S, Ishibashi Y, et al. Role of enhanced visibility in evaluating polyposis syndromes using a newly developed contrast image capsule endoscope. Gut Liver. 2012;6(2):218–22.

269. Riegler G, Esposito I, Esposito P, Bennato R, Bassi M, Ursillo A, et al. Wireless capsule enteroscopy (Given) in a case of Cowden syndrome. Dig Liver Dis. 2006;38(2):151–2.

270. Lens M, Bataille V, Krivokapic Z. Melanoma of the small intestine. Lancet Oncol. 2009;10:516–21.

271. Albert JG, Fechner M, Fiedler E, et al. Algorithm for detection of small-bowel metastasis in malignant melanoma of the skin. Endoscopy. 2011;43:490–8.

272. Nakamura M, Ohmiya N, Hirooka Y, et al. Endoscopic diagnosis of follicular lymphoma with small-bowel involvement using video capsule endoscopy and double-balloon endoscopy: a case series. Endoscopy. 2013;45:67–70.

273. Takata K, Okada H, Ohmiya N, et al. Primary gastrointestinal follicular lymphoma involving the duodenal second portion is a distinct entity: a multicenter, retrospective analysis in Japan. Cancer Sci. 2011;102:1532–6.

274. Al-Taie O, Dietrich CG, Flieger D, Katzenberger T, Fischbach W. Is there a role for capsule endoscopy in the staging work-up of patients with gastric marginal zone B-cell lymphoma of MALT? Z Gastroenterol. 2013;51:727–32.

275. Cerwenka H. Neuroendocrine liver metastases: contributions of endoscopy and surgery to primary tumor search. World J Gastroenterol. 2012;18:1009–14.

276. van Tuyl SA, van Noorden JT, Timmer R, et al. Detection of small-bowel neuroendocrine tumors by video capsule endoscopy. Gastrointest Endosc. 2006;64:66–72.

277. Johanssen S, Boivin M, Lochs H, Voderholzer W. The yield of wireless capsule endoscopy in the detection of neuroendocrine tumors in comparison with CT enteroclysis. Gastrointest Endosc. 2006;63:660–5.

278. Ronchi CL, Coletti F, Fesce E, et al. Detection of small bowel tumors by videocapsule endoscopy in patients with acromegaly. J Endocrinol Invest. 2009;32:495–500.

279. Bardan E, Nadler M, Chowers Y, Fidder H, Bar-Meir S. Capsule endoscopy for the evaluation of patients with chronic abdominal pain. Endoscopy. 2003;35:688–9.

280. Fry LC, Carey EJ, Shiff AD, et al. The yield of capsule endoscopy in patients with abdominal pain or diarrhea. Endoscopy. 2006;38:498–502.

281. Spada C, Pirozzi GA, Riccioni ME, et al. Capsule endoscopy in patients with chronic abdominal pain. Dig Liver Dis. 2006;38:696–8.

282. May A, Manner H, Schneider M, Ipsen A, Ell C. Prospective multicenter trial of capsule endoscopy in patients with chronic abdominal pain, diarrhea and other signs and symptoms (CEDAP-Plus Study). Endoscopy. 2007;39:606–12.

283. Shim KN, Kim YS, Kim KJ, et al. Abdominal pain accompanied by weight loss may increase the diagnostic yield of capsule endoscopy: a Korean multicenter study. Scand J Gastroenterol. 2006;41:983–8.

284. Valle J, Alcantara M, Perez-Grueso MJ, et al. Clinical features of patients with negative results from traditional diagnostic work-up and Crohn's disease findings from capsule endoscopy. J Clin Gastroenterol. 2006;40:692–6.

285. Fidder HH, Nadler M, Lahat A, et al. The utility of capsule endoscopy in the diagnosis of Crohn's disease based on patient's symptoms. J Clin Gastroenterol. 2007;41:384–7.

286. Cheifetz AS, Lewis BS. Capsule endoscopy retention: is it a complication? J Clin Gastroenterol. 2006;40:688–91.

287. Varadarajan P, Dunford LM, Thomas JA, et al. Seeing what's out of sight: wireless capsule endoscopy's unique ability to visualize and accurately assess the severity of gastrointestinal graft-versus-host-disease. Biol Blood Marrow Transplant. 2009;15:643–8.

288. Wu D, Hockenberry DM, Brentnall TA, et al. Persistent nausea and anorexia after marrow transplantation: a prospective study of 78 patients. Transplantation. 1998;66:1319–24.

289. Neumann S, Schoppmeyer K, Lange T, et al. Wireless capsule endoscopy for diagnosis of acute intestinal graft-versus-host disease. Gastrointest Endosc. 2007;65:403–9.

290. Shapira M, Adler SN, Jacob H, et al. New insights into the pathophysiology of gastrointestinal graft-

versus-host disease using capsule endoscopy. 2005. p. 1003–4.

291. Yakoub-Agha I, Maunoury V, Wacrenier A, et al. Impact of small bowel exploration using video-capsule endoscopy in the management of acute gastrointestinal graft-versus-host disease. Transplantation. 2004;78:1697–701.

292. Kim HM, Kim YJ, Kim HJ, et al. A pilot study of capsule endoscopy for the diagnosis of radiation enteritis. Hepatogastroenterology. 2011;58:459–64.

293. Rosa-e-Silva L, Gerson LB, Davila M, Triadafilopoulos G. Clinical, radiologic, and manometric characteristics of chronic intestinal dysmotility: the Stanford experience. Clinical Gastroenterol Hepatol: Official Clin Pract J Am Gastroenterol Assoc. 2006;4:866–73.

294. Bassotti G, Villanacci V, Battaglia E. Small bowel motility from videocapsule endoscopy: beware of false prophets! Dig Dis Sci. 2013;58:1161–2.

295. Malagelada C, De Iorio F, Azpiroz F, et al. New insight into intestinal motor function via noninvasive endoluminal image analysis. Gastroenterology. 2008;135:1155–62.

296. Hoog CM, Lindberg G, Sjoqvist U. Findings in patients with chronic intestinal dysmotility investigated by capsule endoscopy. BMC Gastroenterol. 2007;7:29.

297. Park SC, Chun HJ, Kang CD, Sul D. Prevention and management of non-steroidal anti-inflammatory drugs-induced small intestinal injury. World J Gastroenterol. 2011;17:4647–53.

298. Goldstein JL, Eisen GM, Lewis B, et al. Small bowel mucosal injury is reduced in healthy subjects treated with celecoxib compared with ibuprofen plus omeprazole, as assessed by video capsule endoscopy. Aliment Pharmacol Ther. 2007;25:1211–22.

299. Adebayo D, Bjarnason I. Is non-steroidal anti-inflammaory drug (NSAID) enteropathy clinically more important than NSAID gastropathy? 2006. p. 186–91.

300. Wallace JL. Mechanisms, prevention and clinical implications of nonsteroidal anti-inflammatory drug-enteropathy. World J Gastroenterol. 2013;19:1861–76.

301. Maiden L, Thjodleifsson B, Theodors A, Gonzalez J, Bjarnason I. A quantitative analysis of NSAID-induced small bowel pathology by capsule enteroscopy. Gastroenterology. 2005;128:1172–8.

302. Endo H, Higurashi T, Hosono K, et al. Efficacy of Lactobacillus casei treatment on small bowel injury in chronic low-dose aspirin users: a pilot randomized controlled study. J Gastroenterol. 2012;46:894–905.

303. Fujimori S, Seo T, Gudis K, et al. Prevention of nonsteroidal anti-inflammatory drug-induced small-intestinal injury by prostaglandin: a pilot randomized controlled trial evaluated by capsule endoscopy. Gastrointest Endosc. 2009;69:1339–46.

304. Watari I, Oka S, Tanaka S, et al. Effectiveness of polaprezinc for low-dose aspirin-induced small-bowel mucosal injuries as evaluated by capsule endoscopy: a pilot randomized controlled study. BMC Gastroenterol. 2013;13:108.

305. Ito Y, Sasaki M, Funaki Y, et al. Nonsteroidal anti-inflammatory drug-induced visible and invisible small intestinal injury. J Clin Biochem Nutr. 2013;53:55–9.

306. Racz I, Szalai M, Kovacs V, et al. Mucosal healing effect of mesalazine granules in naproxen-induced small bowel enteropathy. World J Gastroenterol. 2013;19:889–96.

307. Meltzer AC, Ali MA, Kresiberg RB, et al. Video capsule endoscopy in the emergency department: a prospective study of acute upper gastrointestinal hemorrhage. Ann Emerg Med. 2013;61(438–43):e1.

308. Aoyama T, Oka S, Aikata H, et al. Small bowel abnormalities in patients with compensated liver cirrhosis. Dig Dis Sci. 2013;58:1390–6.

309. Demongeot C, Moulonguet I, Georges P, Bagot M, Flageul B. Gastric sarcoidosis revealed by cutaneous follicular sarcoidosis. Ann Dermatol Venereol. 2011;138:116–9.

310. Shkolnik LE, Shin RD, Brabeck DM, Rothman RD. Symptomatic gastric sarcoidosis in a patient with pulmonary sarcoidosis in remission. BMJ Case Rep. 2012.

311. Fleming RH, Nuzek M, McFadden DW. Small intestinal sarcoidosis with massive hemorrhage: report of a case. Surgery. 1994;115:127–31.

312. Marie I, Sauvetre G, Levesque H. Small intestinal involvement revealing sarcoidosis. QJM. 2010;103:60–2.

313. Esaki M, Matsumoto T, Nakamura S, et al. GI involvement in Henoch-Schonlein purpura. Gastrointest Endosc. 2002;56:920–3.

314. Keuchel M, Baltes P, Stövesand-Ruge, Steinbrück I, Hagenmüller F. Henoch-Schoenlein Purpura. Video J Encycl GI Endosc. 2013;1:235–6.

315. Skogestad E. Capsule endoscopy in Henoch-Schonlein purpura. Endoscopy. 2005;37:189.

316. Hamdulay SS, Cheent K, Ghosh C, et al. Wireless capsule endoscopy in the investigation of intestinal Behcet's syndrome. Rheumatology (Oxford). 2008;47:1231–4.

317. Neves FS, Fylyk SN, Lage LV, et al. Behcet's disease: clinical value of the video capsule endoscopy for small intestine examination. Rheumatol Int. 2009;29:601–3.

318. Sugimori S, Watanabe T, Tabuchi M, et al. Evaluation of small bowel injury in patients with rheumatoid arthritis by capsule endoscopy: effects of anti-rheumatoid arthritis drugs. Digestion. 2008;78:208–13.

319. Makary R, Davis C, Shuja S. Medium- and small-vessel vasculitis with large bowel infarction in systemic lupus erythematosus: a case report. Am J Gastroenterol. 2009;104:1859–60.
320. Endo H, Kondo Y, Kawagoe K, et al. Lupus enteritis detected by capsule endoscopy. Intern Med. 2007;46:1621–2.
321. Mandelli G, Radaelli F, Amato A, et al. The spectrum of small-bowel lesions of AL-type amyloidosis at capsule endoscopy. Endoscopy. 2009;41(Suppl 2):E51–2.
322. Cowan AJ, Skinner M, Seldin DC, et al. Amyloidosis of the gastrointestinal tract: a 13-year, single-center, referral experience. Haematologica. 2013;98:141–6.
323. Hokama A, Kishimoto K, Nakamoto M, et al. Endoscopic and histopathological features of gastrointestinal amyloidosis. World J Gastrointest Endosc. 2011;3:157–61.
324. Yoshii S, Mabe K, Nosho K, et al. Submucosal hematoma is a highly suggestive finding for amyloid light-chain amyloidosis: two case reports. World J Gastrointest Endosc. 2012;4:434–7.
325. Radzi M, Rihan N, Vijayalakshmi N, Pani SP. Diagnostic challenge of gastrointestinal tuberculosis: a report of 34 cases and an overview of the literature. Southeast Asian J Trop Med Public Health. 2009;40:505–10.
326. Sefr R, Rotterova P, Konecny J. Perforation peritonitis in primary intestinal tuberculosis. Dig Surg. 2001;18:475–9.
327. Loureiro AI, Pinto CS, Oliveira AI, et al. Ulcerated lesion of the cecum as a form of presentation of gastrointestinal tuberculosis. Acta Med Port. 2011;24:371–4.
328. Kim ES, Keum B, Jeen YT, Chun HJ. Isolated small bowel tuberculosis with stricture diagnosed by capsule endoscopy. Digestive and liver disease : official journal of the Italian Society of Gastroenterology and the Italian Association for the Study of the Liver. 2012;44:84.
329. Chang DK, Kim JJ, Choi H, et al. Double balloon endoscopy in small intestinal Crohn's disease and other inflammatory diseases such as cryptogenic multifocal ulcerous stenosing enteritis (CMUSE). Gastrointest Endosc. 2007;66:S96–8.
330. Matsumoto T, Kudo T, Esaki M, et al. Prevalence of non-steroidal anti-inflammatory drug-induced enteropathy determined by double-balloon endoscopy: a Japanese multicenter study. Scand J Gastroenterol. 2008;43:490–6.
331. Oette M, Stelzer A, Gobels K, et al. Wireless capsule endoscopy for the detection of small bowel diseases in HIV-1-infected patients. Eur J Med Res. 2009;14:191–4.
332. Schneider T, Moos V, Loddenkemper C, et al. Whipple's disease: new aspects of pathogenesis and treatment. Lancet Infect Dis. 2008;8:179–90.
333. de Roulet J, Hassan MO, Cummings LC. Capsule endoscopy in Whipple's disease. Clin Gastroenterol Hepatol: Official Clin Pract J Am Gastroenterol Assoc. 2013.
334. Mateescu BR, Bengus A, Marinescu M, et al. First Pillcam Colon 2 capsule images of Whipple's disease: case report and review of the literature. World J Gastrointest Endosc. 2012;4:575–8.
335. Dzirlo L, Blaha B, Muller C, et al. Capsule endoscopic appearance of the small-intestinal mucosa in Whipple's disease and the changes that occur during antibiotic therapy. Endoscopy. 2007;39(Suppl 1):E207–8.
336. Kakugawa Y, Kim SW, Takizawa K, et al. Small intestinal CMV disease detected by capsule endoscopy after allogeneic hematopoietic SCT. Bone Marrow Transplant. 2008;42:283–4.
337. Michalopoulos N, Triantafillopoulou K, Beretouli E, et al. Small bowel perforation due to CMV enteritis infection in an HIV-positive patient. BMC Res Notes. 2013;6:45.
338. Papadimitriou G, Koukoulaki M, Vardas K, et al. Small bowel obstruction caused by inflammatory cytomegalovirus tumor in a renal transplant recipient: report of a rare case and review of the literature. Transpl Infect Dis: Official J Transpl Soc. 2012;14:E111–5.
339. Sakai E, Endo H, Tokoro C, et al. Cytomegalovirus-induced small-bowel bleeding detected by capsule endoscopy. Gastrointest Endosc. 2011;73:1058–60.
340. Aldeman NL, Guimaraes LM, Cabral MM. Atypical duodenal mycobacteriosis in a patient with AIDS. Braz J Infect Dis: Official Publ Braz Soc Infect Dis. 2012;16:209–10.
341. Tzimas D, Wan D. Small bowel perforation in a patient with AIDS. Diagnosis: small bowel infection with Cryptococcus neoformans. Gastroenterology. 2011;140(1882):2150.
342. Cello JP, Day LW. Idiopathic AIDS enteropathy and treatment of gastrointestinal opportunistic pathogens. Gastroenterology. 2009;136:1952–65.
343. Sriram PV, Rao GV, Reddy DN. Wireless capsule endoscopy: experience in a tropical country. J Gastroenterol Hepatol. 2004;19:63–7.
344. Yamashita ET, Takahashi W, Kuwashima DY, Langoni TR, Costa-Genzini A. Diagnosis of Ascaris lumbricoides infection using capsule endoscopy. World J Gastrointest Endosc. 2013;5:189–90.
345. Kalli T, Karamanolis G, Triantafyllou K. Hookworm infection detected by capsule endoscopy in a young man with iron deficiency. Clin Gastroenterol Hepatol: Official Clin Pract J Am Gastroenterol Assoc. 2011;9:e33.
346. Wu IC, Lu CY, Wu DC. Acute hookworm infection revealed by capsule endoscopy. Endoscopy. 2007;39(Suppl 1):E306.

347. Urgesi R, Riccioni ME, Spada C, Pelecca G, Costamagna G. Enterobius vermicularis, the small human pinworm: a chronic infestation diagnosed by Pillcam. Incidental observation on capsule endoscopy. BMJ Case Rep. 2010.

348. Hosoe N, Imaeda H, Okamoto S, et al. A case of beef tapeworm (Taenia saginata) infection observed by using video capsule endoscopy and radiography (with videos). Gastrointest Endosc. 2011;74:690–1.

349. Yang SQ, Huang R, Zhang LN, Hu JG, Yang L. Tapeworm infection identified on capsule endoscopy. J Interv Gastroenterol. 2012;2:19.

350. Hagel AF, de Rossi TM, Zopf Y, et al. Small-bowel capsule endoscopy in patients with gastrointestinal food allergy. Allergy. 2012;67:286–92.

351. Freeman HJ, Nimmo M. Intestinal lymphangiectasia in adults. World J Gastrointest Oncol. 2011;3:19–23.

352. Kim HH, Kim YS, Ok KS, et al. Chronic non-granulomatous ulcerative jejunoileitis assessed by wireless capsule endoscopy. Korean J Gastroenterol. 2010;56:382–6.

353. Soergel KH. Nongranulomatous chronic idiopathic enterocolitis: a primary histologically defined disease. Dig Dis Sci. 2000;45:2085–90.

354. Pungpapong S, Stark ME, Cangemi JR. Protein-losing enteropathy from eosinophilic enteritis diagnosed by wireless capsule endoscopy and double-balloon enteroscopy. Gastrointest Endosc. 2007;65:917–8.

355. Harish K, Gokulan C. Selective amyloidosis of the small intestine presenting as malabsorption syndrome. Trop Gastroenterol. 2008;29:37–9.

356. Werlin SL, Benuri-Silbiger I, Kerem E, et al. Evidence of intestinal inflammation in patients with cystic fibrosis. J Pediatr Gastroenterol Nutr. 2010;51:304–8.

357. Antao B, Bishop J, Shawis R, Thomson M. Clinical application and diagnostic yield of wireless capsule endoscopy in children. J Laparoendosc Adv Surg Tech A. 2007;17:364–70.

358. Fritscher-Ravens A, Scherbakov P, Bufler P, et al. The feasibility of wireless capsule endoscopy in detecting small intestinal pathology in children under the age of 8 years: a multicentre European study. Gut. 2009;58:1467–72.

359. Liao Z, Gao R, Xu C, Li ZS. Indications and detection, completion and retention rates of small bowel capsule endoscopy: a systematic review. Gastrointest Endosc. 2010;7(2):280–6.

360. Rondonotti E, Soncini M, Girelli C, et al. Small bowel capsule endoscopy in clinical practice: a multicentre 7 year survey. Eur J Gastroenterol Hepatol. 2010;22:1380–6.

361. Storch I, Barkin S. Contraindications to capsule endoscopy: do any still exist? Gastrointest Endosc Clin N Am. 2006;16:329–36.

362. Wax JR, Pinette MG, Cartin A, et al. Cavernous transformation of the portal vein complicating pregnancy. Obstet Gynecol. 2006;108(3 Pt 2):782–4.

363. Hogan RB, Ahmad N, Hogan RB III, et al. Video capsule endoscopy detection of jejunal carcinoid in life threatening haemorrhage, first trimester pregnancy. Gastrointest Endosc. 2007;66(1):205–7.

364. Shellock FG, Spinazzi A. MRI safety update 2008: Part 2, screening patients for MRI. Am J Roentgenol. 2008;185(4):1048–50.

365. Anderson BW, Liang JJ, DeJesus RS. Capsule endoscopy device retention and magnetic resonance imaging. Proc Bayl Univ Med Cent. 2013;26(3):270–1.

366. Berry PA, Srijaaskanthan R, Anderson SH. An urgent call to the magnetic resonance scanner: potential dangers of capsule endoscopy. Clin Gastroenterol Hepatol. 2010;8(5):A26.

367. Gaba RC, Schlesinger PK, Wilbur AC. Endoscopic video capsules: radiologic findings of spontaneous entrapment in small intestinal diverticula. Am J Roentgenol. 2005;185(4):1048–50.

368. De Luca L, Di George P, Rivellini G, et al. Capsule endoscopy experience: experience in southern Italy. 2nd International Conference on Capsule Endoscopy, Berlin. March 2003.

369. Cave D, Legnani P, De Franchis R, et al. ICCE Consensus for capsule retention. Endoscopy. 2005;37:1065–7.

370. Goldstein JL, Eisen GM, Lewis B, et al. Video capsule endoscopy to prospectively assess small bowel injury with celecoxib, naproxen plus omeprazole and placebo. Clin Gastroenterol Hepatol. 2005;3:133–41.

371. Cheifetz AS, Kornbluth AA, Legnani P, et al. The risk of retention of the capsule endoscope in patients with known or suspected Crohn's disease. Am J Gastroenterol. 2006;101(10):2218–22.

372. Cheon JH, Kim YS, Lee IS, et al. Can we predict spontaneous capsule passage after retention? A nationwide study to evaluate incidence and clinical outcomes of retention. Endoscopy. 2007;39:1046–52.

373. Li F, Gurudu SR, De Petris G, et al. Retention of the capsule endoscope: a single centre experience of 1000 capsule endoscopy procedures. Gastrointest Endosc. 2008;68:174–80.

374. Rondonotti E, Herrerias JM, Pennazio M, et al. Complications, limitations and failures of capsule endoscopy: a review of 733 cases. Gastrointest Endosc. 2005;62(5):712–6.

375. Sears DM, Avots-Avonis A, Culp K, et al. Frequency and clinical outcome of capsule retention during capsule endoscopy for GI bleeding of obscure origin. Gastrointest Endosc. 2004;60:822–7.

376. Horiuchi A, Nakayama Y, Kajiyama M, et al. Video capsule retention in a Zenker Diverticulum. Case Rep Gastroenterol. 2011;5:361–5.

377. Courcoutsakis N, Pitiakodis M, Mimidis K, et al. Capsule retention in a giant Meckel's diverticulum containing multiple enteroliths. Endoscopy. 2011;43(suppl 42 UCTN):E308–9.

378. Gortzak Y, Lantsberg L, Odes HS. Video capsule entrapped in a Meckels diverticulum. J Clin Gastroenterol. 2003;37:270–1.

379. Yu WK, Yang RD. M2A video capsule lodged in the Meckel's diverticulum. Gastrointest Endosc. 2006;63:1071–2.

380. Ferreira F, Bastos P, Cardoso H, et al. Retention of endoscopic capsule in an umbilical hernia. Endoscopy. 2011;43(Suppl 2):E111–2.

381. De Franchis R, Avesani EM, Abbiati C, et al. Unsuspected ileal stenosis causing obscure GI bleeding in patients with previous abdominal surgery-diagnosis by capsule endoscopy: a report of two cases. Dig Liver Dis. 2003;35:577–84.

382. Xin L, Liao Z, Du YQ, et al. Retained capsule endoscopy causing intestinal obstruction—endoscopic retrieval by retrograde single balloon enteroscopy. J Interv Gastroenterol. 2012;2(1):15–8.

383. Levsky JM, Milikow DL, Rosenbilt AM. Small bowel obstruction due to an impacted endoscopy capsule. Abdom Imaging. 2008;33:579–81.

384. Rammohan A. Capsule endoscopy: new technology, old complication. J Surg Tech Case Rep. 2011;3(2):91–3.

385. De Palma G, Masone S, Persico M, et al. Capsule impaction presenting as acute small bowel perforation: a case series. J Med Case Rep. 2012;6(1):121.

386. Gonzalez Carro P, Picazo Yuste J, Fernández Díez S, et al. Intestinal perforation due to retained capsule endoscope. Endoscopy. 2005;37:684.

387. Lin OS, Brandabur JJ, Schembre DB. Acute symptomatic small bowel obstruction due to capsule impaction. Gastrointest Endosc. 2007;65:725–8.

388. Parikh DA, Parikh JA, Albers GC, et al. Acute small bowel perforation after wireless capsule endoscopy in a patient with Crohn's disease: a case report. Cases J. 2009;2:7607.

389. Repici A, Barbon V, De Angelis C. Acute small bowel perforation secondary to capsule endoscopy. Gastrointest Endosc. 2008;67:180–3.

390. Um S, Poblete H, Zavotsky J. Small bowel perforation caused by an impacted endocapsule. Endoscopy. 2008;40:E122–3.

391. Yadav A, Heigh RI, Hara AK, et al. Performance of the patency capsule compared with nonenteroclysis radiologic examinations in patients with known or suspected intestinal strictures. Gastrointest Endos. 2011;74(4):834–9.

392. Buchman AL, Miller FH, Wallin A. Videocapsule endoscopy versus barium contrast studies for the diagnosis of Crohn's disease recurrence involving the small intestine. Am J Gastroenterol. 2004;99:2171–7.

393. Caunedo A, Rodriguez-Tellez M, Garcia-Montes JM. Usefulness of capsule endoscopy in patients with suspected small bowel disease. Rev Esp Enferm Dig. 2004;96:10–21.

394. Otterson MF, Lundeen SJ, Spinelli KS, et al. Radiographic underestimation of small bowel stricturing Crohn's disease: a comparison with surgical findings. Surgery. 2004;136:854–60.

395. Soncini M, Rondonotti E, Girelli CM, et al. Small bowel capsule endoscopy (SBCE) complications: frequency, management and policy to prevent them. Prospective data from a regional registry: Registro Lombardo delle complicanze (abstract). Dig Liver Dis. 2013;45(S135–S136).

396. Voderholzer WA, Beinhoelzl J, Rogalla P, et al. Small bowel involvement in Crohn's disease: a prospective comparison of wireless capsule endoscopy and computed tomography enteroclysis. Gut. 2005;54:369–73.

397. Spada C, Spera G, Ricconi M, et al. A novel diagnostic tool for detecting functional patency of the small bowel: the Given Patency Capsule. Endoscopy. 2005;37:793–800.

398. Perowne R, Parker C, Davison C, et al. Abdominal Xray is the most useful tool initial screening tool in determining position of 'retained' patency capsule (abstract). Gut. 2011;60:A197–8. doi:10.1136/gut.2011.239301.416.

399. Postgate AJ, Burling D, Gupta A, et al. Safety, reliability and limitations of the Given Patency Capsule in patients at risk of capsule retention: a 3 year technical review. Dig Dis Sci. 2008;53:2732–8. doi:10.1007/s10620-008-0210-5.

400. Sidhu R, Blakeborough A, McAlindon ME. A novel and accurate single assessment patency capsule screening protocol (abstract). Gut. 2010;59(Suppl 1):A47–8.

401. Gay G, Delvaux M, Laurent V, et al. Temporary intestinal occlusion induced by a patency capsule in a patient with Crohn's disease. Endoscopy. 2005;37:174–7.

402. Boivin ML, Lochs H, Voderholzer WA. Does passage of a patency capsule indicate small bowel patency? A prospective clinical trial? Endoscopy. 2005;37:808–15.

403. Caunedo-Alvarez A, Romero-Vazquez J, Herrerias-Gutierrez JM. Patency and agile capsules. World J Gastroenterol. 2008;14(34):5269–73.

404. Cohen SA, Gralnek IM, Ephrath H, et al. The use of a patency capsule in pediatric Crohn's disease: a prospective evaluation. Dig Dis Sci. 2011;56:860–5.

405. Signorelli C, Rondonotti E, Villa F, et al. Use of the Given patency system for the screening of patients at high risk for capsule retention. Dig and Liv Dis. 2006;38:326–30.

406. Spada C, Shah SK, Riccioni ME, et al. Video capsule endoscopy in patients with known or suspected small bowel stricture previously tested with the dissolving patency capsule. J Clin Gastroenterol. 2007;41(6):576–82.

407. DeSilva PS, Baldwin L, Miao YM. Failure of patency capsules—a district general hospital experience in the UK (abstract). Gastroenterology. 2010;138(5 SUPPL 1, S670).

408. Yang XY, Chen CX, Zhang BL, et al. Diagnostic effect of capsule endoscopy in 31 cases of subacute small bowel obstruction. World J Gastroenterol. 2009;15:2401–5.

409. May A, Nachbar L, Ell C, et al. Extraction of entrapped capsules from the small bowel by means of push and pull enteroscopy with the double balloon technique. Endoscopy. 2005;37:591–3.

410. Al-Toma A, Hadithi M, Heine D, et al. Retrieval of video capsule endoscope by using a double balloon endoscope. Gastrointest Endosc. 2005;62:613.

411. Lee BI, Choi H, Choi KY, et al. Retrieval of retained capsule by double balloon enteroscopy. Gastronintest Endosc. 2005;62:463–5.

412. Tanaka S, Mitsui K, Shirakawa K, et al. Successful retrieval of video capsule endoscopy retained at ileal stenosis of Crohns disease using double-balloon endoscopy. J Gastroenterol Hepatol. 2006;21:922–3.

413. Weyenberg SJ, Turenhout ST, Bouma G, et al. Double Balloon Endoscopy as a primary method for small bowel video capsule endoscope retrieval. Gastrointest Endosc. 2010;71(3):535–41.

414. Baichi MM, Arifuddin RM, Mantry PS. What we have learned from 5 cases of permanent capsule retention. Gastrointest Endosc. 2006;64:283–7.

415. Mason M, Swain J, Matthews BD, et al. Use of video capsule endoscopy in the setting of Recurrent Sub-acute small bowel obstruction. J Laparoendosc Adv Surg Tech. 2008;18(5):713–6.

416. Dominguez EP, Choi Y, Raijman IL, et al. Laparoscopic approach for the retrieval of retained video capsule. JSLS. 2006;10:496–8.

417. Lucendo AJ, Gonzalez-Castillo S, Fernandez-Fuente M, et al. Tracheal aspiration of a capsule endoscope: a new case report and literature compilation of an increasingly reported complication. Dig Dis Sci. 2011;56(9):2758–62.

418. Schneider AR, Hoepffner N, Rosch W, et al. Aspiration of an M2A capsule. Endoscopy. 2003;35(8):713.

419. Koulaouzidis A, Douglas S, Plevris JN. Tracheal aspiration of capsule endoscopes: completing a case compilation. Dig Dis Sci. 2011;56(10):3101–2.

420. Simmons DT, Baron TH. Endoscopic retrieval of a capsule endoscope from a Zenker's diverticulum. Dis Esophagus: Official J Int Soc Dis Esophagus. 2005;18(5):338–9.

421. Holden JP, Dureja P, Pfau PR, et al. Endoscopic placement of the small-bowel video capsule by using a capsule endoscope delivery device. Gastrointest Endos. 2007;65(6):842–77.

422. Carey EJ, Heigh RI, Fleischer DE. Endoscopic capsule endoscope delivery for patients with dysphagia, anatomical abnormalities, or gastroparesis. Gastrointest Endos. 2004;59(3):423–6.

423. Buchkremer F, Herrmann T, Stremmel W. Mild respiratory distress after wireless capsule endoscopy. Gut. 2004;53(3):472.

424. Pezzoli A, Fusetti N, Carella A, et al. Asymptomatic bronchial aspiration and prolonged retention of a capsule endoscope: a case report. J Med Case Rep. 2011;5:341.

425. Tabib S, Fuller C, Daniels J, et al. Asymptomatic aspiration of a capsule endoscope. Gastrointest Endos. 2004;60(5):845–8.

426. Kelly OB, O'Donnell S, O'Morain CA. A case of achalasia diagnosed first on capsule endoscopy: find that hard to swallow? Eur J Gastroenterol Hepatol. 2010;22(8):1013–4.

427. Despott EJ, O'Rourke A, Anikin V, et al. Tracheal aspiration of capsule endoscopes: detection, management, and susceptibility. Dig Dis Sci. 2012;57(7):1973–4.

428. Gomez V, Cheesman AR, Heckman MG, et al. Safety of capsule endoscopy in the octogenarian as compared with younger patients (abstract). Gastrointest Endosc. 2013. doi:10.1016/j.gie.2013.05.004.

429. Choi HS, Kim JO, Kim HG, et al. A case of asymptomatic aspiration of a capsule endoscope with a successful resolution. Gut and Liver. 2010;4(1):114–6.

430. Guy T, Jouneau S, D'Halluin PN, et al. Asymptomatic bronchial aspiration of a video capsule. Interact CardioVasc Thorac Surg. 2009;8(5):568–70.

431. Parker C, Davison C, Panter S. Tracheal aspiration of a capsule endoscope: not always a benign event. Dig Dis Sci. 2012;57(6):1727–8.

432. Girdhar A, Usman F, Bajwa A. Aspiration of capsule endoscope and successful bronchoscopic extraction. J Bronchol Intervent Pulmonol. 2012;19(4):328–31.

433. Depriest K, Wahla AS, Blair R, et al. Capsule endoscopy removal through flexible bronchoscopy. Respir Int Rev Thorac Dis. 2010;79(5):421–4.

434. Hall JJ, Fischer UM, Shah SK, et al. Video endoscope removal from the right main bronchus using a flexible esophagogastroduodenoscope. Am Surg. 2013;79(5):E185–6.

435. Bass LM, Misiewicz L. Use of a real-time viewer for endoscopic deployment of capsule endoscope in the pediatric population. J Pediatr Gastroenterol Nutr. 2012;55(5):552–5.

436. Lai LH, Wong GL, Lau JY, et al. Initial experience of real-time capsule endoscopy in monitoring progress of the videocapsule through the upper GI tract. Gastrointest Endosc. 2007;66(6):1211–4.

437. Westerhof J, Weersma RK, Koornstra JJ. Risk factors for incomplete small bowel capsule endoscopy. Gastrointest Endosc. 2009;1:74–80.

438. Chen JM, Zhong DD, Xie CG, et al. Effect of metoclopramide on capsule endoscopy examination: a randomized study. Zhejiang da xue xue bao. Yi xue ban J Zhejiang Univ Med Sci. 2012;41(2):206–9.

439. Postgate A, Tekkis P, Patterson N, et al. Are bowel purgatives and prokinetics useful for small-bowel capsule endoscopy? A prospective randomized controlled study. Gastrointest Endosc. 2009;69(6):1120–8.

440. Selby W. Complete small-bowel transit in patients undergoing capsule endoscopy: determining factors and improvement with metoclopramide. Gastrointest Endosc. 2005;61(1):80–5.

441. Ben-Soussan E, Savoye G, Antoniette M, et al. Factors that affect gastric passage of video capsule. Gastrointest Endosc. 2005;62:785–90.

442. Fireman Z, Paz D, Kopelman Y, et al. Capsule endoscopy: improving transit time and image view. World Gastroenterol. 2005;11:5863–6.

443. Iwamoto J, Mizokami Y, Shimokobe K, et al. The effect of metoclopramide in capsule endoscopy. Hepatogastroenterol. 2010;57:1356–9.

444. Keuchel M, Volderholzer WA, Schenk G, et al. Domperidone shortens gastric transit time of videocapsule endoscopy (VCE) abstract. Gastrointest Endosc. 2003;57:AB163.

445. Leung WK, Chan FKL, Fung SSL, et al. Effect of oral erythromycin on gastric and small bowel transit time of capsule endoscopy. World J Gastroenterol. 2005;11:4865–8.

446. Zhang JS, Ye LP, Zhang JL, et al. Intramuscular injection of metoclopramide decreases the gastric transit time and does not increase the complete examination rate of capsule endoscopy: a prospective randomized controlled trial. Hepatogastroenterol. 2011;58:1618–21.

447. Ogata H, Kumai K, Imaeda H, et al. Clinical impact of a newly developed capsule endoscope: usefulness of a real-time image viewer for gastric transit abnormality. J Gastroenterol. 2008;43(3):186–92.

448. Hollerbach S, Kraus K, Willert J, et al. Endoscopically assisted video capsule endoscopy of the small bowel in patients with functional gastric outlet obstruction. Endoscopy. 2003;35(3):226–9.

449. Bandorski D, Jakobs R, Bruck M, et al. Capsule endoscopy in patients with cardiac pacemakers and implantable cardioverter defibrillators: (Re)evaluation of the current state in Germany, Austria, and Switzerland 2010. Gastroenterol Res Pract. 2012;2012:717408.

450. Bandorski D, Diehl KL, Jaspersen D. Capsule endoscopy in patients with cardiac pacemakers: current situation in Germany. Z Gastroenterol. 2005;43(8):715–8.

451. Cuschieri JR, Osman MN, Wong RC, et al. Small bowel capsule endoscopy in patients with cardiac pacemakers and implantable cardioverter defibrillators: outcome analysis using telemetry review. World J Gastrointest Endosc. 2012;4(3):87–93.

452. Wei W, Ge ZZ, Gao YJ, et al. An analysis of failure and safety profiles of capsule endoscopy. Zhonghua nei ke za zhi (Chin J Intern Med). 2008;47(1):19–22.

453. Bandorski D, Lotterer E, Hartmann D, et al. Capsule endoscopy in patients with cardiac pacemakers and implantable cardioverter-defibrillators—a retrospective multicenter investigation. J Gastrointest Liver Dis. 2011;20(1):33–7.

454. Dirks MH, Costea F, Seidman EG. Successful videocapsule endoscopy in patients with an abdominal cardiac pacemaker. Endoscopy. 2008;40(1):73–5.

455. Bandorski D, Irnich W, Bruck M, et al. Capsule endoscopy and cardiac pacemakers: investigation for possible interference. Endoscopy. 2008;40(1):36–9.

456. Payeras G, Piqueras J, Moreno VJ, et al. Effects of capsule endoscopy on cardiac pacemakers. Endoscopy. 2005;37(12):1181–5.

457. Ladas SD, Triantafyllou K, Spada C, et al. European Society of Gastrointestinal Endoscopy (ESGE): recommendations (2009) on clinical use of video capsule endoscopy to investigate small-bowel, esophageal and colonic diseases. Endoscopy. 2010;42(3):220–7.

458. Spera G, Spada C, Riccioni ME, et al. Video capsule endoscopy in a patient with a Billroth II gastrectomy and obscure bleeding. Endoscopy. 2004;36(10):931.

459. Pfeiffer RF. Gastrointestinal dysfunction in Parkinson's disease. Lancet Neurol. 2003;2(2):107–16 (Review).

460. Marie I, Gourcerol G, Leroi AM, Ménard JF, Levesque H, Ducrotté P. Delayed gastric emptying determined using the 13C-octanoic acid breath test in patients with systemic sclerosis. Arthritis Rheum. 2012;64(7):2346–55.

461. Sharma A, Jamal MM. Opioid induced bowel disease: a twenty-first century physicians' dilemma. Considering pathophysiology and

treatment strategies. Curr Gastroenterol Rep. 2013;15(7):334.

462. Parkman HP, Trate DM, Knight LC, Brown KL, Maurer AH, Fisher RS. Cholinergic effects on human gastric motility. Gut. 1999;45(3):346–54.

463. Inamori M, Iida H, Endo H, Hosono K, Akiyama T, Yoneda K, Fujita K, Iwasaki T, Takahashi H, Yoneda M, Goto A, Abe Y, Kobayashi N, Kubota K, Nakajima A. Aperitif effects on gastric emptying: a crossover study using continuous real-time 13C breath test (BreathID System). Dig Dis Sci. 2009;54(4):816–8.

464. Eliakim R, Fischer D, Suissa A, et al. Wireless capsule video endoscopy is a superior diagnostic tool in comparison to barium follow-through and computerized tomography in patients with suspected Crohn's disease. Eur J Gastroenterol Hepatol. 2003;15:363–7.

465. Fireman Z, Mahajna E, Broide E, et al. Diagnosing small bowel Crohn's disease with wireless capsule endoscopy. Gut. 2003;52:390–2.

466. Herrerias JM, Caunedo A, Rodriguez-Tellez M, et al. Capsule endoscopy in patients with suspected Crohn's disease and negative endoscopy. Endoscopy. 2003;35:564–8.

467. Mow WS, Lo SK, Targan SR. Initial experience with wireless capsule endoscopy in the diagnosis and management of inflammatory bowel disease. Clin Gastroenterol Hepatol. 2004;2:31–40.

# Oesophageal Capsule Endoscopy

**4**

Anastasios Koulaouzidis, Sarah Douglas and John N. Plevris

**Abstract**

To date, only one system is available for wireless examination of the oesophagus (PillCam®ESO 2; Given Imaging®Ltd, Yoqneam, Israel). Tethered examination of the oesophagus has been attempted with both PillCam and OMOM® (Chongqing Jinshan Science and Technology Group Co., Ltd, Beijing, China). Although a useful alternative to conventional endoscopy for anxious patients, evidence on the validity of oesophageal capsule endoscopy in Barrett's oesophagus, oesophagitis and oesophageal varices is less favourable. In this chapter, we present the technical specifications of the oesophageal capsule, the ingestion protocol, indications and contraindications for its use, potential alternatives and on-going projects.

**Keywords**

Obscure gastrointestinal bleeding · Iron deficiency anaemia · Capsule endoscopy · Device-assisted enteroscopy · Outcomes

## 4.1 Oesophageal Capsule

The oesophageal capsule endoscopy (ECE) device (PillCam®ESO; Given®Imaging, Ltd., Yoqneam, Israel) consists of a capsule

A. Koulaouzidis (✉) · S. Douglas · J. N. Plevris
Centre for Liver and Digestive Disorders, The Royal Infirmary of Edinburgh, 51 Little France Crescent, Edinburgh, EH164SA, Scotland
e-mail: akoulaouzidis@hotmail.com

S. Douglas
e-mail: sarah.douglas@luht.scot.nhs.uk

J. N. Plevris
e-mail: j.plevris@ed.ac.uk

11 × 26 mm with cameras in both ends (heads) that can acquire images much faster than its small-bowel counterpart at a rate (per head) of 9 frames/s (fps) i.e. total of 18 fps. Although the oesophageal capsule works for approximately 30 min i.e. until battery is exhausted, it passes through the entire gut and it is naturally excreted [1]. The angle of view (for each head) is 169°, the optics is improved (three lenses instead of one in its predecessor ESO1) and there is automated adjustable light source control [1].

Initially cleared by the US food and drug administration (FDA) in November 2004 (Pill-Cam®ESO1), and as happens with disruptive technology, its successor (PillCam®ESO2) received FDA clearance and was available as

Z. Li et al. (eds.), *Handbook of Capsule Endoscopy*,
DOI: 10.1007/978-94-017-9229-5_4, © Springer Science+Business Media Dordrecht 2014

early as 2007 [1]. Advantages of ECE include the elimination of the need for conscious sedation and intubation i.e. the minimally invasive nature of the test, and the ability to obtain high-resolution images of the upper part of the gastrointestinal (GI) tract (Fig. 4.1a).

## 4.2    Ingestion Protocol

Small-bowel and colon capsules are typically ingested whilst the patient is sitting upright and water is given to aid passage of the capsule through the gastro-oesophageal junction (GEJ). Due to the inherent function of the oesophagus to act as efficient conduit into the stomach, it was necessary to develop a modified ingestion protocol for ECE. Normal solid oesophageal transit time is between 4 and 8 s [2] and, as such, too rapid to allow enough number of images for meaningful interpretation. Table 4.1 details the original ingestion protocol used in clinical trials and early ECE/ESO1 studies. This protocol resulted in highly variable oesophageal transit times between 6 and 1,200 s [1, 3] with a mean oesophageal transit time of 189 s. It should be noted that use of a real-time viewer is essential during ECE studies.

Pendlebury et al. [4] further modified this protocol in an attempt to enhance imaging of the gastric lumen. An extra stage between stage 5 and 6 was added involving the patient lying flat and then rolling onto their left and right sides for 2 min each. The patient was then allowed to sit upright whilst the test completed. This group also employed the use of prokinetics (Metoclopramide or Domperidone) to increase visualisation of the duodenum during ECE studies, however results were mixed.

Unfortunately effective image visualisation of the oesophagus and GEJ remained an issue prompting Gralnek et al. [1, 5] to develop a simplified ingestion protocol (SIP). This protocol has the patient ingesting the capsule whilst lying in the right lateral position. Sips of 15 ml of water are given every 30 s from a syringe

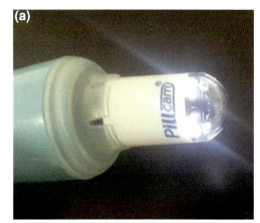
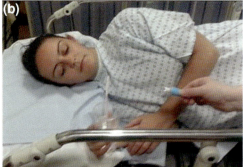
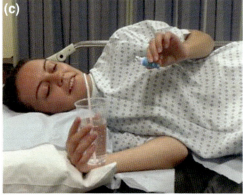
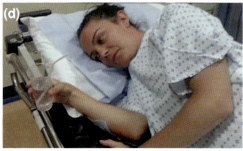

**Fig. 4.1**  **a** PillCamESO2. **b, c, d** Current ESO ingestion protocol as per text

**Table 4.1** Original ECE ingestion protocol

| Protocol stage | Duration | Angle of elevation |
|---|---|---|
| 1. Ingestion of 100 ml water whilst in upright position | 5 s | N/A |
| 2. Ingestion of capsule in supine position with 20 ml water | 2 min | 0° |
| 3. First elevation of back position | 2 min | 30° |
| 4. Second elevation of back position | 2 min | 60° |
| 5. Sip of water | 2 min | 60° |
| 6. Sit upright | 20 min | 90° |

(or via a straw) until the capsule enters the stomach (Fig. 4.1b–d).

SIP improved on the original protocol by significantly extending oesophageal transit time (mean 3 m 45 s vs. 0 min 38 s; $p = 0.0001$) and improving visualisation of the GEJ but with no change in the number of GEJ frames captured [1]. De Jonge et al. (2008) [6] reported that SIP increased complete visualisation rate of the GEJ in a group of patients with Barrett's and reflux oesophagitis when compared to the original protocol (93 vs. 68 % $p = 0.04$) and improved sensitivity in the diagnosis of these disorders. SIP has now been adopted as the protocol of choice for ECE in clinical centres [1, 7].

## 4.3 Clinical Use of Oesophageal Capsule Endoscopy

### 4.3.1 Barrett's Oesophagus Screening

Gastro-oesophageal reflux disease (GERD) is a common problem [8] and a risk factor for developing Barrett's oesophagus which occurs in 5–15 % of patients with symptomatic GERD [7]. Barrett's oesophagus is associated with 0.5 % annual incidence of high-grade dysplasia or oesophageal adenocarcinoma [7, 9]. Therefore, efforts to curb its incidence have been

focused on the use of selective screening of high risk (for developing Barrett's oesophagus) individuals [10]. Although there are currently no controlled trials to examine the validity of this surveillance strategy, esophagogastroscopy (EGD) remains the gold standard for the examination of the oesophagus [7]. EGD though is invasive, often uncomfortable and may be poorly tolerated; moreover, sedation carries risks that are not negligible, especially with increasing age [1, 11, 12].

Therefore, ECE seems to be a prime alternative candidate for this task. Several studies have been conducted since the first report of the use of PillCam®ESO1 in the diagnosis of oesophageal disorders that involved a small group 17 patients with GERD symptomatology [3, 13]. The first systematic assessment was a meta-analysis in 2009 [14]. This was carried out in order to calculate the pooled sensitivity/specificity of ECE for the diagnosis of Barrett's oesophagus. Subgroup analyses were performed based on the reference standard used. Nine studies, comprising a total of 618 patients, were included. In the majority of included studies, PillCam®ESO1 was used [15–19], whilst in one study [20] the current model (ESO2) was utilised. The PillCam® SB on a string was also used in another study [21]. Allowing for this heterogeneity, the pooled sensitivity and specificity for the diagnosis of Barrett's oesophagus was 77 and 86 %, respectively. In subgroup analyses, when EGD and histopathology-confirmed intestinal metaplasia was taken as reference standard, pooled sensitivity/specificity of ECE was 78/90 % and 78/73 %, respectively. Furthermore, ECE was found to be safe and had a high rate of patient preference. However, on the basis of ECE moderate sensitivity/specificity for the diagnosis of Barrett's, the authors concluded that in patients with GERD, conventional EGD remains the modality of choice for evaluation of suspected Barrett's (Fig. 4.2a–d).

Interestingly, despite the fact that oesophageal inspection with single-head viewing capsules is disappointing [22–24], due to the rapid movement of the capsule and low capture frame rate together with the upright swallowing protocol, the string-

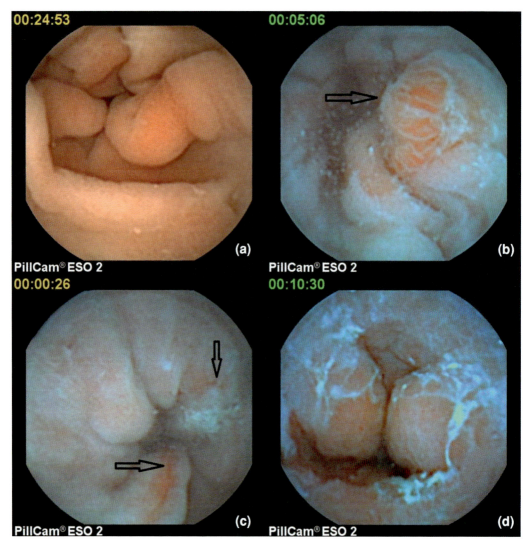

**Fig. 4.2** **a** Normal gastro-oesophageal junction (*GEJ*) (under *white light*), **b** inflammatory nodule at the GEJ (under *blue mode*), **c** oesophagitis (under *blue mode*), **d** fibrous ring and bleeding at the GEJ (under *blue mode*)

capsule endoscopy devised by Ramirez et al. [21] and later modified by Liao et al. [25], allow converting a purely passive process to an operator-controlled procedure (Fig. 4.3) [26, 27]. With this simple modification, dwell time in the oesophagus is increased and real-time monitoring of the images on a standard real-time viewer is feasible. Furthermore, after high-level of glutaraldehyde disinfection [25] or disposal of the removable latex sheath, the capsules can be reused multiple times, thus allowing significant cost-effectiveness (Fig. 4.4). Despite the aforementioned advantages, it should be noted that tethered capsule endoscopy has not received official approval (FDA or CE), therefore its use cannot be recommended.

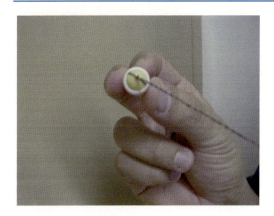

**Fig. 4.3** A string-capsule endoscope. Reprint with permission from Gastrointest Endosc [56]

## 4.4 Oesophageal Varices Screening

The most common cause of portal hypertension is liver cirrhosis. It is estimated that cirrhosis accounts for more than 25,000 deaths and 373,000 hospital discharges in 1998 [28]. The rise in portal pressure is associated with the development of collateral circulation (varices) [29]. Cirrhotic patients develop varices at a rate of 8 % per year [29]. The risk of variceal rupture/haemorrhage increases with the size of varices [29]. The average mortality of the first episode of variceal bleeding is ∼ 50 % [30]. Since primary prophylactic treatment (band ligation or non-selective beta-blockade) in cirrhotic patients with medium/large size varices reduces the risk of bleeding and mortality, current guidelines stress the importance of variceal screening [29]. The gold standard in the diagnosis of varices is EGD. Endoscopic screening is recommended for every 1–3 years, depending with the size of varices on index endoscopy [3, 30].

In 2006, pilot studies from the States and France [3, 31, 32] reported high sensitivity and specificity (81–100 % and 89–100 %, respectively) in the detection of varices. Since then, an increasing evidence base allowed 2 meta-analyses. In the first meta-analysis (2010), Lu et al. included seven studies [33], all comparing the yield of ECE and EGD in patients diagnosed or suspected of having oesophageal varices. All were performed with the first ESO model (Pill-Cam®ESO1). In a total of 446 patients, the pooled sensitivity and specificity of ECE for detecting oesophageal varices was 85.8 and 80.5 %, respectively. In subgroup analyses, the pooled sensitivity/specificity in patients undergoing oesophageal varices screening and in those under surveillance was 82.7/54.8 % and 87.3/84.7 %, respectively. A year later, Guturu et al. [34, 35] presented a meta-analysis of 9 studies, comprising a total of 631 patients, comparing the use of ECE and EGD in screening and surveillance of oesophageal varices. In 619 patients (they were 12 capsule failures), the pooled sensitivity and specificity of Pill-Cam®ESO 1 (as compared to conventional EGD) was 83 and 85 %, respectively. Pooled likelihood ratios (LR) for the detection of oesophageal varices by ECE were also calculated. It is accepted that LR > 5 and < 0.2 give strong diagnostic evidence. The pooled positive likelihood and negative likelihood ratios were 4.09 and 0.25, respectively. Therefore, the authors concluded that ECE can only be an acceptable alternative in certain situations, but it cannot be recommended as replacement option for conventional EGD (Fig. 4.5).

The string/tethered PillCam®SB seem to perform similarly well to its ESO counterpart. In a feasibility study [36] by Ramirez et al., 30 patients with clinical liver cirrhosis were enroled, 19 for surveillance and 11 for screening purposes. The procedure was safe (no strings were disrupted and no capsule was lost). The mean recording time was 5.8 min, the accuracy 96.7 % with only minimal discomfort. The majority (83.3 %) of patients preferred string-capsule endoscopy to EGD. A follow-up study was published in 2012 [37]; 100 patients (33 for screening and 67 for surveillance) were enroled. The sensitivity and specificity of tethered capsule endoscopy for clinically significant varices was 82 and 90 %, respectively with a PPV of 84 % and NPV of 89 %.

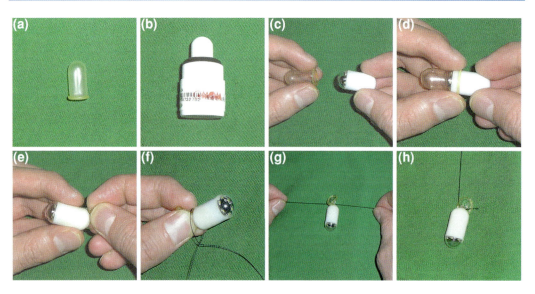

**Fig. 4.4** The procedure of sleeve string-capsule endos-copy. **a**. The latex sleeve. **b** The OMOM® capsule endoscope. **c**, **d**, **e** Enclosing the capsule with the sleeve. **f**, **g**, **h** The string attachment. Reprint with permission from Gastrointest Endosc [25]

**Fig. 4.5** Varices as seen with ESO

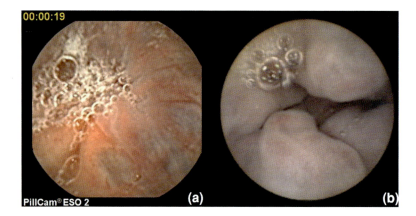

## 4.5 Contraindications and Complications

It should not be forgotten that ECE, despite its reduced battery life, has to traverse the rest of the GI tract to be excreted. Therefore, the same contraindications that apply for small-bowel capsule endoscopy e.g. known and/or suspected critical bowel stenosis, pregnancy and/or prior complex abdominal surgery, apply for ECE. Moreover, ECE is contraindicated in patients with oesophageal achalasia and/or known oesophageal diverticulae [38–40]. Furthermore, the patients with known oropharyngeal dysfunction (due to high risk of aspiration) should be discouraged. Such group includes often elderly patients with oesophageal dysmotility problems. To date, unlike SBCE, there is no recorded case of aspiration of PillCam®ESO but this may be related to the frequency of its use [41]. Of course, some of the above contraindications are obsolete, in case the tethered capsule is used.

## 4.6 Alternatives

Minimally invasive alternatives for examining the oesophagus and the stomach include the trans-nasal endoscopy with ultrathin scopes and/or single use endoscopes [42, 43] (Fig. 4.6). Moreover, the advent of a magnetically controlled capsule will theoretically allow an accurate (wireless) examination of the upper digestive tract [44–47]. Swain et al. [44] modified a capsule endoscope to include neodymium-iron-boron magnets. The capsule's magnetic switch was replaced with a thermal one that turns on by hot water. One imager was removed from the PillCam® colon and the available space was used to house the magnets. In the first-in-human study, a handheld external magnet used to manipulate this capsule in the oesophagus of a volunteer. The capsule was swallowed and observed in the oesophagus by using a gastroscope. Capsule images were viewed on a real-time viewer. The capsule was manipulated in the oesophagus for 10 min. Furthermore, Hale et al. [45] showed that examination of the upper gastrointestinal tract is feasible in a porcine model using a magnet and positional change. Using a handheld magnet, Mirocam Navi (Intromedic Ltd), positional changes and a "real-time" viewer hey showed satisfactory marker recognition (Fig. 4.7).

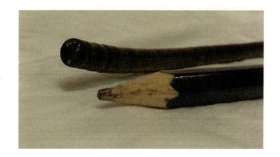

**Fig. 4.6** Transnasal endoscpe (Fujinon Corp)

Using PillCam®ESO1, Di Biase et al. [48] showed that 8/88 post-RFA patients had oesophageal lesions anatomically consistent with the location of the ablation catheter. PillCam®ESO was well tolerated and provided satisfactory oesophageal images without potential risk related to insufflation with regular EGD. Furthermore, anti-acid therapy can be rationalised this way [48].

Patients with haemophilia or other coagulation defects such as von Willebrand's disease are at risk of harbouring variant Creutzfeldt-Jakob disease (vCJD), hence at risk transmission to others in cases of "invasive" procedure with conventional endoscopes [49]. Data from our hospital show that the preferential use of ECE in this patient cohort is cost-effective, well tolerated and provides satisfactory oesophageal surveillance and [50, 51] diagnostic yield in this subgroup of patient with high pretest probability of varices due to previous, transfusion-related infections such as hepatitis C.

## 4.7 Specialised Groups

Although the use of ECE is not currently recommended as a first line test for screening of GERD or cirrhosis-related complications in relevant guidelines by scientific societies, there is certainly a niche for ECE in cases of patients who are either unwilling or unable to tolerate conventional upper GI endoscopy, patients with possible oesophageal injury due to a prior left atrial radiofrequency ablation (RFA) and patients with haemophilia.

Oesophageal injury can result from left atrial RFA therapy and it can potentially lead to the development of atrial-oesophageal fistulae.

## 4.8 Capsule Options for the Future

Magnetically controlled capsule endoscopes have been into the development phase for quite a whilst now. External control of the capsule movement holds promise for reliable wireless gastroscopy [44–47], whilst the recent advent of tethered capsule endomicroscopy which involves swallowing an optomechanically engineered pill that captures cross-sectional microscopic images of the gut wall at 30 μm

**(a)**

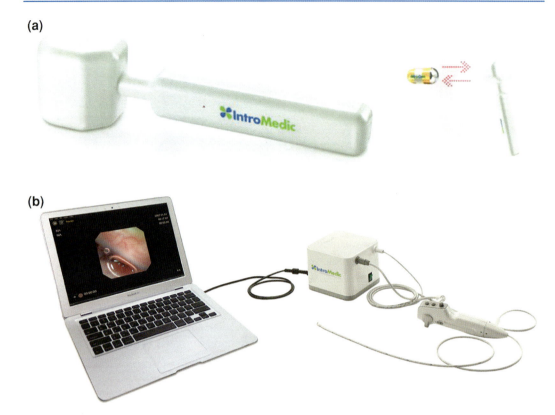

**(b)**

**Fig. 4.7** **a** Handheld magnet for control of the MiroCam Navi (courtesy of Intromedic Ltd.). **b** EG scan, a novel disposable endoscopy for transnasal application with system (*right*) and screen (*left*) (courtesy of IntroMedic Co Ltd)

(lateral) × 7 µm (axial) resolution as it travels through the digestive tract [52–55]. Results in human subjects show that this technique rapidly provides three-dimensional, microstructural images of the upper gastrointestinal tract in a simple and painless procedure, opening up new opportunities for screening for internal diseases [52].

**Conflict of Interest Statement** Anastasios Koulaouzidis has received research Grant from Given®Imaging Ltd., Germany (ESGE-Given®Imaging Research Grant 2011) and material support for capsule endoscopy research from SYNMED©, both unrelated to the present work. Ms. S. Douglas and Prof J.N. Plevris has previously received research support from Fujinon Corp for a research fellow.

## References

1. Waterman M, Gralnek IM. Capsule endoscopy of the esophagus. J Clin Gastroenterol. 2009;43:605–12.
2. Eriksen CA, Holdsworth RJ, Sutton D, Kennedy N, Cuschieri A. The solid bolus oesophageal egg transit test: its manometric interpretation and usefulness as a screening test. Br J Surg. 1987;74:1130–3.
3. Gerson LB. Screening for esophageal varices: is esophageal capsule endoscopy ready for prime time? J Clin Gastroenterol. 2009;43:899–901.
4. Pendlebury J, Douglas S, Plevris JN. Wireless oesophageal video capsule endoscopy: preliminary experience in seven patients. Gut. 2006;55:A65.
5. Gralnek IM, Rabinovitz R, Afik D, Eliakim R. A simplified ingestion procedure for esophageal capsule endoscopy: initial evaluation in healthy volunteers. Endoscopy. 2006;38:913–8.

6. De Jonge PJ, Van Eijck BC, Geldof H, Bekkering FC, Essink-Bot ML, Polinder S, Kuipers EJ, Siersema PD. Capsule endoscopy for the detection of oesophageal mucosal disorders: a comparison of two different ingestion protocols. Scand J Gastroenterol. 2008;43:870–7.

7. http://www.bsg.org.uk/images/stories/docs/clinical/guidelines/oesophageal/Barretts_Oes.pdf.

8. Kahrilas PJ. Clinical practice. Gastroesophageal reflux disease. N Engl J Med. 2008;359:1700–7.

9. Atkinson M, Chak A. Screening for Barrett's esophagus. Tech Gastrointest Endosc. 2010;12:62–6.

10. Spechler SJ. Barrett esophagus and risk of esophageal cancer: a clinical review. JAMA. 2013;310:627–36.

11. Romero-Vázquez J, Jiménez-García VA, Herrerías-Gutiérrez JM. Esophageal capsule endoscopy and Barrett's esophagus: where are we in 2013? Rev Gastroenterol Mex. 2013;78:55–6.

12. Sharma VK, Eliakim R, Sharma P. Faigel D; ICCE. ICCE consensus for esophageal capsule endoscopy. Endoscopy. 2005;37:1060–4.

13. Eliakim R, Yassin K, Shlomi I, Suissa A, Eisen GM. A novel diagnostic tool for detecting oesophageal pathology: the PillCam oesophageal video capsule. Aliment Pharmacol Ther. 2004;20:1083–9.

14. Bhardwaj A, Hollenbeak CS, Pooran N, Mathew A. A meta-analysis of the diagnostic accuracy of esophageal capsule endoscopy for Barrett's esophagus in patients with gastroesophageal reflux disease. Am J Gastroenterol. 2009;104:1533–9.

15. Eliakim R, Sharma VK, Yassin K, et al. A prospective study of the diagnostic accuracy of PillCam ESO esophageal capsule endoscopy versus conventional upper endoscopy in patients with chronic gastroesophageal reflux diseases. J Clin Gastroenterol. 2005;39:572–8.

16. Koslowsky B, Jacob H, Eliakim R, et al. PillCam ESO in esophageal studies: improved diagnostic yield of 14 frames per second (fps) compared with 4 fps. Endoscopy. 2006;38:27–30.

17. Sharma P, Wani S, Rastogi A, et al. The diagnostic accuracy of esophageal capsule endoscopy in patients with gastroesophageal reflux disease and Barrett's esophagus: a blinded, prospective study. Am J Gastroenterol. 2008;103:525–32.

18. Lin OS, Schembre DB, Mergener K, et al. Blinded comparison of esophageal capsule endoscopy versus conventional endoscopy for a diagnosis of Barrett's esophagus in patients with chronic gastroesophageal reflux. Gastrointest Endosc. 2007;65:577–83.

19. Galmiche JP, Sacher-Huvelin S, Coron E, et al. Screening for esophagitis and Barrett's esophagus with wireless esophageal capsule endoscopy: a multicenter prospective trial in patients with reflux symptoms. Am J Gastroenterol. 2008;103:538–45.

20. Gralnek IM, Adler SN, Yassin K, et al. Detecting esophageal disease with second-generation capsule endoscopy: initial evaluation of the PillCam ESO 2. Endoscopy. 2008;40:275–9.

21. Ramirez FC, Akins R, Shaukat M. Screening of Barrett's esophagus with string-capsule endoscopy: a prospective blinded study of 100 consecutive patients using histology as the criterion standard. Gastrointest Endosc. 2008;68:25–31.

22. Fernandez-Urien I, Borobio E, Elizalde I, Irisarri R, Vila JJ, Urman JM, Jimenez J. Z-line examination by the PillCam SB: prospective comparison of three ingestion protocols. World J Gastroenterol. 2010;16:63–8.

23. Koulaouzidis A. Upper oesophageal images and Z-line detection with 2 different small-bowel capsule systems. World J Gastroenterol. 2012;18:6003–4.

24. Koulaouzidis A, Douglas S, Plevris JN. Identification of the ampulla of Vater during oesophageal capsule endoscopy: two heads and viewing speed make a difference. Eur J Gastroenterol Hepatol. 2011;23:361.

25. Liao Z, Gao R, Xu C, Xu DF, Li ZS. Sleeve string capsule endoscopy for real-time viewing of the esophagus: a pilot study (with video). Gastrointest Endosc. 2009;70:201–9.

26. Hale W. Esophageal capsule endoscopy: the string is the thing. Gastrointest Endosc. 2009;70:210–1.

27. Weston AP. String capsule endoscopy: a viable method for screening for Barrett's esophagus? Gastrointest Endosc. 2008;68:32–4.

28. Rondonotti E, Villa F, Dell' Era A, Tontini GE, de Franchis R. Capsule endoscopy in portal hypertension. Clin Liver Dis. 2010;14:209–20.

29. http://www.bsg.org.uk/images/stories/docs/clinical/guidelines/liver/vari_hae.pdf.

30. http://www.aasld.org/practiceguidelines/documents/bookmarked%20practice%20guidelines/prevention%20and%20management%20of%20gastro%20varices%20and%20hemorrhage.pdf.

31. Eisen GM, Eliakim R, Zaman A, et al. The accuracy of PillCam ESO capsule endoscopy versus conventional upper endoscopy for the diagnosis of esophageal varices: a prospective three-center pilot study. Endoscopy. 2006;38:31–5.

32. Lapalus MG, Dumortier J, Fumex F, et al. Esophageal capsule endoscopy versus esophagogastroduodenoscopy for evaluating portal hypertension: a prospective comparative study of performance and tolerance. Endoscopy. 2006;38:36–41.

33. Lu Y, Gao R, Liao Z, Hu LH, Li ZS. Meta-analysis of capsule endoscopy in patients diagnosed or suspected with esophageal varices. World J Gastroenterol. 2009;15:1254–8.

34. Ahn D, Guturu P. Meta-analysis of capsule endoscopy in patients diagnosed or suspected with esophageal varices. World J Gastroenterol. 2010;16:785–6.

35. Guturu P, Sagi SV, Ahn D, Jaganmohan S, Kuo YF, Sood GK. Capsule endoscopy with PILLCAM ESO for detecting esophageal varices: a meta-analysis. Minerva Gastroenterol Dietol. 2011;57:1–11.

36. Ramirez FC, Hakim S, Tharalson EM, Shaukat MS, Akins R. Feasibility and safety of string wireless capsule endoscopy in the diagnosis of esophageal varices. Am J Gastroenterol. 2005;100:1065–71.

37. Stipho S, Tharalson E, Hakim S, Akins R, Shaukat M, Ramirez FC. String capsule endoscopy for screening and surveillance of esophageal varices in patients with cirrhosis. J Interventional Gastroenterol. 2012;2:54–60.

38. Ziachehabi A, Maieron A, Hoheisel U, Bachl A, Hagenauer R, Schöfl R. Capsule retention in a Zenker's diverticulum. Endoscopy 2011;43 Suppl 2 UCTN:E387.

39. Kropf JA, Jeanmonod R, Yen DM. An unusual presentation of a chronic ingested foreign body in an adult. J Emerg Med. 2013;44:82–4.

40. Kelly OB, O'Donnell S, O'Moráin CA. A case of achalasia diagnosed first on capsule endoscopy: find that hard to swallow? Eur J Gastroenterol Hepatol. 2010;22:1013–4.

41. Koulaouzidis A, Rondonotti E, Karargyris A. Small-bowel capsule endoscopy: a ten-point contemporary review. World J Gastroenterol. 2013;19:3726–46.

42. Alexandridis EG, Trimble K, Hayes P, Plevris JN. OC-045 Randomised prospective trial of transnasal versus standard upper diagnostic endoscopy under local anaesthetic: interim analysis of endoscopy quality, patient acceptability and tolerability. Gut. 2012;61:A19–20.

43. http://www.intromedic.com/eng/sub_products_3. html.

44. Keller J, Fibbe C, Volke F, Gerber J, Mosse AC, Reimann-Zawadzki M, RabinovitzE, Layer P, Swain P. Remote magnetic control of a wireless capsule endoscope in the esophagus is safe and feasible: results of a randomized, clinical trial in healthy volunteers. Gastrointest Endosc 2010;72:941–6.

45. Hale MF, Drew K, Baldacchino T, Anderson S, Sanders DS, Riley SA, Sidhu R, McAlindon ME. Gastroscopy without a gastroscope! feasibility in a porcine model using a magnetic capsule. Gut. 2013;62:A156.

46. Rey JF, Ogata H, Hosoe N, Ohtsuka K, Ogata N, Ikeda K, Aihara H, Pangtay I, Hibi T, Kudo S, Tajiri H. Feasibility of stomach exploration with a guided capsule endoscope. Endoscopy. 2010;42:541–5.

47. Carpi F, Kastelein N, Talcott M, Pappone C. Magnetically controllable gastrointestinal steering of video capsules. IEEE Trans Biomed Eng. 2011;58:231–4.

48. Di Biase L, Dodig M, Saliba W, Siu A, Santisi J, Poe S, Sanaka M, Upchurch B, Vargo J, Natale A. Capsule endoscopy in examination of esophagus for lesions after radiofrequency catheter ablation: a potential tool to select patients with increased risk of complications. J Cardiovasc Electrophysiol. 2010;21:839–44.

49. http://www.bsg.org.uk/clinical-guidelines/endoscopy/ guidelines-for-decontamination-of-equipment-for-gastrointestinal-endoscopy.html.

50. Koulaouzidis A, Douglas S, Plevris JN. Refining the indications for oesophageal capsule endoscopy in a tertiary referral centre in Scotland. Endoscopy 2008;40:A 308.

51. Ang YL, Koulaouzidis A, Douglas S, Plevris JN. PTH-068 the use of oesophageal capsule endoscopy in patients with haemophilia. Experience from a tertiary centre. Gut. 2013;62:A238–9.

52. Gora MJ, Sauk JS, Carruth RW, Lu W, Carlton DT, Soomro A, Rosenberg M, Nishioka NS, Tearney GJ. Unsedated imaging of human upper GI tract using tethered capsule endomicroscopy. Gastroenterology 7 Aug 2013. (Epub ahead of print).

53. Gora MJ, Sauk JS, Carruth RW, Gallagher KA, Suter MJ, Nishioka NS, Kava LE, Rosenberg M, Bouma BE, Tearney GJ. Tethered capsule endomicroscopy enables less invasive imaging of gastrointestinal tract microstructure. Nat Med. 2013;19:238–40.

54. Ray K. Tethered capsule endomicroscopy of the oesophagus–an easy pill to swallow. Nat Rev Gastroenterol Hepatol. 2013;10:129.

55. Fillon SA, Harris JK, Wagner BD, Kelly CJ, Stevens MJ, Moore W, Fang R, Schroeder S, Masterson JC, Robertson CE, Pace NR, Ackerman SJ, Furuta GT. Novel device to sample the esophageal microbiome–the esophageal string test. PLoS ONE. 2012;7:e42938.

56. Khan B, Ramirez FC, Shaukat M, et al. String capsule endoscopy: a novel application for the preoperative identification of a small-bowel obscure GI bleeding source (with video). Gastrointest Endosc. 2011;73(2):403–5.

# Colon Capsule Endoscopy

**5**

## Cristiano Spada and Samuel Adler

Colon capsule endoscopy (CCE) is a noninvasive, painless, swallowed endoscopic technique that is able to explore the colon without requiring sedation and gas insufflation. The CCE system includes a colon capsule (PillCam Colon Capsule 2—CCE-2), a data recorder and a software for video processing and viewing (Fig. 5.1). The colon capsule is 11.6 x 31.5 mm in size. It has 2 optical domes with an angle of view of 172° for each imager, allowing nearly 360° coverage of the colon. In order to enhance colon visualization and to save battery energy, the capsule is equipped with an adaptive frame rate [1, 2]. CCE captures up to 35 images/s when in motion and as few as 4 images/s when it is stationary. This advanced system for the control of capsule image rate is the result of a bidirectional communication between the colon capsule and the data recorder that, besides storing the images transmitted from the capsule, also controls the capsule image rate in real time, analyzing the capsule images. To further save battery energy, as well as to allow automatic identification of the small-bowel, colon capsule endoscopy works at a low rate of only 14 images/min after swallowing until small-bowel images are detected, then it switches into the adaptive frame rate. The automatic small-bowel detection is able to recognize when the capsule enters the small bowel. At this point, the data recorder buzzes and vibrates and displays instructions on its liquid crystal diode (LCD) screen to alert the patient to continue the preparation protocol, assisting and guiding the physician and the patient through the procedure.

## 5.1 Regimen of Preparation and Procedure

During CCE, as the capsule is not equipped to insufflate the colon, aspirate liquids, wash the mucosal surface and move actively along the gut, the cleansing protocol cannot be restricted to the time before the procedure but has to be continued during it. The cleansing protocol for CCE aims at (a) adequately cleansing the colonic mucosa, (b) filling the colon lumen with clear liquids to improve mucosal visualization and to decrease the number of air bubbles and (c) facilitating capsule progression so that it reaches the anal verge before battery life ends. Therefore, before capsule ingestion, patients are invited to follow a regimen of preparation specifically designed for CCE (Table 5.1) [2, 3].

As for conventional colonoscopy, a low residue diet is often recommended during the 3–5 days before the bowel cleansing protocol

C. Spada (✉)
Digestive Endoscopy Unit, Catholic University, Rome, Italy
e-mail: cristianospada@gmail.com

S. Adler
Department of Gastroenterology, Shaare Zedek Medical Center, Jerusalem, Israel

Z. Li et al. (eds.), *Handbook of Capsule Endoscopy*,
DOI: 10.1007/978-94-017-9229-5_5, © Springer Science+Business Media Dordrecht 2014

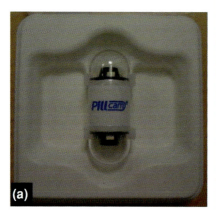
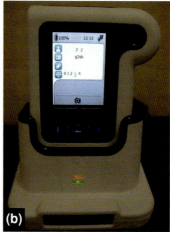
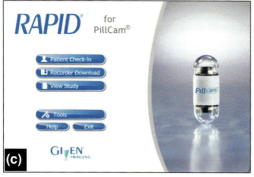
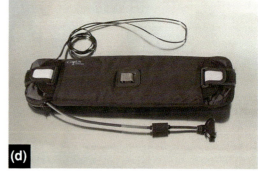

**Fig. 5.1** The new generation of colon capsule endoscopy system. **a** The second generation colon capsule (PillCam colon 2, given Imaging, Israel) is 11.6 x 31.5 mm in size and has 2 optical domes with an angle of view of 172° for each imager. The data recorder (**b**) besides storing the images transmitted from the capsule also (i) controls the capsule image rate in real time, analyzing the capsule images, (ii) it is provided with an LCD for real viewing and (iii) acts also as regimen reminder alerting the patient with an audible and vibrating signal during the day of procedure. A new software (rapid 8) (**c**) improves report and study manager usability. Sensor arrays can be replaced by a more comfortable sensor belt (**d**)

**Table 5.1** Regimen of preparation

| Schedule | | Intake |
|---|---|---|
| Day-2 | All day | At least 10 glasses of water |
| | Bedtime | Four senna tablets, 12 mg each |
| Day-1 | All day | Clear liquid diet |
| | Evening | 2 L PEG |
| Exam Day | Morning | 2 L PEG |
| | ∼ 10 a.m | Capsule ingestion[a] |
| | 1st boost *upon small-bowel detection* | 40 ml NaP and 1 L water |
| | 2nd boost[b] *3 h after 1st boost* | 15–25 ml NaP and 0.5 L water |
| | Suppository *2 h after 2nd boost* | 10 mg Bisacodyl |

[a] 20 mg domperidone tablet if capsule delayed in stomach >1 h
[b] Only if capsule not excreted yet

itself. The aim was to decrease the amount of solid stool in the colon and thus reinforce the lavage effect of polyethylene glycol (PEG) solutions. On the other hand, when CCE is considered, the recent experience seems to suggest that a clear liquid diet prescribed on the day before the procedure might improve the quality of bowel cleansing and consequently the diagnostic yield of CCE. Therefore, diet recommendations (i.e., liquid diet the day before, low residue diet 3–5 days before colon capsule endoscopy) have generally been adopted in the studies published so far.

Starting from the experience with bowel cleansing for colonoscopy, lavage solutions with large volumes (4L) of polyethylene glycol (PEG) solutions have been used in most studies with colon capsule endoscopy. Very little experience with lower doses of PEG is currently available and, therefore, low-dose of PEG is not recommended. Studies demonstrating the equivalence of lower volumes cleansing and PEG protocols for conventional colonoscopies can not be extended to CCE.

A split regimen of PEG is recommended: 2 L of PEG on the day before and 2 L on the day of CCE. This split $(2 + 2)$ regimen of preparation seems to be more acceptable by the patients and equally effective in terms of colon cleanliness [3].

To meet the specific goals of bowel cleansing for colon capsule discussed above, phosphate (NaP) boosters have been added to the classical PEG and diet recommendations used for conventional colonoscopy. The role of boosters administered during capsule progression is not limited to increase and/or maintain colonic cleanliness but includes also a propulsive effect by means of a volume effect allowing the capsule to move in a watery environment. The propulsive effect of NaP boosters results in an effective colon capsule transit along the small and large bowels with a higher rate of capsule expulsion within the limited operating time of the capsule battery. A low NaP dose (total, 45 or 55 mL) is recommended: usually 30 ml of NaP at the small-bowel detection (1st booster) and 15–25 ml of NaP (2nd booster) 2 h after the 1st booster [3].

Prokinetics have been added to the protocol of bowel preparation of CCE mainly to stimulate the progression of the capsule in the upper gut, especially the stomach. Administration of prokinetics should be limited to cases where the capsule had not entered the small bowel within 1 h after ingestion [3].

One of the main advantages of CCE for patients is the option of out-of-clinic colonoscopy. This is possible because the data recorder can be programmed to synchronize with the prescribed regimen to alert the patient with an audible and vibrating signal to view the number displayed on its LCD screen. The "home procedure" was recently evaluated in a prospective study in which 41 patients with known or suspected colonic diseases were offered CCE to be performed as an out-of clinic procedure [4]. According to data recorder-registered alerts, 14 patients (34 %) required a single booster only, 27 patients (66 %) required two boosters and 13 patients (32 %) required a suppository. Patient compliance to data recorder alerts was 100 %. During the procedure, 16 patients (39 %) called the physician/clinic from home for doubts and/or need of explanations. In all the cases, the reason for the call was managed by telephone. In 85 % of the cases, the colon capsule was excreted within the battery operating time. The results of this study suggest that as an out-of-clinic procedure, CCE is feasible and easily performed. A home-based procedure may be associated with better acceptability and potentially with increased adherence to colorectal cancer screening.

## 5.2   Indications and Contraindications

CCCE is feasible, safe and appears to be accurate when used in average risk subjects [3]. Patients with non-alarm symptoms do not appear to be at increased risk of colorectal neoplasia. For this reason, noninvasive tests may be proposed in this setting as an alternative to colonoscopy. Among noninvasive tests, however, imaging tests might be preferred over

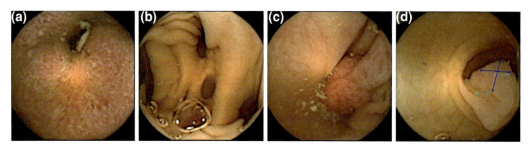

**Fig. 5.2** Findings at colon capsule endoscopy. A typical image of ulcerative colitis (**a**) and diverticulae (**b**). A pedunculated polyp (**c**) and a 9 mm polyp in the sigmoid (**d**). The new software for CCE includes a tool for polyp size estimation. One can place the mouse cursor at one end of the polyp and drag the cursor to the other end. The software immediately calculates the distance and shows the dimension of the polyp in millimeters

nonimaging tests (i.e., fecal tests), because of the ability to detect non-neoplastic conditions that may be regarded as clinically useful (e.g., vascular malformations). Among noninvasive imaging tests, CCE may be applicable to this setting for the considerations of its feasibility, safety and accuracy.

Patients at high risk for colorectal cancer should be referred for colonoscopy, since a test with a very high sensitivity is desirable as the primary option. In this setting, the role of capsule endoscopy should be limited to those patients not compliant with colonoscopy.

The role of CCE in patients with a previous incomplete conventional colonoscopy has been evaluated in several trials [5–7] all showing that the colon capsule is feasible, safe and accurate in visualizing segments unexplored by the previous incomplete colonoscopy, suggesting that incomplete colonoscopy is an indication for CCE [3, 5–7].

To date, there is insufficient data to support the use of CCE in the diagnostic work-up or in the surveillance of patients with suspected or known inflammatory bowel disease [3]. Based on preliminary data, CCE may be useful to monitor inflammation in ulcerative colitis, which may help to guide therapy. In this setting, the first generation of colon capsule has been compared to colonoscopy [8] with the aim to evaluate its accuracy in monitoring colonic inflammation in patients with suspected or known ulcerative colitis. In this preliminary experience, CCE yielded encouraging results for detecting active ulcerative colitis (i.e., sensitivity, 77 %; specificity, 78 %) and substantial agreement with colonoscopy [8]. A study performed on 40 patients with histological confirmed diagnosis of UC using the new generation of colon capsule confirms that colon capsule might be feasible for assessing the severity of mucosal inflammation in patients with ulcerative colitis [9] (Fig. 5.2).

The role of colon capsule endoscopy in colorectal cancer screening is still unclear since no data are available in this setting nor on the possible adherence to CCE in a screening setting [3]. A previous cost-effectiveness analysis has compared the first generation of CCE with colonoscopy in a screening setting. Although CCE was not a cost-effective alternative when assuming an equal adherence, it became an efficient option when assuming that adherence to CCE was higher compared to colonoscopy for colorectal cancer screening, a feature which has not been demonstrated yet using the second generation capsule [10, 11]

Regarding the contraindication for CCE, these are similar to those of small-bowel capsule endoscopy. However, since the procedure includes also sodium phosphate-based boosters, it should be remembered that the use of sodium phosphate should be avoided in patients at increased risk of sodium phosphate toxicity [3].

## 5.3 Results

The accuracy of the second generation of CCE for significant finding (polyps or masses ≥6 mm and ≥10 mm) was evaluated in prospective comparative trials with conventional colonoscopy as gold standard. In an Israeli study [1, 2, 12], per-patient sensitivity for polyps ≥6 and ≥10 mm was 89 % (95 % CI, 70–97 %) and 88 % (95 % CI, 56–98 %), with specificities of 76 % (95 % CI, 72–78 %) and 89 % (95 % CI, 86–90 %), respectively [1] (Fig. 5.1).

Similarly, in a European study [2], per-patient sensitivity for polyps ≥6 and ≥10 mm was 84 % (95 % CI, 74–95 %) and 88 % (95 % CI, 76–99 %), with specificities of 64 % (95 % CI, 52–76 %) and 95 % (95 % CI, 90–100 %), respectively [2].

The relatively low specificity observed in both the series was mainly related to a high number of false-positive polyps because of size mismatch (i.e., capsule detected a polyp ≥6 or ≥10 mm that was <6 or <10 mm by colonoscopy). In the European study [2], the authors reported that 20 (80 %) of the 25 false-positive cases at CCE (6–9 mm, 21 cases; ≥10 mm, 4 cases) were because of size mismatching. Actually, both the CCE and conventional colonoscopy detected polyps. The difference in the polyp size estimation between CCE and colonoscopy represented the main problem that led some of the polyps to be misclassified as false positive. After the unblinding, if these misclassified polyps are considered as true positive results, specificity for any polyp would be as high as 92 % [2].

Recently, CCE was compared in a sixteen-center study [12] with colonoscopy in a cohort of patients classified as average risk per the US Multi-Society Task Force guidelines on colorectal cancer screening. When compared to the Israeli and European trials [1, 2], this study has some peculiarities: (1) the recorded capsule video was reviewed by one of 5 central readers and blinded colonoscopy was performed 4–6 weeks post-colon capsule procedure; (2) the colonoscopist unblinded the capsule report at the end of the colonoscopy and repeated the procedure when the capsule reported "false positive" lesion ≥6 mm. The capsule sensitivity for detecting subjects with adenomas ≥6 and ≥10 mm was 88 % (95 % CI, 82–93) and 92 % (95 % CI, 82–97) respectively, and the specificity was 82 % (95 % CI, 80–83) and 95 % (95 % CI, 94–95). The capsule sensitivity for detecting subjects with any polyp ≥6 and ≥10 mm was 81 % (95 % CI, 77–84) and 80 % (95 % CI, 74–86), respectively, and the specificity was 93 % (95 % CI, 91–95) and 97 % (95 % CI, 96–98) [12].

Interestingly, all trials show similar results in terms of accuracy [1, 2, 10] and when the unblinding is performed routinely [12] the specificity is high. This might suggest that apart the problem of the size mismatch, the low specificity observed in the first trials (i.e., where the unblinding was not included in the design of the trials) was also related to cases that erroneously were classified as false positive at colon capsule and at least some of these cases should be reclassified as false negative cases at colonoscopy rather than colon capsule false-positive cases. In fact, lesions initially classified as colon capsule false positive were actually detected during colonoscopy after the unblinding [12]. In this sense, the presence of a significant finding at colon capsule might serve as a guide during the following colonoscopy and might prompt the endoscopist to perform a very careful colonoscopy.

Recently in a prospective, blinded trial colon capsule was compared to CT-colonography (CTC) in patients with incomplete colonoscopy [5]. To evaluate the incremental value of colon capsule and CTC, the efficacy analysis was performed considering significant findings (polyps/masses ≥6 mm) in segments not visualized during first colonoscopy. In case of significant findings and/or discrepancies, a second colonoscopy (gold standard) was performed. In this trial, 100 patients were enrolled. Colon capsule and CTC were able to complete colonic evaluation in 98 % of cases (i.e., colon capsule and CTC were able to visualize colonic segments which could not have been explored by the previous incomplete colonoscopy). Regarding the diagnostic yield limited to the unexplored segments, colon capsule detected 18 patients [18 % (95 % CI 12–27 %)] with at least a ≥6 mm polyp, while CTC detected 6 patients [6 % (95 % CI 4–13 %)] with at least a ≥6 mm polyp ($p = 0.004$). In the group of patients with at least a polyp ≥10 mm, colon capsule was positive in 7 out of 98 patients [7 % (95 % CI 4–14)] and CTC in 4 [4 % (95 % CI 2–10 %)] ($p = 0.549$). Both the procedures show a high positive predictive value (PPV). In the group of patients with polyps ≥6 mm, the colon capsule results were confirmed in 18 out of 19 patients [95 % (95 % CI 74–100 %)] while the CTC results were confirmed in 6 out of 7 patients [86 % (95 % CI 42–100 %)]. In the group of patients with polyps ≥10 mm, the colon capsule results were confirmed in 7 out of 8 patients [87 % (95 % CI 47–100 %)] while the CTC results were confirmed in 4 out of 4 patients [100 % (86 % CI 40–100 %)]. Results of this study suggest that both, colon capsule endoscopy and CTC, are effective to complete incomplete colonoscopy, but CCE diagnostic yield is significantly higher than CTC for significant polyps in segment unexplored by the previous incomplete colonoscopy.

## 5.4    Safety and Feasibility

CCE is a safe procedure without major complication being reported in over 2,000 procedures; and feasible with a very low rate of technical failures (i.e., 3 %) and a high excretion rate (i.e., over 90 %) [3].

## 5.5    Conclusions

CCCE is a safe, sensitive, noninvasive technique for colon exploration. When coupling this evidence with the feasibility, safety and tolerability, CCE may be considered as an adequate tool to visualize the colorectal mucosa. Colon capsule is not an alternative, but complementary to conventional colonoscopy in average risk subjects or in case of incomplete colonoscopy, when conventional colonoscopy is contraindicated, or in patients who are unwilling to undergo colonoscopy.

## References

1. Eliakim R, Yassin K, Niv Y, Metzger Y, Lachter J, Gal E, Sapoznikov B, Konikoff F, Leichtmann G, Fireman Z, Kopelman Y, Adler SN. Prospective multicenter performance evaluation of the second-generation colon capsule compared with colonoscopy. Endoscopy. 2009;41:1026–31.
2. Spada C, Hassan C, Munoz-Navas M, Neuhaus H, Deviere J, Fockens P, Coron E, Gay G, Toth E, Riccioni ME, Carretero C, Charton JP, Van Gossum A, Wientjes CA, Sacher-Huvelin S, Delvaux M, Nemeth A, Petruzziello L, de Frias CP, Mayershofer R, Amininejad L, Dekker E, Galmiche JP, Frederic M, Johansson GW, Cesaro P, Costamagna G. Second-generation colon capsule endoscopy compared with colonoscopy. Gastrointest Endosc. 2011;74:581–9.
3. Spada C, Hassan C, Galmiche JP, Neuhaus H, Dumonceau JM, Adler S, Epstein O, Gay G, Pennazio M, Rex DK, Benamouzig R, de Franchis R, Delvaux M, Devière J, Eliakim R, Fraser C, Hagenmuller F, Herrerias JM, Keuchel M, Macrae F, Munoz-Navas M, Ponchon T, Quintero E, Riccioni ME, Rondonotti E, Marmo R, Sung JJ, Tajiri H, Toth E, Triantafyllou K, Van Gossum A, Costamagna G. European society of gastrointestinal endoscopy. Colon capsule endoscopy: European society of gastrointestinal endoscopy (ESGE) guideline. Endoscopy 2012; 44:527–36.
4. Adler SN, Hassan C, Metzger Y, Sompolinsky Y, Spada C. Second-generation colon capsule endoscopy is feasible in the out-of-clinic setting. Surg Endosc. 17 Sep 2013. (Epub ahead of print).
5. Spada C, Hassan C, Cesaro P, Barbaro B, Iafrate F, Petruzziello L, Minelli Grazioli L, Alvaro G, Salsano M, Laghi A, Bonomo L, Costamagna G. Prospective trial of pillcam colon capsule (CCE) versus CT-colonography (CTC) in the evaluation of patients with incomplete conventional colonoscopy (CC): an interim analysis. Gastroint est Endosc. 2013; 77:AB163.
6. Alarcón-Fernández O, Ramos L, Adrián-de-Ganzo Z, Gimeno-García AZ, Nicolás-Pérez D, Jiménez A, Quintero E. Effects of colon capsule endoscopy on medical decision making in patients with incomplete colonoscopies. Clin Gastroenterol Hepatol. 2013;11: 534–40.
7. Pioche M, de Leusse A, Filoche B, Dalbiès PA, Adenis Lamarre P, Jacob P, Gaudin JL, Coulom P,

Letard JC, Borotto E, Duriez A, Chabaud JM, Crampon D, Gincul R, Levy P, ben-Soussan E, Garret M, Lapuelle J, Saurin JC. Prospective multicenter evaluation of colon capsule examination indicated by colonoscopy failure or anesthesia contraindication. Endoscopy 2012; 44:911–6.

8. Sung J, Ho KY, Chiu HM, Ching J, Travis S, Peled R. The use of Pillcam Colon in assessing mucosal inflammation in ulcerative colitis: a multicenter study. Endoscopy. 2012;44:754–8.

9. Hosoe N, Matsuoka K, Naganuma M, Ida Y, Ishibashi Y, Kimura K, Yoneno K, Usui S, Kashiwagi K, Hisamatsu T, Inoue N, Kanai T, Imaeda H, Ogata H, Hibi T. Applicability of second-generation colon capsule endoscope to ulcerative colitis: a clinical feasibility study. J Gastroenterol Hepatol. 2013;28:1174–9.

10. Hassan C, Benamouzig R, Spada C, Ponchon T, Zullo A, Saurin JC, Costamagna G. Cost effectiveness and projected national impact of colorectal cancer screening in France. Endoscopy. 2011;43:780–93.

11. Hassan C, Zullo A, Winn S, Morini S. Cost-effectiveness of capsule endoscopy in screening for colorectal cancer. Endoscopy. 2008;40:414–21.

12. Rex DK, Adler S, Aisenberg J, et al. Accuracy of PillCam colon 2 for detecting subjects with adenomas 6 mm. Gastrointest Endosc. 2013; 77:AB29.

# Non-imaging Capsule Endoscopy: The Wireless Motility Capsule to Assess Gut Motility

**6**

Anton Emmanuel

### Abstract

The wireless motility capsule (WMC) is an ambulatory, minimally invasive diagnostic modality that allows continuous assessment of intraluminal pH, temperature, and pressure during its transit through the gastrointestinal (GI) tract. The technology allows for both measurement of transit times in multiple regions of the upper and lower GI tract, as well as pressure profiles in the antro-duodenum. The standardized equipment and procedures in WMC test allow the comparisons of data across multiple sensors. The role of the technology has been best established in the evaluation of patients with suspected gastroparesis and suspected chronic constipation. This review summarizes approximately 50 publications about WMC generated in the last 5 years.

## 6.1 Introduction

Disturbed gut motility and altered visceral sensitivity are thought to be key physiological determinants of the symptoms of the functional gastrointestinal disorders (FGID) such as irritable bowel syndrome, chronic constipation, and gastroparesis [17]. Most patients with FGIDs can be managed by lifestyle and first line pharmacological therapies and do not require specialist physiological investigation [30]. When motility is tested, usually in specialist institutions, it is focused on investigation of the gut region consistent with the chief complaint [27].

However, this may be an insufficient assessment: a majority of patients with slow transit constipation also have abnormal esophageal motility and delayed gastric emptying [1]. These tests often require intrusive intubation or exposure to ionizing radiation. An additional limitation of current testing is that the reproducibility and symptom correlation of motility measurement is poor [4].

## 6.2 Methodology

The wireless motility capsule (WMC) allows measurement of both whole gut and regional transit time in an ambulatory test. Initially, the capsule is calibrated and activated. The $26 \times 13$ mm capsule bears sensors that continuously measure pH, pressure, and temperature

A. Emmanuel (✉)
GI Physiology Unit, University College London, 235 Euston Road, London, NW1 2BU, UK
e-mail: a.emmanuel@ucl.ac.uk

Z. Li et al. (eds.), *Handbook of Capsule Endoscopy*,
DOI: 10.1007/978-94-017-9229-5_6, © Springer Science+Business Media Dordrecht 2014

for up to 5 days after activation. Following an overnight fast and discontinuation of medications that could potentially alter gastric pH and gastrointestinal motility, the capsule is swallowed, followed by a standardized 260-kcal nutrient bar (SmartBar, which consists of 66 % carbohydrate, 17 % protein, 2 % fat, and 3 % fiber) and 120 mL of water. Alternative test meals such as an egg-substitute meal and jam and toast have also been studied, but are less reproducible [15, 25]. The patient abstains from meals for 6 h post-WMC ingestion in order to obtain a standardized measurement of gastric emptying. At that point patients ingest 250 ml Ensure (250 kcal, protein 9 g, carbohydrates 40 g, fat 6 g, fiber 0 g—Abbott Laboratories, Illinois, USA). The fed response to the Ensure manifests as an increase in contraction frequency and/or average amplitude [2]. Thereafter, the patient can eat as normal while the WMC moves through the gut, relaying information telemetrically to a data recorder which must be kept within five feet of his or her body during the testing period. The patient is instructed to record activities such as meals, sleep, and bowel movements by pushing an event button on the data recorder. Strenuous exertion, alcohol, and smoking are prohibited. After 5 days (limit of battery life), or sooner if the capsule is visibly passed in the stools, the patient returns to return the data recorder. Most WMC software generates an automated report including regional transit times; alternatively, the data can be manually reviewed.

## 6.3 Measurement Parameters

### 6.3.1 Transit

Temperature and pH are used to define gut anatomy and hence gut regional transit times. Figure 6.1 shows a sample trace to demonstrate the events and phases as described below:

- Capsule ingestion can be accurately identified as there is marked by a sudden rise in temperature profile.

- Gastric emptying time (GET) is identified as the time from ingestion of the WMC to the abrupt pH rise (>3 pH units) when the WMC leaves the acidic for the duodenum [9].
- Small bowel transit time (SBTT) is defined as the time from capsule ingestion until the abrupt pH drop (>1 pH unit), observed at least 30 min after GET and persisting for a minimum of 10 min, signifying entry into the cecum [34].
- Body exit time is identified as an acute temperature drop when the ambient temperature, rather than body temperature, is sensed.
- Colonic transit time (CTT) is defined as the time from the pH-defined entry of the WMC to the cecum until the temperature-defined body exit time.

### 6.3.2 Pressure

The WMC has a single pressure sensor that records (1) the amplitude and (2) frequency of contractions. It does not identify peristaltic wave propagation since there is a single sensor. Kloetzer et al. [12] have completed normal reference ranges for stomach and proximal small bowel.

Automated software provides the following measurements:
- frequency of contractions (Ct)
- amplitude of contractions, defined as area under the curve (AUC)
- motility index (MI), calculated as the sum of amplitudes × number of contractions + 1).

## 6.4 Clinical Utility

The clinical utility of WMC depends on it (1) offering an improvement over current motility methodologies, (2) providing reproducible results, and (3) correlating with symptoms. Since WMC measurements depend on anatomical identification of landmarks by pH, it is important to know whether the widespread use of proton pump inhibitors (PPI) interferes with measurement. It has been found that although

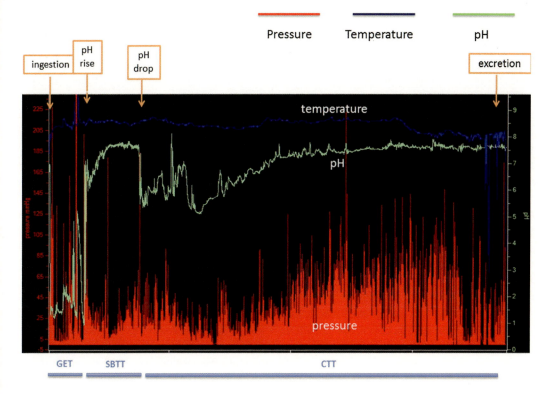

**Fig. 6.1** Sample trace to demonstrate the events and phases

PPI use attenuates the magnitude of pH rise as the WMC leaves the stomach, compared to non-PPI users, there is still a definable pH increase >0.5 units [20], meaning the measurement holds validity in this situation.

### 6.4.1 Gastric Transit

Radio-isotope gastric emptying studies represent the current standard methodology to quantify gastric emptying after a test meal. A wide range of test meals is available, and although widely available the test is poorly standardized [4]. Alternative methodologies to assess gastric emptying include use of radio-opaque markers, breath testing, and gastric ultrasound—however, these are less studied with less well-established reproducibility and clinical correlation.

The WMC provides an indirect measure of meal emptying, since it depends on the gastric housekeeping contractions to remove the indigestible capsule, the assumption being that such motor activity follows meal digestion [33]. This assumption was found to be justified, with strong correlation between meal and capsule emptying [6, 15]. In healthy controls, the WMC cleared the stomach after 97 % of the test meal had cleared the stomach [6]. When gastroparesis patients defined by symptoms and a documented delayed gastric isotope emptying test within the past 2 years, there was a strong correlation between capsule—and isotope-measured transit [15]. The methodology for defining delayed emptying with the WMC uses a 5 h cutoff to signify delayed gastric emptying [15]. However, for the isotope study, Tougas et al. [15] demonstrated that after test meal ingestion in healthy subjects, the 95th percentile gastric emptying at 4 h is >90 % of the meal [31]. Interestingly, only 44 % of gastroparesis patients had a positive repeat isotope test while 65 % had a positive WMC test. This reflects both the poor reproducibility of the isotope study as well as the fact that it measures only fasting gastric emptying, whereas WMC measures fasting and fed emptying.

## 6.4.2  Small Bowel Transit

There is no standard measurement modality to assess small bowel transit. Radiology contrast series provide nonrepresentative data (fasting conditions, non-physiologic "meal") with no normal transit ranges available and exposure to ionizing radiation. Small bowel scintigraphy, breath testing and latterly MRI, have also been used to evaluate SBTT but there is poor standardization of techniques [19].

Using the pH profiling described, the WMC technology allows for determination of SBTT. A small healthy volunteer study comparing SBTT values obtained from scintigraphy with WMC reported good correlation [3, 18]. The clinical correlation of symptoms and slow small bowel transit require further determination, especially with the emerging data on the possible significance of small intestinal bacterial overgrowth in patients with IBS [26].

## 6.4.3  Colonic Transit Time

Of all established motility measurements, CTT is the one with a proven utility, namely in patients with chronic constipation, especially when refractory to conservative therapy [8]. Marker studies (comprising abdominal X-ray after ingestion of capsules containing tiny radio-opaque shapes) are the most widely used methodology, and this is a relatively noninvasive methodology of segmental as well as whole colonic transit. It is, however, poorly standardized (Metcalf et al. 1987). A less widely available alternative is whole gut radio-isotope scintigraphy, which can more accurately assess segmental transit time, but is hindered by expense and exposure to radiation [13].

Colonic transit data generated by the WMC correlate well with radio-opaque marker study data both in control subjects and patients with constipation [5, 23].

## 6.4.4  Gastric Pressure Profile

The existing standard for measurement of antroduodenal motility is ambulatory solid-state manometry. This is undertaken following nasal intubation of the antroduodenum with a catheter bearing multiple pressure transducers allowing simultaneous recording of contractions at multiple sites. However, it is an invasive investigation, requiring fluoroscopic screening to place the catheter, and considerable expertise to interpret the results.

The single-point measuring technology in WMC has been studied in healthy and gastroparesis subjects [12]. Overall, gastroparetics had a 35–50 % reduction in stomach and small bowel contraction frequency compared with healthy subjects. This was especially true for patients with severe gastroparesis as defined by abnormal isotope gastric emptying, possibly reflecting ineffective migrating motor complexes required to empty the capsule from the stomach [12].

## 6.4.5  Small Bowel Pressure Profile

Ambulatory small bowel manometry has been shown to have a role in the assessment of patients with gastroparesis [21] and in differentiating between visceral myopathy and neuropathy [29]. In essence, patients with enteric neuropathy lose the increased motility response seen after meals. Brun et al. [3] have shown that WMC measured delay in small bowel transit correlates with reduced proximal small bowel contraction frequency and amplitude.

## 6.4.6  Colonic Pressure Profile

Colonic manometry is a classical measurement, but despite being available for many years has failed to find a distinct clinical role. An ambulatory technique is deployed, involving placement of a solid-state catheter with multiple pressure ports via the anus into the colon under endoscopic or radiological guidance after bowel preparation [7]. As such the test is non-physiological.

A key potential advantage of the WMC is that it can yield a colonic pressure profile without bowel preparation. It remains to be seen whether such data can correlate with standardized motility data and symptoms. In a study of healthy controls and patients with chronic constipation (normal and slow transit) and constipation-predominant IBS (c-IBS), Hasler et al. [11] have demonstrated that colonic pressure activity was greater distally than proximally in health and all patient groups except those with slow transit. Physiologically, it is though that the distal contractions have a role in propelling stool into the rectum. The authors also noted elevated pressure amplitudes in patients with C-IBS.

## 6.5 Safety

There are three multicenter clinical trials including 495 subjects [5, 14, 24]. Approximately, one-third was healthy volunteers, and the rest had gastroparesis or constipation. The commonest problem was technical failure in 7 % of subjects—this reflects early prototypes of the capsule and software, and estimates of subsequent technical failure are nearer <1 % [32]. Three patients could not swallow (0.6 %) the WMC. Capsule retention leading to intestinal obstruction is the most serious potential safety concern with WMC, although it is rare, with a reported prolonged capsule retention (i.e., beyond 2 weeks) rate of 0.3 % [32]. All of these resolved with time or after prokinetic (erythromycin) administration or endoscopic removal. The longest retention time was 26 days, and no patient required surgical removal of the WMC.

Practical management of possible retention requires confirmation of expulsion by assessing the temperature profile, and if it is unclear from this whether the WMC has been passed, then the location of the capsule can be determined using pH data. If located in the stomach and small bowel, serial X-rays are required, with potential use of a prokinetic agent or endoscopic removal. If located in the colon, there is a minimal risk of obstruction and so follow-up (beyond symptom monitoring and use of laxatives) is not indicated.

## 6.6 Clinical Applications of the WMC

A recent study has shown that in a tertiary care motility setting, WMC testing eliminated the need for colonic transit studies in 68 % and gastric scintigraphy in 17 % [14]. Furthermore, WMC findings led to use of new medicines in 60 %, altered/initiated nutritional regimens in 14 % and surgical referral in 6 % [14]. In a different specialist center, a similar diagnostic yield of approximately 50 % of referred patients [24].

Specialist neurogastroenterology societies have endorsed WMC testing [24] as assessment in certain circumstances:

(a) Gastric emptying in individuals with suspected gastroparesis. Patients with gastroparesis have been shown to have reduced gastric contraction frequency [12] and attenuated postprandial small bowel response [2].

(b) SBTT in helping identify small bowel dysfunction in patients with generalized motility disorders [16].

(c) Assessment of CTT in subjects with symptoms of chronic constipation refractory to medical therapy especially if being considered for surgery. In such patients, the frequently observed presence of delayed small bowel transit would preclude a surgical option [11].

It is evident that a significant proportion of patients with functional GI disorders have abnormal motility in multiple gut regions [10, 23, 27]. A potential strength of the WMC is to assess the whole GI tract with a single ambulatory investigation. The role for transit data is more intuitively understood, but the potential role for WMC pressure data needs determination.

## 6.7 Limitations

The biggest drawback of current WMC is with regard to the pressure measurements related to the fact that it is a single-point technology. As such, it cannot demonstrate peristalsis, merely display contraction numbers and amplitude in terms of AUC. This needs to be validated and normal ranges defined.

The second chief problem is that the WMC measures total meal emptying and cannot differentiate between solid and liquid emptying. In addition, the WMC measures motility following a test meal of a nutrient bar, rather than a more physiological assessment.

The WMC is not approved for use in children. It is contra-indicated in patients with a history of dysphagia, gastric bezoar, swallowing disorders, suspected intestinal strictures, or fistulae (including active Crohn's disease and diverticulitis), gastrointestinal surgery within the previous 3 months or an implanted electromechanical medical device (e.g., a cardiac pacemaker).

## 6.8 Summary

The WMC is an emerging technology to assess gut transit, and possibly a pressure profile. It is an ambulatory, noninvasive, and well-tolerated technique, with no exposure to ionizing radiation. The capsule measures luminal pH and temperature permitting anatomical localization and thus giving values for gastric, small bowel, colon, and whole GI transit. The capsule bears a pressure sensor, and so after a standard meal, it allows for an indirect assessment of motility. The WMC has comparable diagnostic accuracy with gastric scintigraphy and has good sensitivity in diagnosing gastroparesis. The WMC is comparable to radio-opaque marker studies in diagnosing slow transit constipation.

## References

1. Agrawal A, Houghton IA, Reilly B, Morris J, Whorwell PJ. Bloating and distension in irritable bowel syndrome: the role of gastrointestinal transit. Am J Gastroenterol. 2009;104:1998–2004.
2. Brun M, Michalek W, McCallum R, Kock KL, Sitrin MD, Wo JM, et al. Comparison of small bowel postprandial response in healthy, gastroparetic and constipated subjects as measured by wireless motility capsule (WMC). Gastroenterology. 2010;138:S-459.
3. Brun M, Michalek W, Surjanhata B, Kuo B. Small bowel transit time (SBTT) by wireless motility capsule (WMC): normal values and analysis of pressure profiles in different subgroups of patients with slow SBTT. Gastroenterology. 2011;140:S-865.
4. Camilleri M, Hasler WL, Parkman HP, Quigley EM, Soffer E. Measurement of gastrointestinal motility In the GI laboratory. Gastroenterology. 1998;115:747–62.
5. Camilleri M, Thorne NK, Ringel Y, Hasler WL, Kuo B, Esfandyari T, et al. Wireless pH-motility capsule for colonic transit: prospective comparison with radiopaque markers in chronic constipation. Neurogastroenterol Motil. 2010;22: 874–882; e233. [PMC free article].
6. Cassilly D, Kantor S, Knight LC, Maurer AH, Fisher RS, Semler J, et al. Gastric emptying of a non-digestible solid: assessment with simultaneous smartpill pH and pressure capsule, antroduodenal manometry, gastric emptying scintigraphy. Neurogastroenterol Motil. 2008;20:311–9.
7. De Schryver A, Samsom M, Smout A. In search of objective manometric criteria for colonic high-amplitude propagated pressure waves. Neurogastroenterol Motil. 2002;14:375–81.
8. Emmanuel A. Current management strategies and therapeutic targets in chronic constipation. Therap Adv Gastroenterol. 2011;4:37–48.
9. Evans DF, Pye G, Bramley R, Clark AG, Dyson TJ, Hardcastle JD. Measurement of gastrointestinal pH profiles in normal ambulant human subjects. 1988;Gut 29:1035–1041. [PMC free article].
10. Hasler WL, Coleski R, Chey WD, Koch KL, McCallum RW, Wo JM, et al. Differences in intragastric pH in diabetic vs. idiopathic gastroparesis: relation to degree of gastric retention. Am J Physiol Gastrointest Liver Physiol. 2008;294:G1384–91.
11. Hasler WL, Saad RJ, Rao SS, Wilding GE, Parkman HP, Koch KL, et al. Heightened colon motor activity measured by a wireless capsule in patients with constipation: relation to colon transit and IBS. Am J Physiol Gastrointest Liver Physiol. 2009;297:G1107–14.

12. Kloetzer L, Chey WD, McCallum RW, Koch KL, Wo JM, Sitrin M, et al. Motility of the antroduodenum in healthy and gastroparetics characterized by wireless motility capsule. Neurogastroenterol Motil 2010;22: 527–533; e117.

13. Knowles CH, Dinning PG, Pescatori M, Rintala R, Rosen H. Surgical management of constipation. Neurogastroenterol Motil. 2009;21(Suppl 2):62–71.

14. Kuo B, Maneerattanaporn M, Lee AA, Baker JR, Wiener SM, Chey WD, et al. Generalized transit delay on wireless motility capsule testing in patients with clinical suspicion of gastroparesis, small intestinal dysmotility, or slow transit constipation. Dig Dis Sci. 2011;56:2928–38.

15. Kuo B, McCallum RW, Koch KL, Sitrin MD, Wo JM, Chey WD, et al. Comparison of gastric emptying of a nondigestible capsule to a radio-labelled meal in healthy and gastroparetic subjects. Aliment Pharmacol Ther. 2008;27:186–96.

16. Lee A, Michalek W, Kuo B. The SmartPill trial group. Variable upper gastrointestinal tract pathophysiological motility in gastroparesis. Neurogastroenterol Motil. 2009;21:73.

17. Longstreth GF, Thompson WG, Chey WD, Houghton LA, Mearin F, Spiller RC. Functional bowel disorders. Gastroenterology. 2006;124:1480–91.

18. Maqbool S, Parkman HP, Friedenberg FK. Wireless capsule motility: comparison of the smartpill GI monitoring system with scintigraphy for measuring whole gut transit. Dig Dis Sci. 2009;54:2167–74.

19. Menys A, Taylor SA, Emmanuel A, Ahmed A, Plumb AA, Odille F, Alam A, Halligan S, Atkinson D. Global small bowel motility: assessment with dynamic MR imaging. Radiology. 2013 (epub ahead of print).

20. Michalek W, Semler JR, Kuo B. Impact of acid suppression on upper gastrointestinal pH and motility. Dig Dis Sci. 2011;56:1735–42.

21. Parkman HP. Assessment of gastric emptying and small-bowel motility: scintigraphy, breath tests, manometry, and SmartPill. Gastrointest Endosc Clin N Am. 2009;19:49–55.

22. Rao SS. Constipation: evaluation and treatment of colonic and anorectal motility disorders. Gastrointest Endosc Clin N Am. 2009;19:117–39.

23. Rao SS, Kuo B, McCallum RW, Chey WD, Dibaise JK, Hasler WL, et al. Investigation of colonic and whole-gut transit with wireless motility capsule and radiopaque markers in constipation. Clin Gastroenterol Hepatol. 2009;7:537–44.

24. Rao SS, Camilleri M, Hasler WL, Maurer AH, Parkman HP, Saad R, et al. Evaluation of gastrointestinal transit in clinical practice: position paper of the American and European Neurogastroenterology and Motility Societies. Neurogastroenterol Motil. 2011;23:8–23.

25. Saad RJ, Hasler WL. A technical review and clinical assessment of the wireless motility capsule. Gastroenterol Hepatol (NY). 2011;7:795–804.

26. Sachdev AH, Pimentel M. Gastrointestinal bacterial overgrowth: pathogenesis and clinical significance. Ther Adv Chronic Dis. 2013;4:223–31.

27. Sarosiek I, Selover KH, Katz LA, Semler JR, Wilding GE, Lackner JM, et al. The assessment of regional gut transit times in healthy controls and patients with gastroparesis using wireless motility technology. Aliment Pharmacol Ther. 2010;31:313–22.

28. Scott S. Manometric techniques for the evaluation of colonic motor activity: current status. Neurogastroenterol Motil. 2003;15:483–513.

29. Scott SM, Picon L, Knowles CH, Fourquet F, Yazaki E, Williams NS, Lunniss PJ, Wingate DL. Automated quantitative analysis of nocturnal jejunal motor activity identifies abnormalities in individuals and subgroups of patients with slow transit constipation. Am J Gastroenterol. 2003;98:1123–34.

30. Spiller R, Aziz Q, Creed F, Emmanuel A, Houghton L, Hungin P, Jones R, Kumar D, Rubin G, Trudgill N, Whorwell P. Clinical Services Committee of The British Society of Gastroenterology. Guidelines on the irritable bowel syndrome: mechanisms and practical management. Gut. 2007;56:1770–98.

31. Tougas G, Eaker EY, Abell TL, Abrahamsson H, Boivin M, Chen J, et al. Assessment of gastric emptying using a low fat meal: establishment of international control values. Am J Gastroenterol. 2000;95:1456–62.

32. Tran K, Brun R, Kuo B. Evaluation of regional and whole gut motility using the wireless motility capsule: relevance in clinical practice. Therap Adv Gastroenterol. 2012;5:249–60.

33. Worsøe J, Fynne L, Gregersen T, Schlageter V, Christensen LA, Dahlerup JF, Rijkhoff NJ, Laurberg S, Krogh K. Gastric transit and small intestinal transit time and motility assessed by a magnet tracking system. BMC Gastroenterol. 2011;29(11):145.

34. Zarate N, Mohammed SD, O'Shaughnessy E, Newell M, Yazaki E, Williams NS, et al. Accurate localization of a fall in pH within the ileocecal region: validation using a dual-scintigraphic technique. Am J Physiol Gastrointest Liver Physiol. 2010;299:G1276–86.

# Capsule Endoscopy in Pediatrics

**7**

Salvatore Oliva and Stanley Cohen

## 7.1 Small Bowel Capsule Endoscopy in Pediatrics

### 7.1.1 Introduction

Small bowel capsule endoscopy (SBCE) becomes particularly valuable for pediatric patients because it does not require the ionizing radiation, deep sedation, or general anesthesia usually employed by other imaging modalities. In light of these features supportive data, the US Food and Drug Administration (FDA) expanded the role of SBCE for use in children aged 2 years and older and approved the use of a patency capsule (PC) for this age group [1].

### 7.1.2 Indications

Indications for SBCE have been developed by the American Society for Gastrointestinal Endoscopy [2]. However, the relative frequency of indications in compiled pediatric reports differs from that in data regarding adults. In

pediatric patients, 60 % of CEs have been for CD, 15 % for obscure gastrointestinal bleeding (OGIB), 10 % for abdominal pain/diarrhea, and 8 % for polyposis. In adults, 66 % of CEs have been for OGIB including iron deficiency anemia (IDA); 11 % for clinical symptoms only (e.g., pain, diarrhea, and weight loss without OGIB); 10 % for CD; and the balance (13 %) for other indications [3–22].

The most common indications for SBCE in pediatric patients are the suspicion of CD and evaluation of existing inflammatory bowel disease (IBD) accounting for 63 % of the total indications [13]. More than half of the procedures for IBD indications are related to evaluation of CD and colitis, with 44 % due to the suspicion of CD, 16 % related to evaluation of known CD, 2 % to indeterminate colitis (IC), and 1 % to ulcerative colitis (UC). Abdominal pain and diarrhea account for another 10 %.

These clinical indications are age-stratified (Table 7.1). In a review of 83 procedures in children aged 1.5–7.9 years (for whom CD is less prevalent), the most common indication for CE was OGIB, accounting for 30 (36 %) procedures, with positive yields in 16 (53 %) [20]. Suspicion of CD accounted for 20 (24 %) procedures, with positive findings in 11 (55 %). Abdominal pain accounted for another 12 procedures (14 %), and CD was the indication in 3 patients. CD was found in 14 (31 %) of the patients where a positive diagnosis was made. Investigation of malabsorption and protein loss required 12 and 9 procedures (14 and 11 %),

S. Oliva (✉)
Pediatric Gastroenterology and Liver Unit, Sapienza University of Rome, Rome, Italy
e-mail: salvatore.oliva@uniroma1.it

S. Cohen
Children's Center for Digestive Health Care, Atlanta, GA, USA

Z. Li et al. (eds.), *Handbook of Capsule Endoscopy*,
DOI: 10.1007/978-94-017-9229-5_7, © Springer Science+Business Media Dordrecht 2014

$P = 0.4247$) [3, 4, 5, 13]. Endoscopy was used to remove five capsules including four from the stomach [8, 14] and one from an ileal pouch [3]; 13 were retrieved surgically while taking appropriate measures to mitigate the cause of the retention [6, 8, 11, 12, 14]. A retained capsule was successfully evacuated by bowel prep at 22 days post-ingestion [8].

The highest risk factors for capsule retention include known IBD (5.2 % risk), previous SBFT demonstrating small bowel CD (35.7 % risk) and a body mass index below the fifth percentile combined with known IBD (43 % risk), although retention has occurred despite the absence of stricture on SBFT [12]. Among four patients with CD having capsule passage lasting longer than 5 days (with three continuing on to retention), there was a difference in age being significant ($18.8 \pm 0.9$ vs. $14.6 \pm 3.5$), but not height or weight compared to patients who did not have retention [14]. Retention rates for indications of OGIB, CD, and neoplastic lesions were 1.2 % (95 %  CI = 0.9–1.6 %;  $P = 0.6014$), 2.6 % (95 %  CI = 1.6–3.9 %), and 2.1 % (95 % CI = 0.7–4.3 %), respectively, with a pooled rate of 1.4 % (95 % CI = 1.2–1.6 %) for those procedures [42]. On a per-procedure basis, this pattern is in adults, where retention in OGIB, CD, and polyps occurs at rate of 1.4, 2.2, and 1.2 %, respectively. Thus, it appears that the risk of retention is dependent on the clinical indication and not age. Rare cases of perforation, aspiration, or small bowel obstruction have been reported in adults but none have been reported in children. Minor mucosal trauma has occurred in children in which capsules were placed with the Roth net [18]. A specific capsule placement device is now available (AdvanCE, US Endsocopy, Mentor, OH [45]).

### 7.1.6 The Patency Capsule: Rationale, Procedure, and Findings in Pediatric Patients

The majority of capsule retentions have occurred in patients with normal small bowel radiological studies, yet functional patency may be present in patients with radiologically documented strictures. An identically sized capsule containing a mixture of barium and lactose and radiofrequency identity tag was developed to test functional patency and gradually implode intact PC passage does not occur within 30 h.

A retrospective study reviewed 23 patients with known (n = 14) or suspected (n = 9) pediatric CD who underwent evaluation with the PC prior to using the video capsule [3]. Of the 19 who were evaluable, patency was established and subsequent CE was performed successfully in all but one who had a retained capsule from CE the following week.

In a single-center prospective pediatric trial that evaluated 18 patients (age 10–16 years) who ingested the PC, 15 excreted an intact PC (mean 34.5 h) [46]. The 18 cases included five known CD, three IC, one UC, and nine suspected CD. CD was eventually diagnosed in all patients having PC transit of more than 40 h and in 9 of 12 who passed the PC in 40 h or less. There were no capsule retentions or adverse events. Thus, the PC can serve as a useful guide and may lessen the likelihood of CE retention, particularly in known CD where the risk of retention is greatest.

### 7.1.7 Conclusion

SBCE is a useful diagnostic tool that has particular benefit in pediatrics, because it is an imaging modality that does not require the ionizing radiation, deep sedation, or general anesthesia. The risk of retention appears to be dependent on indication rather than age and parallels the adult experience by indication, making SBCE a relatively safe procedure with a significant diagnostic yield.

### 7.2 The Esophageal Capsule in Pediatric Patients

Esophageal capsule endoscopy (ECE) was approved by the US FDA and introduced for clinical use in 2004. A second iteration of the capsule, Pillcam ESO 2 (Given Imaging), widened the field of view; increased the frame rate to 18 images per second; and improved the image quality with two additional lenses, higher spatial resolution and a wider dynamic range, was approved by the US FDA in 2007.

However, its use in pediatrics—or at least in clinical trials and the retrospective reporting of that use—have been limited. Only two small pediatric trials of the first ECE capsule have been reported. Both focused on portal hypertension [47, 48]. In the first trial, which also included young adults, 27 of the 28 ECEs were complete, each averaging a total recording time of 20 min and a mean esophageal transit of 192 s (range, 4–631) [47]. Esophageal varices were small in 10 (37 %), medium to large in 4 (17 %), and negative in 13 (48 %), with gastric varices in 10 (37 %). Of note, other esophageal and duodenal findings also identified.

In the other study, the ECE was successful in 10 of 11 patients [48]. The mean esophageal transit was 45 s (range, 9–171). Varices were small in four, small and large in four, multiple/large in one, and negative in one. Again, other findings were present in the esophagus.

Although the first study did not report how the varices were graded, the second study appraised the size of the varix as a fraction of the circumference. A cut-point of 25 % differentiated small versus large varices. The lack of insufflation with ECE required a grading system that differed from that used for traditional endoscopy [49].

## 7.3 The Colon Capsule in Pediatric Patients

Colon capsule endoscopy (CCE; Given Imaging Ltd, Yoqneam, Israel) is a novel minimally invasive and painless endoscopic technique allowing exploration of the colon without need for sedation, rectal intubation, and gas insufflation [50, 51]. A second-generation CCE device (CCE-2), recently released provides a higher number of images per second and a larger viewing angle [52–54].

Consensus guidelines of ESGE on CCE have established that CCE-2 may be useful to monitor inflammation in UC, which may help guide therapy [55]. To date, there have been only a few studies on this topic, showing that CCE is a safe procedure to monitor mucosal status and healing in UC, while it cannot replace conventional colonoscopy. These studies have all been conducted in adults, with one using second generation of CCE [56–59].

There is only one study using CCE-2 in 29 pediatric UC, and its results are going to be published [60]. In this pilot study, sensitivity of CCE-2 in detecting disease activity was 96 % [95 % CI = 79–99] and specificity was 100 % [95 % CI = 61–100], corresponding to an overall accuracy of 97 % [95 % CI = 90–100]. The positive and negative predictive values were 100 % [95 % CI = 85–100] and 85 % [95 % CI = 49–97], respectively. To this data, CCE-2 seems to be able to play an important role in monitoring mucosal inflammation in pediatric UC without invasiveness and discomfort, also providing a good level of diagnostic accuracy and tolerability. However, future multicenter studies are recommended and mandatory before considering CCE-2 as an alternative technique in the follow-up of pediatric UC.

## References

1. U.S. Food and Drug Administration, Center for Devices and Radiological Health. PC Patency system and pillcam platform with pillcam SB capsules. Available at: http://www.accessdata.fda.gov/cdrh_docs/pdf9/K090557.pdf. Accessed 10 Feb 2010.
2. Mishkin DS, Chuttani R, Croffie J, et al. ASGE technology status evaluation report: wireless capsule endoscopy. Gastrointest Endosc. 2006;63:539–45.
3. Cohen SA, Klevens AI. Use of capsule endoscopy in diagnosis and management of pediatric patients, based on meta-analysis. Clin Gastroenterol Hepatol. 2011;9:490–6.
4. Cohen SA, Ephrath H, Lewis JD, et al. Pediatric capsule endoscopy: a single center, 5 year retrospective review of small bowel and patency capsules. JPGN. 2012;54:409–13.

5. Gralnek IM, Cohen SA, Ephrath H. Small bowel capsule endoscopy impacts diagnosis and management of pediatric inflammatory bowel disease: a prospective study. Digest Dis Sci. DOI 10.1007/s10620-011-1894-5.

6. Tokuhara D, Watanabe K, Okano Y, et al. Wireless capsule endoscopy in pediatric patients: the first series from Japan. J Gastroenterol. 2010;45:683–91.

7. Guilhon de Araujo Sant'Anna AM, Dubois J, Miron MC, et al. Wireless capsule endoscopy for obscure small-bowel disorders: final results of the first pediatric controlled trial. Clin Gastroenterol Hepatol 2005;3:264–270.

8. Jensen MK, Tipnis NA, Bajorunaite R, et al. Capsule endoscopy performed across the pediatric age range: indications, incomplete studies, and utility in management of inflammatory bowel disease. Gastrointest Endosc. 2010;72:95–102.

9. Antao B, Bishop J, Shawis R, et al. Clilnical application and diagnostic yield of wireless capsule endoscopy in children. J Laparoendosc Adv Surg Tech. 2007;17:364–70.

10. Cohen SA, Gralnek IM, Ephrath H, et al. Capsule endoscopy may reclassify pediatric inflammatory bowel disease: a historical analysis. J Pediatr Gastroenterol Nutr. 2008;47:31–6.

11. de' Angelis GL, Fornaroli F, de' Angeles N, et al. Wireless capsule endoscopy for pediatric small-bowel diseases. Am J Gastroenterol 2007; 102:1749–1757.

12. Atay O, Mahajan L, Kay M, et al. Risk of capsule endoscope retention in pediatric patients: a large single-center experience and review of the literature. J Pediatr Gastroenterol Nutr. 2009;49:1–6.

13. Cohen S. Pediatric capsule endoscopy. Tech Gastrointest Endosc. 2013;15:32–5.

14. Moy L, Levine J. Wireless capsule endoscopy in the pediatric age group: experience and complications. J Pediatr Gastroenterol Nutr. 2007;44:516–20.

15. Ge ZZ, Chen HY, Gao YJ, et al. Clinical application of wireless capsule endoscopy in pediatric patients for suspected small bowel diseases. Eur J Pediatr. 2007;166:825–9.

16. Arguelles-Arias F, Caunedo A, Romero J, et al. The value of capsule endoscopy in pediatric patients with a suspicion of Crohn's disease. Endoscopy. 2004;36:869–73.

17. Urbain D, Tresinie M, De Looze D, et al. Capsule endoscopy in paediatrics: multicentric Belgian study. Acta Gastroenterol Belg. 2007;70:11–4.

18. Barth BA, Donovan K, Fox VL. Endoscopic placement of the capsule endoscope in children. Gastrointest Endosc. 2004;60:818–21.

19. Shamir R, Hino B, Hartman C, et al. Wireless video capsule in pediatric patients with functional abdominal pain. J Pediatr Gastroenterol Nutr. 2007;44:45–50.

20. Fritscher-Ravens A, Scherbakov P, Bufler P, et al. The feasibility of wireless capsule endoscopy in detecting small intestinal pathology in children under the age of 8 years: a multicentre European study. Gut. 2009;58:1467–72.

21. Postgate A, Hyer W, Phillips R, et al. Feasibility of video capsule endoscopy in the management of children with Peutz-Jeghers Syndrome: a blinded comparison with barium enterography for the detection of small bowel polyps. J Pediatr Gastroenterol Nutr. 2009;49:417–23.

22. Thomson M, Fritscher-Ravens A, Mylonaki M, et al. Wireless capsule endoscopy in children: a study to assess diagnostic yield in small bowel disease in pediatric patients. J Pediatr Gastroenterol Nutr. 2007;44:192–7.

23. Werlin SL, Benuri-Silbiger I, Kerem E, et al. Evidence of intestinal inflammation in patients with cystic fibrosis. JPGN. 2010;51:304–8.

24. Cohen SA, Lewis J, Stallworth A, et al. Mucosal healing with the specific carbohydrate diet in pediatric Crohn's disease: preliminary results of a 12 week pilot study. Gastroenterol 2012;142(5):Supp AB Sa1992.

25. Viazis N, Sgouros S, Papaxoinis K, et al. Bowel preparation increases the diagnostic yield of capsule endoscopy: a prospective, randomized, controlled study. Gastrointest Endosc. 2004;60:534–8.

26. Burke CA, Church JM. Enhancing the quality of colonoscopy: the importance of bowel purgatives. Gastrointest Endosc. 2007;66:565–73.

27. de Franchis R, Avgerinos A, Barkin J, et al. ICCE consensus for bowel preparation and prokinetics. Endoscopy. 2005;37:1040–5.

28. Mergener K, Ponchon T, Gralnek I, et al. Literature review and recommendations for clinical application of small-bowel capsule endoscopy, based on a panel discussion by international experts. Consensus statements for small-bowel capsule endoscopy, 2006/2007. Endoscopy. 2007;39:895–909.

29. Dai N, Gubler C, Hengstler P, et al. Improved capsule endoscopy after bowel preparation. Gastrointest Endosc. 2005;61:28–31.

30. Ladas SD, Triantafyllou K, Spada C, et al. ESGE recommendations on VCE in investigation of small-bowel, esophageal, and colonic diseases. Endoscopy. 2010;42:220–7.

31. van Tuyl SA, den Ouden H, Stolk MF, et al. Optimal preparation for video capsule endoscopy: a prospective, randomized, single-blind study. Endoscopy. 2007;39:1037–40.

32. Wei W, Ge ZZ, Lu H, et al. Purgative bowel cleansing combined with simethicone improves capsule endoscopy imaging. Am J Gastroenterol. 2008;103:77–82.

33. Ben Soussan E, Savoye G, Antonietti M, et al. Is a 2-liter PEG preparation useful before capsule endoscopy? J Clin Gastroenterol. 2005;2005(39):381–4.

34. Mishkin DS, Chuttani R, Croffie J, et al. ASGE technology status evaluation report: wireless capsule endoscopy. Gastrointest Endosc. 2006;63:539–45.

35. Faigel DO, Baron TH, Adler DG, et al. ASGE guideline: guidelines for credentialing and granting

privileges for capsule endoscopy. Gastrointest Endosc. 2005;61:503–5.

36. Villa F, Signorelli C, Rondonotti E, et al. Preparations and prokinetics. Gastrointest Endosc Clin N Am. 2006;16:211–20.

37. Spada C, Riccioni ME, Familiari P, et al. Polyethylene glycol plus simethicone in small-bowel preparation for capsule endoscopy. Dig Liver Dis. 2010;42:365–7.

38. Chen H, Huang Y, Che S, et al. Small bowel preparations for capsule endoscopy with mannitol and simethicone: a prospective, randomized, clinical trial. J Clin Gastroenterol. 2011;45:337–41.

39. Oliva S, Cucchiara S, Spada C, et al. Small bowel cleansing for capsule endoscopy in pediatric patients: a prospective randomized single-blinded study. Dig Liver Dis. 2014;45:51–5.

40. Malagelada C, DeIorio F, Azpiroz F, et al. New insight into intestinal motor function via noninvasive endoluminal image analysis. J Gastroenterol. 2008;135:1155–62.

41. Fireman Z, Mahajana E, Broide E, et al. Diagnosing small bowel Crohn's disease with wireless capsule endoscopy. Gut. 2003;52:390–2.

42. Liao Z, Gao R, Xu C, Zhao-Shen L. Indications and detection, completion, and retention rates of small-bowel capsule endoscopy: a systematic review. Gastrointest Endosc. 2010;71:280–6.

43. Gay G, Fassler I, Florent C, Delvaux M. Malabsorption. In: Halpern M, Jacob H, editors. Atlas of capsule endoscopy. Norcross, GA: Given Imaging; 2002. p. 84–90.

44. Murray JA, Rubio-Tapia A, Van Dyke CT, et al. Mucosal atrophy in celiac disease: extent of involvement, correlation with clinical presentation, and response to treatment. Clin Gastroenterol Hepatol. 2008;6:186–93.

45. Uko V, Atay O, Mashajan L, et al. Endoscopic deployment of the wireless capsule using a capsule delivery device in pediatric patients: a case series. Endoscopy. 2009;41:380–2.

46. Cohen SA, Gralnek IM, Ephrath H, et al. The use of a patency capsule in pediatric Crohn's disease: a prospective evaluation. Dig Dis Sci. 2011;56(3):860–5.

47. Fox V. Esophageal capsule endoscopy in children and young adults with portal hypertension. 6th International Conference on Capsule Endoscopy (ICCE) 2006;Madrid:AB887874.

48. Schaible TD, Olive AP, Wilson DS, et al. Use of esophageal capsule endoscopy in pediatric patients with portal hypertension. Gastrointest Endosc. 2010;71(5):M1562.

49. De Franchis R, Eisen GM, Laine L, et al. Esophageal capsule endoscopy for screening and surveillance of esophageal varices in patients with portal hypertension. Hepatology. 2008;47:1595–603.

50. Schoofs N, Deviere J, Van Gossum A, et al. PillCam colon capsule endoscopy compared with colonoscopy for colorectal tumor diagnosis: a prospective pilot study. Endoscopy. 2006;38:971–7.

51. Van Gossum A, Navas MM, Fernandez-Urien I, et al. Capsule endoscopy versus colonoscopy for the detection of polyps and cancer. N Engl J Med. 2009;361:264–70.

52. Eliakim R, Yassin K, Niv Y, et al. Prospective multicenter performance evaluation of the second-generation colon capsule compared with colonoscopy. Endoscopy. 2009;41:1026–31.

53. Spada C, Hassan C, Munoz-NavasMet al. Second-generation colon capsule compared with colonoscopy. Gastrointest Endosc 2011;74:581–589 e1. Erratum in Gastrointest Endosc 2011;74:1174.

54. Spada C, Hassan C, Munoz-NavasMet al. Second-generation colon capsule compared with colonoscopy. Gastrointest Endosc 2011;74:581–589 e1. Erratum in Gastrointest Endosc 2011;74:1174.

55. Spada C, Hassan C, Galmiche JP, et al. Colon capsule endoscopy: European Society of Gastrointestinal Endoscopy (ESGE) Guideline. Endoscopy. 2012;44:527–36.

56. Sung J, Ho KY, Chiu HM, et al. The use of pillcam colon in assessing mucosal inflammation in ulcerative colitis: a multicenter study. Endoscopy. 2012;44:754–8.

57. Ye CA, Gao YJ, Ge ZZ, et al. PillCam colon capsule endoscopy versus conventional colonoscopy for the detection of severity and extent of ulcerative colitis. J Dig Dis. 2013;14:117–24.

58. Meister T, Heinzow HS, Domagk D, et al. Colon capsule endoscopy versus standard colonoscopy in assessing disease activity of ulcerative colitis: a prospective trial. Tech Coloproctol. 2013;17(6):641–6.

59. Hosoe N, Matsuoka K, Naganuma M, et al. Applicability of second generation colon capsule endoscope to ulcerative colitis: a clinical feasibility study. J Gastroenterol Hepatol. 2013;28(7):1174–9.

60. Oliva S, Di Nardo G, Hassan C et al. Second generation colon capsule endoscopy versus colonoscopy in pediatric ulcerative colitis: a pilot study. Endoscopy. 2014;46(6):485–92.

# Comparison of Capsule Endoscopy and Device-Assisted Enteroscopy

# 8

Sung Chul Park and Hoon Jai Chun

**Keywords**

Capsule endoscopy · Device-assisted enteroscopy

## 8.1 Introduction

The development and improvements in endoscopic devices and technique has made it for us to diagnose and treat diseases of the esophagus, stomach, colon, and the parts of the small intestine. However, the small intestine extending from the third part of the duodenum to the ileum has been considered the part where the use of an endoscopic approach is very difficult due to its distance from the mouth or anus, as well as its anatomical structure consisting of numerous flexions and a length exceeding 5 m. To diagnose lesions of the small intestine, radiographic examinations such as small bowel series and enteroclysis, push enteroscopy, sonde enteroscopy, rope-way enteroscopy, and intraoperative enteroscopy were developed, but these examinations have many limitations. Since capsule

S. C. Park
Division of Gastroenterology and Hepatology, Department of Internal Medicine, Kangwon National University Hospital, Kangwon National University School of Medicine, Baengnyeong-ro 156, Chuncheon, Kangwon-do 200-722, South Korea
e-mail: schlp@naver.com

H. J. Chun (✉)
Division of Gastroenterology and Hepatology, Department of Internal Medicine, Korea University Anam Hospital, Korea University College of Medicine, 126-1, Anam-dong 5 ga, Seongbuk-Gu, Seoul 136-705, South Korea
e-mail: drchunhj@chol.com

endoscopy and deep small bowel enteroscopy, which were developed as effective diagnostic methods for direct observation of the entire small intestine, were introduced in clinical use in 2001, these methods have become as the new standard techniques for the diagnosis and treatment of small intestine diseases that are undetectable by other methods [1]. In this chapter, we compare the abilities of capsule endoscopy and device-assisted enteroscopy among the representative endoscopy approaches to observe the small intestine.

### 8.1.1 Capsule Endoscopy

Capsule endoscopy is the most commonly used procedure for examination of the small intestine in clinical practice and is considered the standard assay for small intestine diseases.

Currently used capsule endoscopes for examination of the small intestine include the PillCam SB/SB2 (Given Imaging Co., Yoqneam, Israel), MiroCam (Intromedic, Seoul, South Korea), Endocapsule (Olympus, Tokyo, Japan), and OMOM (Jinshan Science and Technology, Chongqing, China) [2–4].

Capsule endoscopy is non-invasive and is likely to get a picture of the entire small intestine compared to other assays. However, since the capsule moves passively along the small intestine by peristalsis to acquire images, controlling its movements and speed is impossible. Thus, in some parts, the capsule passes very quickly, making it difficult to obtain sufficient information.

Z. Li et al. (eds.), *Handbook of Capsule Endoscopy*,
DOI: 10.1007/978-94-017-9229-5_8, © Springer Science+Business Media Dordrecht 2014

In contrast, if the capsule passes slowly through the gastrointestinal tract, imaging may be terminated without observation of the entire small intestine. Additionally, infusion of air into the lumen and tissue biopsy is not possible. Capsule retention results in cases of intestinal strictures and the capsule might have to be removed [5]. Use of the capsule is relatively safe, but complications such as intra-airway aspiration, intra-diverticulum impaction, capsule fracture, and perforation of the small intestine have been reported [6].

The most common indication for capsule endoscopy is obscure gastrointestinal bleeding (OGIB). Capsule endoscopy has been used to screen cases of suspected Crohn's disease in the small intestine, diagnose small intestinal tumors, visualize mucosal injury in the intestine due to non-steroidal anti-inflammatory drugs, localize abdominal pain of unknown origin, and identify cases of familial adenomatous polyposis (FAP) [7]. Clinical experience with capsule endoscopy in pediatric patients continues to accumulate, and this procedure can now be used in children over 10 years of age with indications [8]. Capsule endoscopy was recently reported to be possible in 3-year-old children [9].

Contraindications for capsule endoscopy include established or suspected obstruction, stricture or fistula in the gastrointestinal tract, dysphasia, intestinal pseudo-obstruction, and cases of implanted artificial heart pacemakers or other electrical medical equipment. Safe use in pregnancy has not yet been established [10].

## 8.1.2 Device-Assisted Enteroscopy

Deep small bowel enteroscopy is designed to allow entry to the small intestine with its many flexures using an overtube or a balloon. Methods currently being used in clinical practice include double-balloon enteroscopy, single-balloon enteroscopy, and spiral enteroscopy with an outer spiral tube. Deep enteroscopy is being used as a means of diagnosis and treatment for various indications including gastrointestinal bleeding. There are a few differences in the indications for capsule endoscopy and deep enteroscopy. The indications for deep enteroscopy include OGIB; inflammatory bowel disease; small intestinal tumors; small intestinal strictures; and cases of a small intestine with structural deformation due to gastrointestinal surgery, unsuccessful endoscopic retrograde cholangiopancreatography, or colonoscopy.

### 8.1.2.1 Double-Balloon Enteroscopy

Fixing the small intestine with a balloon at the end of the outer tube in the endoscope prevents the small intestine from being extended excessively and helps the endoscope move forward easily when the endoscope is inserted into the bowel. If both balloons are used, the flexion of the gastrointestinal tract can be relieved and the length of gastrointestinal tract can be shortened. With this method, the insertion of the endoscope is significantly better than with the existing method of push enteroscopy. The proportion of the entire small intestine that can be observed via the oral and anal approach is 40–80 %, similar to that with capsule endoscopy [11]. Unlike capsule endoscopy however, the infusion of air and washing are possible. Moving the endoscope back and forth enables the close observation of lesions. Further, chromoendoscopy, biopsy, and endoscopic therapy are possible. Therefore, double-balloon enteroscopy is a useful tool for diagnosing and treating various intestinal diseases.

However, double-balloon enteroscopy is somewhat invasive and takes longer than a general endoscopic examination (approximately 1 h). Thus, patients experience much discomfort and endoscopists must invest additional effort. Because observation of the entire small intestine via both oral and anal approaches during a single procedure is difficult, two procedures may be required. A history of Crohn's disease, gastrointestinal surgery, or intestinal adhesions complicates the procedure, and the procedure is often unsuccessful because of insufficient insertion. Practice with approximately 40–60 tests is estimated to be needed for a clinician to develop proficiency in performing double-balloon enteroscopy [12]. A recent multicenter study on the learning curve showed that the average inspection times for the initial 10 examples and for the next 10 examples were 109 and 92 min, respectively, with the procedure time tending to decrease with experience [12]. As the double-balloon enteroscopy for therapy was developed, various endoscopic therapies including hemostasis, balloon angioplasty, and polypectomy became available. However, device insertion and polyp resection are difficult because of the length of the endoscope and intestinal looping. It has been reported that various complications such as perforation, pancreatitis, and ileus occurred in 0.8 % of the diagnostic double-balloon enteroscopy and 4 % of endoscopic therapy, respectively [13].

### 8.1.2.2 Single-Balloon Enteroscopy

The single-balloon endoscope, first introduced in 2006, is similar in structure to a double-balloon enteroscope, but has no balloon mounted at its distal end. The silicone balloon is equipped with an outer tube, and the diameter of the endoscope tip is approximately 0.2 mm thinner. Because the endoscope is fixed into the small intestine using the hooking of the endoscope tip and advancing of the outer tube, the procedure is simpler and features a less steep learning curve than double-balloon enteroscopy, and it can be performed by a single practitioner without assistance [14]. Because a balloon is not mounted at the distal end of the endoscope, preparation time is as short as approximately 6 min [15]. In addition, the incidence of complications associated with examination using single-balloon enteroscopy is only approximately 1 % [16]. Single-balloon enteroscopy is a relatively safe procedure, with safety comparable to that of double-balloon enteroscopy and shows similar efficacy to double-balloon enteroscopy, with a 7–59 % therapeutic yield [17–19]. However, it has a short outer tube and slides easily without fixation. As such, the proportion of the total enteroscopy is lower than that with double-balloon enteroscopy. Double-balloon enteroscopy is able to access 40–80 % of the entire small intestine, whereas single-balloon enteroscopy is able to access only a significantly lower 12–25 % of the entire small intestine [20, 21].

### 8.1.2.3 Spiral Enteroscopy

Spiral enteroscopy, first introduced by Akerman in 2006, involves the use of screws in the outer tube for easier and faster insertion into the deep part of the small intestine. The operator can turn the outer tube in a clockwise direction because of the use of a special type of outer tube with 4.5–5.5-mm spiral bumps (enteroscopy and spiral outward tube inserted) to advance the endoscope to the bottom, creating wrinkles in the small intestine. In an initial study of spiral enteroscopy, the procedure time was lesser and the enteroscope could be inserted to a similar depth compared to balloon enteroscopy [22, 23]. In addition, in a prospective multicenter study, the insertion depth, lesion observation rate, and treatment success rate were similar to those achieved with conventional methods of deep enteroscopy. However, the rate to observe the entire small intestines was significantly lower compared with balloon enteroscopy in a randomized controlled trial and further evaluation is needed. Both oral and anal approaches can be used in the balloon enteroscopy procedures. However, with spiral enteroscopy, only the oral approach can be used [24].

### 8.1.3 Comparison of Endoscopy Methods According to Disease

Indications for the use of capsule endoscopy are not consistent with indications for the use of balloon enteroscopy. However, each can be used to explore conditions such as unexplained gastrointestinal bleeding, small intestinal Crohn's disease, and small intestine tumors. A disease-specific comparative study of each condition has been reported.

### 8.1.3.1 Obscure Gastrointestinal Bleeding

OGIB has various causes. Studies have shown that vascular lesions including angioectasia are the most common causes in western countries, whereas inflammatory mucosal lesions are reported to be the major cause in eastern countries [25, 26].

**Table 8.1** Diagnostic yield of the obscure gastrointestinal bleeding between capsule endoscopy and double-balloon enteroscopy [27, 28]

| Study or subgroup | Positive CE | Positive DBE | DBE yield after positive CE | DBE yield after negative CE |
|---|---|---|---|---|
| Matsumoto et al. [63] | 10/13 (76.9 %) | 6/13 (53.8 %) | – | – |
| Hadithi et al. [34] | 28/35 (80 %) | 21/35 (60 %) | 20/28 (71.5 %) | 1/7 (14.3 %) |
| Mehdizadeh et al. [12] | 63/115 (54.8 %) | 57/115 (49.6 %) | 41/63 (65.1 %) | 16/52 (30.8 %) |
| Nakamura et al. [33] | 17/28(60.7 %) | 12/28 (42.9 %) | 9/17 (52.9 %) | 3/11 (27.3 %) |
| Fujimori et al. [32] | 18/45 (40 %) | 18/36 (50 %) | 16/16 (100 %) | 2/20 (10 %) |
| Ohmiya et al. [31] | 37/74 (50 %) | 39/74 (52.7 %) | – | – |
| Kameda et al. [30] | 23 (71.9 %) | 21 (65.6 %) | 15/23 (65.2 %) | 2/3 (66.7 %) |
| Arakawa et al. [42] | 40/74 (54.1 %) | 40/74 (63.5 %) | 36/40 (90 %) | 11/34 (32.4 %) |
| Fukumoto et al. [29] | 16/42 (38.1 %) | 18/42 (42.9 %) | – | – |
| Marmo et al. [44] | 174/193 (90.2 %) | 132/193 (68.4 %) | 124/174 (71.3 %) | 8/19 (42.1 %) |
| Shisido et al. [27] | 53/118 (44.9 %) | 63/118 (53.4 %) | 51/53 (96.2 %) | 12/65 (18.5 %) |

*CE* capsule endoscopy, *DBE* double-balloon enteroscopy. (Reprint with permission from Journal of Gastroenterology and Hepatology, [28])

It is difficult to perform capsule endoscopy and double-balloon enteroscopy in patients with OGIB at the same time. Thus, the establishment of the preferred method in terms of efficacy and cost-effectiveness will be helpful in the treatment of patients. Table 8.1 summarizes the diagnostic yield of capsule endoscopy and double-balloon enteroscopy in patients with OGIB [27, 28].

A meta-analysis of 10 studies comparing capsule endoscopy with double-balloon enteroscopy yielded a diagnosis rate of 62 % for capsule endoscopy (95 % confidence interval [CI], 47.3–76.1 %) and of 56 % for double-balloon enteroscopy (95 % CI, 48.9–62.1 %) with an odds ratio (OR) of 1.39 (95 % CI, 0.88–2.20, $p = 0.61$) [28]. The diagnosis rate of double-balloon enteroscopy following capsule endoscopy was 75.0 %, whereas the diagnosis rate of double-balloon enteroscopy without capsule endoscopy was 27.5 %.

According to the study by the Korean Gut Image Study Group, the diagnosis rates for capsule endoscopy and double-balloon enteroscopy in cases of OGIB are similar [35]. However, no randomized controlled studies of the two procedures for OGIB have been undertaken. A meta-analysis of six prospective studies and

three retrospective studies showed that the pooled OR for the diagnostic yield was 1.48 (95 % CI, 0.90–2.43). No difference was noted between the two procedures. In patients with OGIB, OR between double-balloon enteroscopy after positive result of capsule endoscopy and double-balloon enteroscopy from the beginning was 1.79 (95 % CI, 1.09–2.96) in a meta-analysis [35]. Generally, capsule endoscopy is more economical than double-balloon enteroscopy. The use of double-balloon enteroscopy based on the capsule endoscopy result is then cost-effective [36].

Particularly, the ability of double-balloon enteroscopy to check the entire small intestine is important in patients with OGIB. Capsule endoscopy facilitates observation of the small intestine without discomfort in 79–90 %. In contrast, the rate to observe the entire small intestine in the double-balloon enteroscopy is reported as 16–86 % [37, 38]. Technical difficulties prevent the observation of the entire intestine using double-balloon enteroscopy. If the cause of bleeding is detected during the procedure, the procedure might not be performed to completion. According to three meta-analyses, the diagnosis rate of double-balloon enteroscopy for OGIB was approximately 60 %, similar to that of capsule endoscopy [13, 28, 39]. Compared to single-insertion (per-anal or per-oral) double-balloon enteroscopy, capsule endoscopy was superior, whereas compared to double-insertion (per-anal and per-oral) double-balloon enteroscopy, capsule endoscopy was comparable [39]. In addition, small bowel lesions were more likely to be found when double-balloon enteroscopy was performed soon after the bleeding episode (for example, <1 month later) as was the case for capsule endoscopy [40, 41].

According to Shishido and colleagues, a total of 118 patients underwent capsule endoscopy and then underwent double-balloon enteroscopy via both anal and oral approaches [27]. The overall diagnosis rates of capsule endoscopy and double-balloon enteroscopy were 44.9 % in 53 patients and 53.4 % in 63 patients ($p = 0.01$), respectively, with good agreement between the two procedures (kappa statistic $= 0.76$). In a study comparing double-balloon enteroscopy and capsule endoscopy in 162 patients with OGIB, double-balloon enteroscopy was superior to capsule endoscopy for the detection of lesions in the Roux-en-Y loop or diverticular disease [42].

Based on many studies, the relationship between capsule endoscopy and double-balloon enteroscopy at least in cases of OGIB seems to be complementary rather than competitive [43, 44]. Double-balloon enteroscopy has the advantage of therapeutic procedure in the cases of persistent bleeding or when the bleeding site is confirmed during capsule endoscopy in OGIB. Bleeding in the small intestine can be treated using various hemostasis methods such as injection therapy, argon plasma coagulation, and hemoclipping.

Many clinical guidelines suggest that a combination of the two endoscopy techniques be used [45–47]. The guidelines also suggest that double-balloon enteroscopy be performed after capsule endoscopy. This makes it possible to select the most efficient approach (per-oral or per-anal) [48, 49]. The use of double-balloon enteroscopy immediately after standard endoscopy is recommended for the diagnosis and treatment of acute massive bleeding. Based on the above results, a flowchart for the diagnosis and management of OGIB is shown in Fig. 8.1.

### 8.1.3.2 Small Intestine Crohn's Disease

Capsule endoscopy has a very high diagnosis rate in patients already diagnosed with or suspected to have Crohn's disease. For Crohn's disease confined to the small intestine, the diagnosis rate of capsule endoscopy was superior (incremental yield = 38 %) to that of push enteroscopy [50]. It was also superior to abdominal computed tomography (CT). Another study also showed that capsule endoscopy has a higher diagnosis rate than other procedures for Crohn's disease confined to the small intestine [51]. A meta-analysis comparing the diagnosis rates between capsule endoscopy and double-balloon enteroscopy showed no difference between the two. However, no study to date has compared the two procedures for suspected Crohn's disease. According to a meta-analysis of 11 studies consisting of 375 patients with suspected small intestine lesions that compared capsule endoscopy and double-balloon enteroscopy, the detection rates of an inflammatory disease of the small intestine were comparable (pooled yield 16 % with double-balloon enteroscopy and 18 % with capsule endoscopy) [13].

Capsule endoscopy is less invasive than balloon enteroscopy and is more likely to facilitate observation of the entire small intestine. Additionally, capsule endoscopy is generally less expensive and less difficult than balloon enteroscopy. In fact, the results of capsule endoscopy can help determine the approach that should be used for balloon enteroscopy. Thus, the use of capsule endoscopy rather than balloon endoscopy is preferred in cases of suspected Crohn's disease [45]. However, capsule endoscopy has two limitations. First, a biopsy cannot be performed. Second, the capsule may be retained within the intestine. The incidence of a capsule remaining in the intestine of healthy subjects and patients with inflammatory bowel disease was 1–6 and 7–13 %, respectively (Table 8.2) [13, 38]. Thus, the presence of stricture in patients with suspected or established Crohn's disease

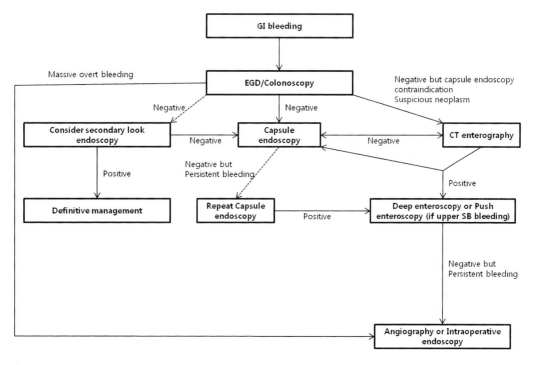

**Fig. 8.1** The chart for the diagnosis and patient management in obscure gastrointestinal bleeding (*dotted line* represents the second best) [35]. *EGD* esophagogastro duodenoscopy, *SB* small bowel, (Reprint from clinical endoscopy [35])

**Table 8.2** Comparison of capsule endoscopy and double-balloon enteroscopy [13, 38]

|  | Capsule endoscopy | Double-balloon enteroscopy |
|---|---|---|
| Sedation requirement | None | Yes |
| Evaluation of the entire SB | 79–90 % | 16–86 % |
| Diagnostic yield of small bowel disease | 60 % | 57 % |
| Risks | Capsule retention, overall 1–6 %, CD 7–13 % | Pancreatitis 1 % Perforation 1 % |

*SB* small bowel, *CD* Crohn's disease

requires confirmation using small bowel series, CT enterography, or MR enterography and then capsule endoscopy should be performed. When capsule enteroscopy or radiological imaging studies reveal positive or suspected results, device-assisted enteroscopy may be conducted

to perform a biopsy. Additionally, in cases of clinically suspected small intestine stricture, device-assisted enteroscopy is more useful for diagnostic and treatment purposes, and the stagnant capsule endoscope due to stricture associated with Crohn's disease can be removed.

In particular, the availability of balloon enteroscopy in patients already diagnosed with Crohn's disease places greater emphasis on treatment. In a prospective study, 11 patients with small bowel strictures due to Crohn's disease underwent balloon angioplasty via balloon enteroscopy. As a result, the patients' subjective symptoms improved significantly despite the fact that only a small number of patients were studied [52]. However, balloon enteroscopy is unlikely to facilitate examination of the entire small intestine compared to imaging studies or capsule endoscopy. The disadvantages of balloon enteroscopy also include patient discomfort due to the long procedure time, high cost, and the risk of complications such as perforation or pancreatitis.

**Fig. 8.2** Flowchart for the diagnosis of Crohn's disease. *SBCD* small bowel Crohn's disease, *SBFT* small bowel follow through, *CTE* computed tomography enterography, *MRE* magnetic resonance enterography

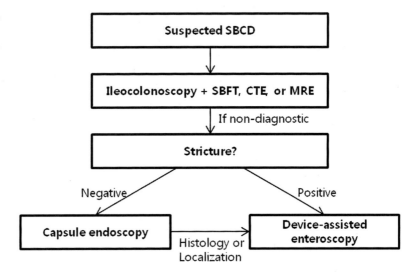

Capsule endoscopy and device-assisted enteroscopy are used in cases of Crohn's disease as shown in the flowchart in Fig. 8.2.

### 8.1.3.3 Small Intestine Tumors

The incidence of primary tumors in the small intestine is very low, accounting for approximately 3–6 % of gastrointestinal tumors and 1–3 % of malignant gastrointestinal tumors [53–56]. The proportion of malignant small intestine cancers among all malignant cancers is 0.3 %. Overall, cancer of the small intestine is rare. Reasons for this are related to the transit time of the contents of the small intestine and the high levels of enzymes that break down carcinogens [56]. Well-developed lymphoid tissues secrete large amounts of immunoglobulin A, while the alkaline digestive fluid inhibits the propagation of bacteria. Additionally, the removal and regeneration cycles of epithelial cells in the intestinal mucosa are very short [57]. The perceived rarity of tumors of the small intestine could be attributable to the lack of appropriate diagnostic tests. However, in studies using capsule endoscopy and enteroscopy that enabled direct observation of the lumen of the small intestine, the incidence of small intestine tumors was 2.4–4.3 % in South Korea and Europe [58, 59]. This finding suggests the possibility that the actual prevalence of small intestine tumors is higher than suspected.

The diagnosis rate of capsule endoscopy for small intestine tumors in the entire population has not yet been conducted. In a retrospective study based on a registry of cases in which capsule endoscopy of the small intestine was used for a variety of clinical indications, the reported diagnosis rate was approximately 4 % [58, 59].

A recent multicenter study in South Korea analyzed the usefulness of the capsule endoscopy in cases limited to small intestine tumors. In that study, 12.3 % of the small intestine tumors identified by the capsule were malignant and were then surgically resected [58]. The overall diagnostic efficiency of balloon enteroscopy in patients with OGIB was 50.0–61.1 %, treatment was possible in 27.8–35.0 %, and the frequency of diagnosed small intestine polyps or tumors was 6–10 % [60]. In a single study on OGIB, the overall diagnostic efficiency reached 45 % and tumors of the small intestine were found in 13 % of cases [61].

In South Korea, cases of all double-balloon enteroscopy procedures were analyzed regardless of indication. In that study, small intestine tumors were found in 13.8 % of cases, similar to the 7–20 % rate reported in studies of other countries [62]. In a study compared double-balloon enteroscopy and capsule endoscopy in nine patients with GI polyposis, double-balloon enteroscopy detected a larger number of polyps than capsule endoscopy [63]. The frequency of the tumor diagnosis with double-balloon enteroscopy was relatively high compared to that with capsule endoscopy (4 %). The main reason for this is that the balloon endoscope was actively manipulated to obtain images of the intestinal lumen and is usually preformed after the other tests compared to the capsule endoscope. The possibility of operator manipulation lends an advantage to enteroscopy over capsule endoscopy for diagnosing tumors of the small intestine.

A total of 18 cases diagnosed using double-balloon enteroscopy were analyzed, one-third of which were detected by capsule endoscopy, whereas four cases of small intestine adenocarcinomas were missed [64]. Double-balloon enteroscopy is useful for the diagnosis and treatment of patients with familial adenomatous polyposis FAP and Peutz-Jegher syndrome (PJS), groups at high risk of developing adenomatous polyps in the small intestine [65, 66].

Deep small bowel enteroscopy is useful in the diagnosis of causative diseases by facilitating observation and biopsy of neoplastic lesions in the small intestine. Further, this procedure can help perform surgical treatment through impacting the extent of surgery by enabling submucosal injection in the area of the lesion and disclosing the lesion's exact location [67, 68]. In addition, if hemorrhage associated with the tumor is detected, hemostasis is possible. Deep enteroscopy is also a useful therapeutic tool in the treatment of polyps [69].

## 8.2    Conclusion

A variety of enteroscopy methods have been developed to diagnose and treat diseases of the small intestine. Of these, the application of capsule endoscopy and balloon enteroscopy has greatly impacted the diagnosis and treatment of small intestine diseases that were previously difficult. According to the results of several studies, these two procedures are able to improve the diagnosis rate of diseases of the small intestine, affect the clinical course and

treatment, and play a complementary role in the their management.

Capsule endoscopy is likely to be non-invasive and enables the observation of the entire small intestine. As such, it can be used in cases in which common endoscopic examination is difficult. Balloon enteroscopy is available for various purposes in addition to diagnosis, such as tissue biopsy and endoscopic therapy. Double- and single-balloon enteroscopy are currently being used in clinical practice and do not differ significantly in terms of lesion observation rates and success rates. Of the 2 techniques, double-balloon enteroscopy is considered deep small bowel endoscopy that can be selected to examine the entire small intestine given that it has the highest observation rate of the entire small intestine.

Once we understand the complementary roles of these two endoscopies and apply them in clinical practice, management of small intestinal diseases can be expected to improve.

## References

1. Kwon JG. Indications and choice of small bowel endoscopy. The 48th Korean Society of gastrointestinal endoscopy seminar. 2013. p. 216–220.
2. Bang S, Park JY, Jeong S, Kim YH, Shim HB, Kim TS, Lee DH, Song SY. First clinical trial of the "MiRo" capsule endoscope by using a novel transmission technology: electric-field propagation. Gastrointest Endosc. 2009;69:253–9. doi:10.1016/j.gie.2008.04.033 (PMID: 18640676).
3. Cave DR, Fleischer DE, Leighton JA, Faigel DO, Heigh RI, Sharma VK, Gostout CJ, Rajan E, Mergener K, Foley A, Lee M, Bhattacharya K. A multicenter randomized comparison of the Endocapsule and the Pillcam SB. Gastrointest Endosc. 2008;68:487–94. doi:10.1016/j.gie.2007.12.037 (PMID: 18410941).
4. Liao Z, Gao R, Li F, Xu C, Zhou Y, Wang JS, Li ZS. Fields of applications, diagnostic yields and findings of OMOM capsule endoscopy in 2400 Chinese patients. World J Gastroenterol: WJG. 2010;16:2669–76 (PMID: 20518090).
5. Liao Z, Gao R, Xu C, Li ZS. Indications and detection, completion, and retention rates of small-bowel capsule endoscopy: a systematic review. Gastrointest Endosc. 2010;71:280–6. doi:10.1016/j.gie.2009.09.031 (PMID: 20152309).
6. Mishkin DS, Chuttani R, Croffie J, Disario J, Liu J, Shah R, Somogyi L, Tierney W, Song LM, Petersen

BT. ASGE technology status evaluation report: wireless capsule endoscopy. Gastrointest Endosc. 2006;63:539–45.        doi:10.1016/j.gie.2006.01.014 (PMID: 16564850).

7. D'Halluin PN, Delvaux M, Lapalus MG, Sacher-Huvelin S, Ben Soussan E, Heyries L, Filoche B, Saurin JC, Gay G, Heresbach D. Does the "suspected blood indicator" improve the detection of bleeding lesions by capsule endoscopy? Gastrointest Endosc. 2005; 61:243–249 (PMID: 15729233).

8. Guilhon de Araujo Sant'Anna AM, Dubois J, Miron MC, Seidman EG. Wireless capsule endoscopy for obscure small-bowel disorders: final results of the first pediatric controlled trial. Clin Gastroenterol Hepatol: Official Clin Pract J Am Gastroenterol Assoc. 2005;3:264–270 (PMID: 15765446).

9. Kavin H, Berman J, Martin TL, Feldman A, Forsey-Koukol K. Successful wireless capsule endoscopy for a 2.5-year-old child: obscure gastrointestinal bleeding from mixed, juvenile, capillary hemangioma-angiomatosis of the jejunum. Pediatrics. 2006;117:539–543. doi: 10.1542/peds. 2005-0710 (PMID: 16452379).

10. Barkin JS, O'Loughlin C. Capsule endoscopy contraindications: complications and how to avoid their occurrence. Gastrointest Endosc Clin N Am. 2004;14:61–5.        doi:10.1016/j.giec.2003.10.016 (PMID: 15062381).

11. May A, Nachbar L, Ell C. Double-balloon enteroscopy (push-and-pull enteroscopy) of the small bowel: feasibility and diagnostic and therapeutic yield in patients with suspected small bowel disease. Gastrointest Endosc. 2005;62:62–70 (PMID: 15990821).

12. Mehdizadeh S, Ross A, Gerson L, Leighton J, Chen A, Schembre D, Chen G, Semrad C, Kamal A, Harrison EM, Binmoeller K, Waxman I, Kozarek R, Lo SK. What is the learning curve associated with double-balloon enteroscopy? Technical details and early experience in 6 U.S. tertiary care centers. Gastrointest Endosc. 2006;64:740–50. doi:10.1016/j. gie.2006.05.022 (PMID: 17055868).

13. Pasha SF, Leighton JA, Das A, Harrison ME, Decker GA, Fleischer DE, Sharma VK. Double-balloon enteroscopy and capsule endoscopy have comparable diagnostic yield in small-bowel disease: a meta-analysis. Clin Gastroenterol Hepatol: Official Clin Pract J Am Gastroenterol Assoc. 2008;6:671–6. doi:10.1016/j.cgh.2008.01.005 (PMID: 18356113).

14. Upchurch BR, Vargo JJ. Single-balloon enteroscopy. Gastrointest Endosc Clin N Am. 2009;19:335–47. doi:10.1016/j.giec.2009.04.010 (PMID: 19647643).

15. May A, Nachbar L, Schneider M, Ell C. Prospective comparison of push enteroscopy and push-and-pull enteroscopy in patients with suspected small-bowel bleeding. Am J Gastroenterol. 2006;101:2016–24. doi:10.1111/j.1572-0241.2006.00745.x        (PMID: 16968508).

16. Aktas H, de Ridder L, Haringsma J, Kuipers EJ, Mensink PB. Complications of single-balloon

enteroscopy: a prospective evaluation of 166 procedures. Endoscopy. 2010;42:365–8. doi:10. 1055/s-0029-1243931 (PMID: 20178072).

17. Kawamura T, Yasuda K, Tanaka K, Uno K, Ueda M, Sanada K, Nakajima M. Clinical evaluation of a newly developed single-balloon enteroscope. Gastrointest Endosc. 2008;68:1112–6. doi:10.1016/ j.gie.2008.03.1063 (PMID: 18599052).

18. May A, Farber M, Aschmoneit I, Pohl J, Manner H, Lotterer E, Moschler O, Kunz J, Gossner L, Monkemuller K, Ell C. Prospective multicenter trial comparing push-and-pull enteroscopy with the single- and double-balloon techniques in patients with small-bowel disorders. Am J Gastroenterol. 2010;105:575–81. doi:10.1038/ajg.2009.712 (PMID: 20051942).

19. Upchurch BR, Sanaka MR, Lopez AR, Vargo JJ. The clinical utility of single-balloon enteroscopy: a single-center experience of 172 procedures. Gastrointest Endosc. 2010;71:1218–23. doi:10.1016/ j.gie.2010.01.012 (PMID: 20409544).

20. Pohl J, Blancas JM, Cave D, Choi KY, Delvaux M, Ell C, Gay G, Jacobs MA, Marcon N, Matsui T, May A, Mulder CJ, Pennazio M, Perez-Cuadrado E, Sugano K, Vilmann P, Yamamoto H, Yano T, Zhong JJ. Consensus report of the 2nd international conference on double balloon endoscopy. Endoscopy. 2008;40:156–160. doi: 10.1055/ s-2007-966994 (PMID: 18253908).

21. Tsujikawa T, Saitoh Y, Andoh A, Imaeda H, Hata K, Minematsu H, Senoh K, Hayafuji K, Ogawa A, Nakahara T, Sasaki M, Fujiyama Y. Novel single-balloon enteroscopy for diagnosis and treatment of the small intestine: preliminary experiences. Endoscopy. 2008;40:11–5. doi:10.1055/ s-2007-966976 (PMID: 18058613).

22. Buscaglia JM, Dunbar KB, Okolo PI, 3rd, Judah J, Akerman PA, Cantero D, Draganov PV. The spiral enteroscopy training initiative: results of a prospective study evaluating the Discovery SB overtube device during small bowel enteroscopy (with video). Endoscopy. 2009;41:194–199. doi: 10. 1055/s-0028-1119602 (PMID: 19280530).

23. Khashab MA, Lennon AM, Dunbar KB, Singh VK, Chandrasekhara V, Giday S, Canto MI, Buscaglia JM, Kapoor S, Shin EJ, Kalloo AN, Okolo PI 3rd. A comparative evaluation of single-balloon enteroscopy and spiral enteroscopy for patients with mid-gut disorders. Gastrointest Endosc. 2010;72:766–72. doi:10.1016/j.gie.2010.04.043 (PMID: 20619404).

24. Messer I, May A, Manner H, Ell C. Prospective, randomized, single-center trial comparing double-balloon enteroscopy and spiral enteroscopy in patients with suspected small-bowel disorders. Gastrointest Endosc. 2013;77:241–9. doi:10.1016/j. gie.2012.08.020 (PMID: 23043851).

25. Jeon SR, Kim JO, Kim HG, Lee TH, Kim WJ, Ko BM, Cho JY, Lee JS, Lee MS. Changes over time in indications, diagnostic yield, and clinical effects of double-balloon enteroscopy. Clin Gastroenterol

Hepatol: Official Clin Prac J Am Gastroenterol Assoc. 2012;10:1152–6. doi:10.1016/j.cgh.2012.06. 024 (PMID: 22801056).

26. Xin L, Liao Z, Jiang YP, Li ZS. Indications, detectability, positive findings, total enteroscopy, and complications of diagnostic double-balloon endoscopy: a systematic review of data over the first decade of use. Gastroint Endosc. 2011;74:563–70. doi:10.1016/j.gie.2011.03.1239 (PMID: 21620401).

27. Shishido T, Oka S, Tanaka S, Aoyama T, Watari I, Imagawa H, Yoshida S, Chayama K. Diagnostic yield of capsule endoscopy vs. double-balloon endoscopy for patients who have undergone total enteroscopy with obscure gastrointestinal bleeding. Hepatogastroenterology. 2012;59:955–9. doi:10. 5754/hge12242 (PMID: 22580642).

28. Teshima CW, Kuipers EJ, van Zanten SV, Mensink PB. Double balloon enteroscopy and capsule endoscopy for obscure gastrointestinal bleeding: an updated meta-analysis. J Gastroenterol Hepatol. 2011;26:796–801. doi:10.1111/j.1440-1746.2010. 06530.x (PMID: 21155884).

29. Fukumoto A, Tanaka S, Shishido T, Takemura Y, Oka S, Chayama K. Comparison of detectability of small-bowel lesions between capsule endoscopy and double-balloon endoscopy for patients with suspected small-bowel disease. Gastrointest Endosc. 2009;69:857–865 doi:10.1016/j.gie.2008.06.007 (PMID: 19136103)

30. Kameda N, Higuchi K, Shiba M, Machida H, Okazaki H, Yamagami H, Tanigawa T, Watanabe K, Watanabe T, Tominaga K, Fujiwara Y, Oshitani N, Arakawa T. A prospective, single-blind trial comparing wireless capsule endoscopy and double-balloon enteroscopy in patients with obscure gastrointestinal bleeding. J Gastroenterol. 2008;43:434–440 doi:10.1007/s00535-008-2182-9 (PMID: 18600387)

31. Ohmiya N, Yano T, Yamamoto H, Arakawa D, Nakamura M, Honda W, Itoh A, Hirooka Y, Niwa Y, Maeda O, Ando T, Yao T, Matsui T, Iida M, Tanaka S, Chiba T, Sakamoto C, Sugano K, Goto H. Diagnosis and treatment of obscure GI bleeding at double balloon endoscopy. Gastrointest Endosc. 2007;66:S72–77 doi: 10.1016/j.gie.2007.05.041 (PMID: 17709039)

32. Fujimori S, Seo T, Gudis K, Tanaka S, Mitsui K, Kobayashi T, Ehara A, Yonezawa M, Tatsuguchi A, Sakamoto C. Diagnosis and treatment of obscure gastrointestinal bleeding using combined capsule endoscopy and double balloon endoscopy: 1-year follow-up study. Endosc. 2007;39:1053–58 doi: 10. 1055/s-2007-967014 (PMID: 18072055)

33. Nakamura M, Niwa Y, Ohmiya N, Miyahara R, Ohashi A, Itoh A, Hirooka Y, Goto H. Preliminary comparison of capsule endoscopy and double-balloon enteroscopy in patients with suspected small-bowel bleeding. Endosc. 2006;38:59–66 doi:10.1055/s-2005-870446 (PMID: 16429356)

34. Hadithi M, Heine GD, Jacobs MA, van Bodegraven AA, Mulder CJ. A prospective study comparing video capsule endoscopy with double-balloon enteroscopy in patients with obscure gastrointestinal bleeding. Am J Gastroenterol. 2006;101:52–57 doi:10.1111/j.1572-0241.2005.00346.x (PMID: 16405533)

35. Shim KN, Moon JS, Chang DK, Do JH, Kim JH, Min BH, Jeon SR, Kim JO, Choi MG. Guideline for capsule endoscopy: obscure gastrointestinal bleeding. Clin Endosc. 2013;46:45–53. doi:10.5946/ ce.2013.46.1.45 (PMID: 23423225).

36. Gerson LB. Small bowel endoscopy: cost-effectiveness of the different approaches. Best Pract Res Clin Gastroenterol. 2012;26:325–35. doi:10. 1016/j.bpg.2012.01.018 (PMID: 22704574).

37. Gross SA, Stark ME. Initial experience with double-balloon enteroscopy at a U.S. center. Gastrointest Endosc. 2008;67:890–897 doi:10.1016/j.gie.2007.07. 047 (PMID: 18178204)

38. Yamamoto H, Sekine Y, Sato Y, Higashizawa T, Miyata T, Iino S, Ido K, Sugano K. Total enteroscopy with a nonsurgical steerable double-balloon method. Gastrointest Endosc. 2001;53:216–220 (PMID: 11174299)

39. Chen X, Ran ZH, Tong JL. A meta-analysis of the yield of capsule endoscopy compared to double-balloon enteroscopy in patients with small bowel diseases. World J Gastroenterol: WJG. 2007;13:4372–8 (PMID: 17708614).

40. Gerson LB. Outcomes associated with deep enteroscopy. Gastrointest Endosc Clin N Am. 2009;19:481–96. doi:10.1016/j.giec.2009.04.007 (PMID: 19647653).

41. Pennazio M, Santucci R, Rondonotti E, Abbiati C, Beccari G, Rossini FP, De Franchis R. Outcome of patients with obscure gastrointestinal bleeding after capsule endoscopy: report of 100 consecutive cases. Gastroenterology. 2004;126:643–53 (PMID: 14988816).

42. Arakawa D, Ohmiya N, Nakamura M, Honda W, Shirai O, Itoh A, Hirooka Y, Niwa Y, Maeda O, Ando T, Goto H. Outcome after enteroscopy for patients with obscure GI bleeding: diagnostic comparison between double-balloon endoscopy and videocapsule endoscopy. Gastrointest Endosc. 2009;69:866–74. doi:10.1016/j.gie.2008.06.008 (PMID: 19136098).

43. Alexander JA, Leighton JA. Capsule endoscopy and balloon-assisted endoscopy: competing or complementary technologies in the evaluation of small bowel disease? Curr Opi Gastroenterol. 2009;25:433–7. doi:10.1097/MOG.0b013e32832d 641e (PMID: 19461511).

44. Marmo R, Rotondano G, Casetti T, Manes G, Chilovi F, Sprujevnik T, Bianco MA, Brancaccio ML, Imbesi V, Benvenuti S, Pennazio M. Degree of concordance between double-balloon enteroscopy and capsule endoscopy in obscure gastrointestinal bleeding: a multicenter study. Endoscopy. 2009;41:587–92. doi:10.1055/s-0029-1214896 (PMID: 19588285).

45. Bourreille A, Ignjatovic A, Aabakken L, Loftus EV Jr, Eliakim R, Pennazio M, Bouhnik Y, Seidman E, Keuchel M, Albert JG, Ardizzone S, Bar-Meir S, Bisschops R, Despott EJ, Fortun PF, Heuschkel R, Kammermeier J, Leighton JA, Mantzaris GJ, Moussata D, Lo S, Paulsen V, Panes J, Radford-Smith G, Reinisch W, Rondonotti E, Sanders DS, Swoger JM, Yamamoto H, Travis S, Colombel JF, Van Gossum A. Role of small-bowel endoscopy in the management of patients with inflammatory bowel disease: an international OMED-ECCO consensus. Endoscopy. 2009;41:618–37. doi:10.1055/s-0029-1214790 (PMID: 19588292).

46. Fisher L, Lee Krinsky M, Anderson MA, Appalaneni V, Banerjee S, Ben-Menachem T, Cash BD, Decker GA, Fanelli RD, Friis C, Fukami N, Harrison ME, Ikenberry SO, Jain R, Jue T, Khan K, Maple JT, Strohmeyer L, Sharaf R, Dominitz JA. The role of endoscopy in the management of obscure GI bleeding. Gastrointest Endosc. 2010;72:471–9. doi:10.1016/j.gie.2010.04.032 (PMID: 20801285).

47. Sidhu R, Sanders DS, Morris AJ, McAlindon ME. Guidelines on small bowel enteroscopy and capsule endoscopy in adults. Gut. 2008;57:125–36. doi:10.1136/gut.2007.129999 (PMID: 18094205).

48. Keum B, Chun HJ. Capsule endoscopy and double balloon enteroscopy for obscure gastrointestinal bleeding: which is better? J Gastroenterol Hepatol. 2011;26:794–5. doi:10.1111/j.1440-1746.2011.06708.x (PMID: 21488944).

49. Pasha SF, Leighton JA. How useful is capsule endoscopy for the selection of patients for double-balloon enteroscopy? Nature Clin Prac Gastroenterol Hepatol. 2008;5:490–1. doi:10.1038/ncpgasthep1201 (PMID: 18648342).

50. Triester SL, Leighton JA, Leontiadis GI, Gurudu SR, Fleischer DE, Hara AK, Heigh RI, Shiff AD, Sharma VK. A meta-analysis of the yield of capsule endoscopy compared to other diagnostic modalities in patients with non-structuring small bowel Crohn's disease. Am J Gastroenterol. 2006;101:954–64. doi:10.1111/j.1572-0241.2006.00506.x (PMID: 16696781).

51. Dionisio PM, Gurudu SR, Leighton JA, Leontiadis GI, Fleischer DE, Hara AK, Heigh RI, Shiff AD, Sharma VK. Capsule endoscopy has a significantly higher diagnostic yield in patients with suspected and established small-bowel Crohn's disease: a meta-analysis. Am J Gastroenterol. 2010;105:1240–1248; quiz 1249. doi: 10.1038/ajg.2009.713 (PMID: 20029412).

52. Despott EJ, Gupta A, Burling D, Tripoli E, Konieczko K, Hart A, Fraser C. Effective dilation of small-bowel strictures by double-balloon enteroscopy in patients with symptomatic Crohn's disease (with video). Gastrointest Endosc. 2009;70:1030–6. doi:10.1016/j.gie.2009.05.005 (PMID: 19640518).

53. Bilimoria KY, Bentrem DJ, Wayne JD, Ko CY, Bennett CL, Talamonti MS. Small bowel cancer in the United States: changes in epidemiology, treatment, and survival over the last 20 years. Ann Surg. 2009;249:63–71. doi:10.1097/SLA.0b013e31818e4641 (PMID: 19106677).

54. Chow JS, Chen CC, Ahsan H, Neugut AI. A population-based study of the incidence of malignant small bowel tumours: SEER, 1973-1990. Int J Epidemiol. 1996;25:722–8 (PMID: 8921448).

55. Jemal A, Siegel R, Ward E, Hao Y, Xu J, Thun MJ. Cancer statistics, 2009. CA Cancer J Clin. 2009;59:225–49. doi:10.3322/caac.20006 (PMID: 19474385).

56. Neugut AI, Jacobson JS, Suh S, Mukherjee R, Arber N. The epidemiology of cancer of the small bowel. Cancer Epidemiol Biomarkers Prev: Publ Am Assoc Cancer Res Cosponsored Am Soc Prev Oncol. 1998;7:243–51 (PMID: 9521441).

57. Gao C, Wang AY. Significance of increased apoptosis and Bax expression in human small intestinal adenocarcinoma. J Histochem Cytochem: Official J Histochem Soc. 2009;57:1139–48. doi:10.1369/jhc.2009.954446 (PMID: 19729672).

58. Cheung DY, Lee IS, Chang DK, Kim JO, Cheon JH, Jang BI, Kim YS, Park CH, Lee KJ, Shim KN, Ryu JK, Do JH, Moon JS, Ye BD, Kim KJ, Lim YJ, Choi MG, Chun HJ. Capsule endoscopy in small bowel tumors: a multicenter Korean study. J Gastroentero and Hepatol. 2010;25:1079–86 doi:10.1111/j.1440-1746.2010.06292.x (PMID: 20594222)

59. Rondonotti E, Pennazio M, Toth E, Menchen P, Riccioni ME, De Palma GD, Scotto F, De Looze D, Pachofsky T, Tacheci I, Havelund T, Couto G, Trifan A, Kofokotsios A, Cannizzaro R, Perez-Quadrado E, de Franchis R. Small-bowel neoplasms in patients undergoing video capsule endoscopy: a multicenter European study. Endoscopy. 2008;40:488–95. doi:10.1055/s-2007-995783 (PMID: 18464193).

60. Takano N, Yamada A, Watabe H, Togo G, Yamaji Y, Yoshida H, Kawabe T, Omata M, Koike K. Single-balloon versus double-balloon endoscopy for achieving total enteroscopy: a randomized, controlled trial. Gastrointest Endosc. 2011;73:734–9. doi:10.1016/j.gie.2010.10.047 (PMID: 21272875).

61. Godeschalk MF, Mensink PB, van Buuren HR, Kuipers EJ. Primary balloon-assisted enteroscopy in patients with obscure gastrointestinal bleeding: findings and outcome of therapy. J Clin Gastroenterol. 2010;44:e195–200. doi: 10.1097/MCG.0b013e3181dd1110 (PMID: 20505527).

62. Ell C, Remke S, May A, Helou L, Henrich R, Mayer G. The first prospective controlled trial comparing wireless capsule endoscopy with push enteroscopy in chronic gastrointestinal bleeding. Endoscopy. 2002;34:685–9. doi:10.1055/s-2002-33446 (PMID: 12195324).

63. Matsumoto T, Esaki M, Moriyama T, Nakamura S, Iida M. Comparison of capsule endoscopy and enteroscopy with the double-balloon method in patients with obscure bleeding and polyposis. Endoscopy. 2005;37:827–32. doi:10.1055/s-2005-870207 (PMID: 16116533).

64. Ross A, Mehdizadeh S, Tokar J, Leighton JA, Kamal A, Chen A, Schembre D, Chen G, Binmoeller K, Kozarek R, Waxman I, Dye C, Gerson L, Harrison ME, Haluszka O, Lo S, Semrad C. Double balloon enteroscopy detects small bowel mass lesions missed by capsule endoscopy. Dig Dis Sci. 2008;53:2140–3. doi:10.1007/s10620-007-0110-0 (PMID: 18270840).

65. Monkemuller K, Fry LC, Ebert M, Bellutti M, Venerito M, Knippig C, Rickes S, Muschke P, Rocken C, Malfertheiner P. Feasibility of double-balloon enteroscopy-assisted chromoendoscopy of the small bowel in patients with familial adenomatous polyposis. Endoscopy. 2007;39:52–7. doi:10.1055/s-2006-945116 (PMID: 17252461).

66. Plum N, May AD, Manner H. Ell C [Peutz-Jeghers syndrome: endoscopic detection and treatment of small bowel polyps by double-balloon enteroscopy]. Z Gastroenterol. 2007;45:1049–55. doi:10.1055/s-2007-963345 (PMID: 17924301).

67. Iwamoto M, Yamamoto H, Kita H, Sunada K, Hayashi Y, Sato H, Sugano K. Double-balloon endoscopy for ileal GI stromal tumor. Gastrointest Endosc. 2005;62:440–441; discussion 441 (PMID: 16111968).

68. Yamagami H, Oshitani N, Hosomi S, Suekane T, Kamata N, Sogawa M, Okazaki H, Watanabe K, Tominaga K, Watanabe T, Fujiwara Y, Arakawa T. Usefulness of double-balloon endoscopy in the diagnosis of malignant small-bowel tumors. Clin Gastroenterol Hepatol: Official Clin Pract J Am Gastroenterol Assoc. 2008;6:1202–5. doi:10.1016/j.cgh.2008.05.014 (PMID: 18799359).

69. Kita H, Yamamoto H. New indications of double balloon endoscopy. Gastrointest Endosc. 2007;66:S57–59. DOI: 10.1016/j.gie.2007.03.1038 (PMID: 17709033).

# Future Development of Capsule Endoscopy

**9**

Melissa F. Hale and Mark McAlindon

## 9.1 Introduction

Capsule endoscopy (CE) has evolved substantially since its introduction 13 years ago due to a combination of technical innovation and commercial competition. Despite this, it remains a diagnostic tool for mainly small bowel pathologies. Capsules to image the oesophagus and colon are available but as yet do not offer a real alternative to conventional flexible endoscopy due to lower diagnostic yields, extensive bowel preparation (colon capsule), cost issues and their inability to take biopsies or perform therapeutic intervention. However, CE offers a major advantage to patients in that it is well tolerated and in most cases preferred over standard endoscopy. Technology is swiftly progressing in such we may see CE expand its horizons to become a diagnostic and therapeutic modality for the whole gastrointestinal tract. This chapter explores some of the recent advances and future expectations for capsule technology.

M. F. Hale (✉) · M. McAlindon
Directorate of Gastroenterology, Royal Hallamshire Hospital, Sheffield Teaching Hospitals NHS Trust, Glossop Road, Sheffield, S10 2JF, UK
e-mail: melissa.hale@sth.nhs.uk

M. McAlindon
e-mail: mark.mcalindon@sth.nhs.uk

## 9.2 Technical Improvements

### 9.2.1 Hardware

Considerable improvements have been made to the original small bowel capsules. Optical enhancements include the use of multi-element lenses, which allow a wider angle of view and adaptive illumination, an automatic internal analysis of the average illumination of each frame leading to response by the internal LED. Superior quality lenses also contribute to improved picture clarity, and in the future, it is likely pictures will be available in high definition. Power management strategies have increased the duration and performance of capsule endoscopes and are imperative to facilitate other capsule technological advancements.

### 9.2.2 Software and Data Analysis

One of the major drawbacks of CE is the time-consuming process of CE reporting, and therefore, great efforts have been devoted to streamlining this process without jeopardising diagnostic accuracy. The suspected blood indicator highlights frames containing multiple red pixels as an indicator of bleeding or vascular abnormalities but in practice results have been inconsistent, and currently, it can only be recommended as a supportive tool [1, 2]. Quick view aims to reduce CE reading time by selecting 1 frame every X frames (as set by the reader), producing a condensed video for review. This has

Z. Li et al. (eds.), *Handbook of Capsule Endoscopy*,
DOI: 10.1007/978-94-017-9229-5_9, © Springer Science+Business Media Dordrecht 2014

shown promising potential, especially when coupled with other image enhancing software systems [3, 4]. Fujinon intelligent chromoendoscopy (FICE) enhances surface contrast in three specific wavelengths (red, green and blue) and appears to improve image quality and visualisation of small bowel lesions; however, its clinical utility remains unclear [5, 6].

3D reconstruction of the gastrointestinal (GI) tract seems to assist diagnosis at conventional endoscopy by enhancing mucosal textural features and abnormalities [7–9]. A version for CE has been trialled and improved visualisation of a significant proportion of vascular lesions but was less beneficial for inflammatory and protruding lesions [10]. Encouraging results have been reported by investigators using automated tumour recognition software, where the computer aided system achieved a tumour recognition accuracy of 92.4 % [11]. Still in the early stages of development, the future of such field-enhancement techniques remains uncertain.

## 9.3    Novel Indications

The success of small bowel CE and its favourable tolerability profile has led many clinicians and researchers to consider broader indications for its use. The expansion of technology leading to the introduction of oesophageal and colon capsules has also facilitated this process.

### 9.3.1    Upper GI Bleeding

Upper GI haemorrhage is a common cause of Emergency Department (ED) attendance and early therapeutic upper GI endoscopy (OGD), within 24 h, has established benefits [12]. When OGD is performed in ED, up to 46 % of patients can be safely discharged compared to 14 % when OGD is not available [13, 14]. Despite recommendation in UK guidelines [15], many hospitals are unable to meet this demand with one study indicating only 50 % of patients had an OGD within 24 h [16]. Validated scoring

systems [17, 18] exist to enable risk stratification of patients in ED but due to increasing patient age and co-morbidities may ultimately require admission for OGD. Promising results have been achieved using oesophageal CE to risk-stratify patients presenting to the ED with upper GI bleeding in the hope of allowing early discharge. CE detected dyspeptic/inflammatory lesions comparable to OGD in one study [19], while a further reported 88 % sensitivity and 65 % specificity for CE ability to detect fresh blood in the upper GI tract. 25 % of patients with normal OGD in this study had a positive CE suggesting lesions can be overlooked with both techniques [20]. CE appears to be at least as accurate as our traditional scoring systems for upper GI bleeding; however, larger studies are needed to confirm these findings [21]. Poor visualisation of the duodenum due to the lapsed battery life of PillCam Eso was a major factor in lack of concordance between CE and OGD findings; this could potentially be addressed in newer generation capsules. ED physicians appeared to be competent to use the system after a brief training period [22]. Initial cost analyses appear favourable although further studies are required to validate this [20].

### 9.3.2    GAVE

CE could be regarded as a more accurate physiologic representation of the stomach than seen with conventional endoscopy where air insufflation can compress vasculature leading to diminished blood flow. This has been recognised in GAVE, a recognised cause of OGIB that can be successfully treated with APC. Small bowel CE seems to be a useful tool for identifying the condition where standard OGD often fails [23, 24].

### 9.3.3    Gastric Cancer Screening

Due to its acceptability, CE has been considered as an alternative to conventional OGD in order to improve compliance with investigation of the upper GI tract. This is particularly pertinent to countries with high gastric cancer incidence where screening programmes are under consideration. Small bowel CE is unable to examine all areas of the capacious stomach, even with patient positional change strategies. Certain areas are often obscured by large mucosal folds making it of limited use as a sole diagnostic or screening examination for gastric cancer [25]. The first step in order to examine the large volume stomach will be for capsules to have some element of manoeuvrability and work is already underway to this effect.

## 9.4 Novel Directions

### 9.4.1 Manoeuvrability

The first case report of this novel technology, published by Paul Swain et al. in 2010, used a modified Pillcam Colon with one of the cameras replaced by magnetic material. The magnetically manoeuvrable capsule appeared to be easily manipulated in the oesophagus and stomach using a handheld external magnet [26]. This was followed by a series focussing on gastric visualisation and safety of the technique. No adverse events were experienced, and >75 % of the gastric mucosa was visualised in 7 out of 10 patients undergoing the procedure [27].

Further studies have been undertaken using a specially developed magnetically steerable capsule with a magnetic guidance system similar to standard magnetic resonance imagers. In this case, the capsule is manipulated using a joystick rather than a hand-held paddle. Promising results were also achieved with all major areas of the stomach identified in >85 % of examinations. Comparison with conventional upper GI endoscopy was also encouraging with 58.3 % of gastric lesions detected by both modalities, while 14 lesions were missed by magnetically steerable capsule endoscopy (MSCE) and 31 lesions missed by OGD (that were seen on MSCE) [28]. The relative high cost of installing such a system is a major drawback to this technique.

Impaired visualisation due to gastric mucous and debris remained a challenge for both techniques since there is no suction facility. Changing patient position appeared to facilitate movement of these pools allowing better images to be achieved. Ingestion of water, sodium bicarbonate and simethicone have also been used. More studies are required to determine the optimum preparation protocol for patient tolerability, stomach distention and mucosal visualisation. Learning curves were demonstrated with both techniques and not only in terms of manoeuvring the capsule with the associated equipment but also in familiarising oneself with the altered appearance of a more collapsed stomach, particularly the cardia and fundus.

These devices can also be applied to broadening the clinical utility of small bowel, oesophageal and colon CE. If the capsule can be manoeuvred to stop and look more closely at an area of interest, it may improve diagnostic yield or allow targeted biopsy or therapy. Preliminary studies on ex vivo models show promising results but further work in human populations is necessary [29, 30]. Other techniques to manipulate capsules remotely have been trialled but there is limited published data. Capsule with legs [31], paddles [32] and propellers [33] have been tried with some element of success; however, extensive work is required for these to become clinical reality. Work is also underway to enable a two-way interaction with the capsule so it can be commanded to execute certain functions at a time deemed appropriate by the operator [34].

### 9.4.2 Biopsy

This would be a major advance for CE technology, potentially preventing the need for a flexible endoscopy and biopsy when an abnormality is noted at CE reporting. The nano-based capsule endoscopy with molecular imaging and optical biopsy (NEMO) project is a collaboration between academic and industry pioneers to produce a capsule with recognition, anchoring and bio-sensing capabilities to enable accurate pathology detection and diagnosis. Similarly, the Versatile Endoscopic Capsule for gastrointestinal TumOur Recognition and therapy (VECTOR) project, funded by the European Commission, is developing a mini-robot comprising sensors, controls and a human–machine interface aiming to detect and intervene in early GI cancer. Other capsules using a spring-loaded 'Crosby capsule'-type device, protruding barbs and rotational cutting devices are also being tested.

### 9.4.3 Targeted Therapeutics

Capsules have been used in experimental pharmacology to learn more about drug pharmacokinetics for some time. With real-time viewing and external manipulation, the notion of targeted drug delivery becomes feasible. One such prototype can deliver an injection of 1 ml of targeted medication while using a holding mechanism to resist movement by peristalsis [35]. Whereas the iPill (Phillips Research, Eindhoven, the Netherlands) uses bowel transit time and pH sensors to gauge gut location before drug delivery and is currently being trialled in Crohn's disease and colorectal cancer [36].

### 9.5 Conclusion

Capsule endoscopy has enjoyed a meteoric rise to widespread clinical use, and it remains an exciting, innovative field of gastroenterology. As technology progresses, its role as a purely diagnostic tool is likely to evolve to encompass pathology analysis and targeted therapeutics. More advanced diagnostics may be feasible with capsules able to aspirate fluid samples, perform immunological testing and localised ultrasonography. The most important hurdle to overcome is developing capsules with accurate steering ability. Once achieved, this opens up the potential for pan-enteric gut examination alongside targeted diagnostics and therapeutics. Ultimately, a major factor in the success of CE is its excellent patient tolerability profile, and therefore, future innovations in this field are likely to deliver tangible benefits to patients; a worthy goal for any researcher.

## References

1. Liangpunsakul S, Mays L, Rex DK. Performance of given suspected blood indicator. Am J Gastroenterol. 2003;98(12):2676–8.
2. Buscaglia JM, Giday SA, Kantsevoy SV, Clarke JO, Magno P, Yong E, Mullin GE. Performance characteristics of the suspected blood indicator feature in capsule endoscopy according to indication for study. Clin Gastroenterol Hepatol. 2008;6(3):298–301. doi:10.1016/j.cgh.2007.12.029 (Epub 2008 Feb 6).
3. Kyriakos N, Karagiannis S, Galanis P, Liatsos C, Zouboulis-Vafiadis I, Georgiou E, Mavrogiannis C. Evaluation of four time-saving methods of reading capsule endoscopy videos. Eur J Gastroenterol Hepatol. 2012;24(11):1276–80.
4. Koulaouzidis A, Smirnidis A, Douglas S, Plevris JN. QuickView in small-bowel capsule endoscopy is useful in certain clinical settings, but QuickView with blue mode is of no additional benefit. Eur J Gastroenterol Hepatol. 2012;24(9):1099–104. doi:10. 1097/MEG.0b013e32835563ab.
5. Gupta T, Ibrahim M, Deviere J, Van Gossum A. Evaluation of Fujinon intelligent chromo endoscopy-assisted capsule endoscopy in patients with obscure gastroenterology bleeding. World J Gastroenterol. 2011;17(41):4590–5. doi:10.3748/wjg.v17.i41.4590.
6. Nakamura M, Ohmiya N, Miyahara R, Ando T, Watanabe O, Kawashima H, Itoh A, Hirooka Y, Goto H. Usefulness of flexible spectral imaging color enhancement (FICE) for the detection of angiodysplasia in the preview of capsule endoscopy. Hepatogastroenterology. 2012;59(117):1474–7. doi:10.5754/hge10747.
7. Tsutsui A, Okamura S, Muguruma N, Tsujigami K, Ichikawa S, Ito S, Umino K. Three-dimensional reconstruction of endosonographic images of gastric lesions: preliminary experience. J Clin Ultrasound. 2005;33(3):112–8.
8. Bhandari S, Shim CS, Kim JH, Jung IS, Cho JY, Lee JS, Lee MS, Kim BS. Usefulness of three-dimensional, multidetector row CT (virtual gastroscopy and multiplanar reconstruction) in the evaluation of gastric cancer: a comparison with conventional endoscopy, EUS, and histopathology. Gastrointest Endosc. 2004;59(6):619–26.
9. Taylor SA, Halligan S, Slater A, Goh V, Burling DN, Roddie ME, Honeyfield L, McQuillan J, Amin H, Dehmeshki J. Polyp detection with CT colonography: primary 3D endoluminal analysis versus primary 2D transverse analysis with

computer-assisted reader software. Radiology. 2006;239(3):759–67 (Epub 2006 Mar 16).

10. Koulaouzidis A, Karargyris A, Rondonotti E, Noble CL, Douglas S, Alexandridis E, Zahid AM, Bathgate AJ, Trimble KC, Plevris JN. Three-dimensional representation software as image enhancement tool in small-bowel capsule endoscopy: a feasibility study. Dig Liver Dis. 2013; pii: S1590-8658(13)00213-2. doi:10.1016/j.dld.2013.05.013 (Epub ahead of print).

11. Li B, Meng MQ. Tumor recognition in wireless capsule endoscopy images using textural features and SVM-based feature selection. IEEE Trans Inf Technol Biomed. 2012;16(3):323–9. doi:10.1109/TITB.2012.2185807 (Epub 2012 Jan 24).

12. Stanley AJ, Ashley D, Dalton HR, Mowat C, Gaya DR, Thompson E, Warshow U, Groome M, Cahill A, Benson G, Blatchford O, Murray W. Outpatient management of patients with low-risk upper-gastrointestinal haemorrhage: multicentre validation and prospective evaluation. Lancet. 2009;373(9657):42–7. doi:10.1016/S0140-6736(08)61769-9 (Epub 2008 Dec 16).

13. Meltzer AC, Burnett S, Pinchbeck C, Brown AL, Choudhri T, Yadav K, Fleischer DE, Pines JM. Pre-endoscopic Rockall and Blatchford scores to identify which emergency department patients with suspected gastrointestinal bleed do not need endoscopic hemostasis. J Emerg Med. 2013;44(6):1083–7.

14. Bjorkman DJ, Zaman A, Fennerty MB, Lieberman D, Disario JA, Guest-Warnick G. Urgent vs. elective endoscopy for acute non-variceal upper-GI bleeding: an effectiveness study. Gastrointest Endosc. 2004;60(1):1–8.

15. Scottish Intercollegiate Guidelines Network. Management of acute upper and lower gastrointestinal bleeding: a national clinical guideline. 2008. pp. 1–56.

16. Lee JG, Turnipseed S, Romano PS, Vigil H, Azari R, Melnikoff N, Hsu R, Kirk D, Sokolove P, Leung JW. Endoscopy-based triage significantly reduces hospitalization rates and costs of treating upper GI bleeding: a randomized controlled trial. Gastrointest Endosc. 1999;50(6):755–61.

17. Blatchford O, Murray WR, Blatchford M. A risk score to predict need for treatment for upper-gastrointestinal haemorrhage. Lancet. 2000;356(9238):1318–21.

18. Rockall TA, Logan RF, Devlin HB, Northfield TC. Selection of patients for early discharge or outpatient care after acute upper gastrointestinal haemorrhage. National audit of acute upper gastrointestinal haemorrhage. Lancet. 1996;347(9009):1138–40.

19. Gralnek IM, Ching JY, Maza I, Wu JC, Rainer TH, Israelit S, Klein A, Chan FK, Ephrath H, Eliakim R, Peled R, Sung JJ. Capsule endoscopy in acute upper gastrointestinal haemorrhage: a prospective cohort study. Endoscopy. 2013;45(1):12–9.

20. Chandran S, Testro A, Urquhart P, La Nauze R, Ong S, Shelton E, Philpott H, Sood S, Vaughan R, Kemp W, Brown G, Froomes P. Risk stratification of upper GI bleeding with an esophageal capsule. Gastrointest Endosc. 2013;77(6):891–8.

21. Gutkin E, Shalomov A, Hussain SA, Kim SH, Cortes R, Gray S, Judeh H, Pollack S, Rubin M. Pillcam ESO® is more accurate than clinical scoring systems in risk stratifying emergency room patients with acute upper gastrointestinal bleeding. Therap Adv Gastroenterol. 2013;6(3):193–8.

22. Meltzer AC, Pinchbeck C, Burnett S, Buhumaid R, Shah P, Ding R, Fleischer DE, Gralnek IM. Emergency physicians accurately interpret video capsule endoscopy findings in suspected upper gastrointestinal haemorrhage: a video survey. Acad Emerg Med. 2013;20(7):711–5. doi:10.1111/acem.12165.

23. Sidhu R, Sanders DS, McAlindon ME. Does capsule endoscopy recognise gastric antral vascular ectasia more frequently than conventional endoscopy? J Gastrointestin Liver Dis. 2006;15(4):375–7.

24. Ohira T, Hokama A, Kinjo N, Nakamoto M, Kobashigawa C, Kise Y, Yamashiro S, Kinjo F, Kuniyoshi Y, Fujita J. Detection of active bleeding from gastric antral vascular ectasia by capsule endoscopy. World J Gastrointest Endosc. 2013;5(3):138–40.

25. Jun BY, Lim CH, Lee WH, Kim JS, Park JM, Lee IS, Kim SW, Choi MG. Detection of neoplastic gastric lesions using capsule endoscopy: pilot study. Gastroenterol Res Pract. 2013;2013:730261. doi:10.1155/2013/730261 (Epub 2013 May 22).

26. Swain P, Toor A, Volke F, Keller J, Gerber J, Rabinovitz E, Rothstein RI. Remote magnetic manipulation of a wireless capsule endoscope in the esophagus and stomach of humans (with videos). Gastrointest Endosc. 2010;71(7):1290–3.

27. Keller J, Fibbe C, Volke F, Gerber J, Mosse AC, Reimann-Zawadzki M, Rabinovitz E, Layer P, Schmitt D, Andresen V, Rosien U, Swain P. Inspection of the human stomach using remote-controlled capsule endoscopy: a feasibility study in healthy volunteers (with videos). Gastrointest Endosc. 2011;73(1):22–8. doi:10.1016/j.gie.2010.08.053 (Epub 2010 Nov 9).

28. Rey JF, Ogata H, Hosoe N, Ohtsuka K, Ogata N, Ikeda K, Aihara H, Pangtay I, Hibi T, Kudo SE, Tajiri H. Blinded nonrandomized comparative study of gastric examination with a magnetically guided capsule endoscope and standard videoendoscope. Gastrointest Endosc. 2012;75(2):373–81. doi:10.1016/j.gie.2011.09.030 (Epub 2011 Dec 9).

29. Ciuti G, Donlin R, Valdastri P, Arezzo A, Menciassi A, Morino M, Dario P. Robotic versus manual control in magnetic steering of an endoscopic capsule. Endoscopy. 2010;42(2):148–52. doi:10.1055/s-0029-1243808 (Epub 2009 Dec 16).

30. Arezzo A, Menciassi A, Valdastri P, Ciuti G, Lucarini G, Salerno M, Di Natali C, Verra M, Dario P, Morino M. Experimental assessment of a novel robotically-driven endoscopic capsule compared to traditional colonoscopy. Dig Liver

Dis. 2013;45(8):657–62. doi:10.1016/j.dld.2013.01. 025 (Epub 2013 Feb 28).

31. Quirini M, Menciassi A, Scapellato S, Dario P, Rieber F, Ho CN, Schostek S, Schurr MO. Feasibility proof of a legged locomotion capsule for the GI tract. Gastrointest Endosc. 2008;67(7):1153–8. doi:10. 1016/j.gie.2007.11.052.

32. Kim HM, Yang S, Kim J, Park S, Cho JH, Park JY, Kim TS, Yoon ES, Song SY, Bang S. Active locomotion of a paddling-based capsule endoscope in an in vitro and in vivo experiment (with videos). Gastrointest Endosc. 2010;72(2):381–7. doi:10.1016/ j.gie.2009.12.058 (Epub 2010 May 23).

33. Morita E, Ohtsuka N, Shindo Y, Nouda S, Kuramoto T, Inoue T, Murano M, Umegaki E, Higuchi K. In vivo trial of a driving system for a self-propelling capsule endoscope using a magnetic field (with video). Gastrointest Endosc. 2010;72(4):836–40. doi:10.1016/j.gie.2010.06.016.

34. Swain P. At a watershed? Technical developments in wireless capsule endoscopy. J Dig Dis. 2010;11:259–65.

35. Woods SP, Constandinou TG. Wireless capsule endoscope for targeted drug delivery: mechanics and design considerations. IEEE Trans Biomed Eng. 2013;60(4):945–53. doi:10.1109/TBME.2012. 2228647 (Epub 2012 Nov 21).

36. Phillips Technology. Phillips Intelligent Pill Technology. http://www.research.philips.com/newscenter/backgrounders/081111-ipill.html.

# Case Presentations

# 10

Zhuan Liao, Min Tang, Qiang Guo, Bangmao Wang, Qiong He, Fachao Zhi, Mark McAlindon, Dan Carter, Rami Eliakim, Anastasios Koulaouzidis, Sarah Douglas, Wenbin Zou, Zhizheng Ge and Zhaoshen Li

## 10.1 Small Bowel Capsule Endoscopy I

**Case 1. Cavernous hemangioma in jejunum.**

A 74-year-old Chinese woman with recurrent melena for 7 years. Her hemoglobin level was 90 g/L (Fig. 10.1).

**Case 2. Meckel's diverticulum.**

A 21-year-old Chinese woman was admitted for recurrent melena. Gastroscopy and colonoscopy revealed no hemorrhagic lesion. Her hemoglobin level was 115 g/L (Fig. 10.2).

**Case 3. Rupture of ileum venous aneurysm.**

A 49-year-old Chinese woman presented with recurrent melena and hematochezia for a month. Her hemoglobin level was 69 g/L. Colonoscopy found only intraluminal blood with no abnormal mucosa (Fig. 10.3).

Z. Liao (✉) · W. Zou · Z. Li (✉)
Department of Gastroenterology, Changhai Hospital, Second Military Medical University, 168 Changhai Road, Yangpu District, Shanghai, 200433, China
e-mail: liao.zhuan@gmail.com
e-mail:

W. Zou
e-mail: zwbpeak@gmail.com

M. Tang · Q. Guo
Department of Gastroenterology, The First People's Hospital of Yunnan Province, Kunming, China

B. M. Wang
Department of Gastroenterology, General Hospital Affiliated to Tianjin Medical University, Tianjin, China

Q. He
Department of Gastroenterology, The Third Affiliated Hospital of Southern Medical University, Guangzhou, 510630, China

Q. He · F. C. Zhi (✉)
Department of Gastroenterology, Nanfang Hospital, Southern Medical University, Guangzhou, 510515, China

M. McAlindon (✉)
Gastroenterology, Royal Hallamshire Hospital, Sheffield Teaching Hospitals NHS Trust, Glossop Road, Sheffield, S10 2JF, UK
e-mail: mark.mcalindon@sth.nhs.uk

R. Eliakim (✉)
Department of Gastroenterology, Sheba Medical Center, Sackler School of Medicine, Tel-Aviv University, Tel-Aviv, Israel
e-mail: abraham.eliakim@sheba.health.gov.il

A. Koulaouzidis (✉) · S. Douglas
The Royal Infirmary of Edinburgh, Centre for Liver and Digestive Disorders, 51 Little France Crescent, Edinburgh, EH16 4SA, UK
e-mail: akoulaouzidis@hotmail.com

S. Douglas
e-mail: sarah.douglas@luht.scot.nhs.uk

Z. Ge (✉)
Department of Gastroenterology and Hepatology, Digestive Endoscopy Centre, Renji Hospital, School of Medicine, Shanghai Jiao Tong University, Shanghai, China

D. Carter
Department of Gastroenterology, Chaim Sheba Medical Center, 2nd Sheba Road, 52621, Ramat-Gan, Israel
e-mail: dan.carter@sheba.gov.il

Z. Li et al. (eds.), *Handbook of Capsule Endoscopy*,
DOI: 10.1007/978-94-017-9229-5_10, © Springer Science+Business Media Dordrecht 2014

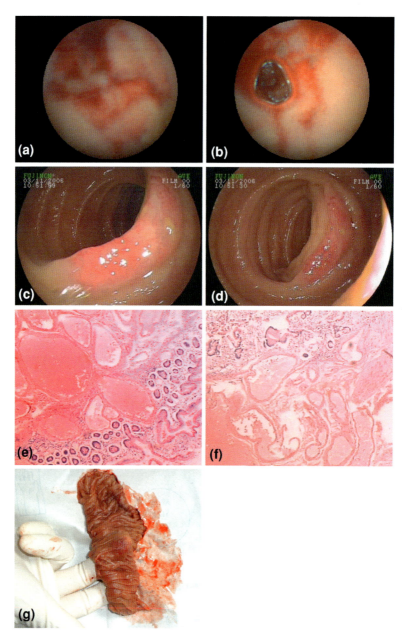

**Fig. 10.1** **a**, **b** SBCE revealed the hemorrhagic lesions in the upper of jejunum; **c**, **d** hemangiomas were suspected under double-balloon enteroscopy in the jejunum; **e**, **f** pathological findings confirmed the diagnosis of cavernous hemangioma of jejunum; and **g** surgical specimens

**Fig. 10.2** **a**, **b** SBCE found ileal ulcers; **c**, **d** double-balloon enteroscopy confirmed Meckel's diverticulum; and **e**, **f** surgical specimen

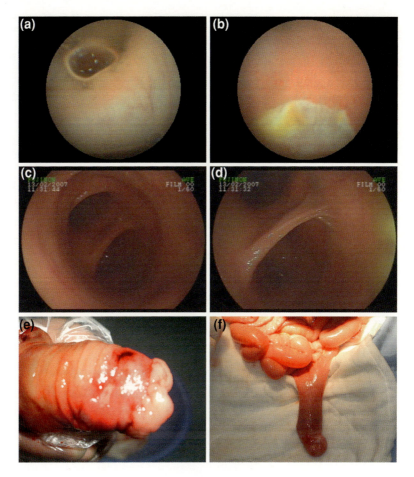

**Case 4. Mucosa-associated B-cell lymphoma in the small intestine.**

A 51-year-old Chinese woman had melena twice. She was admitted for hematochezia (Fig. 10.4).

**Case 5. Jejunum vascular malformation.**

A 15-year-old Chinese boy had melena accompanying with syncope for a week. He was admitted for a sudden severe melena with hemoglobin of 70 g/L, which led to shock (Fig. 10.5).

**Case 6. Hookworms in duodenum.**

A 45-year-old Chinese man had melena for a week (Fig. 10.6).

**Case 7. Taeniasis in small intestine.**

A 58-year-old Chinese man presented with recurrent abdominal pain for three years (Fig. 10.7).

**Case 8. Stromal tumors in mid-ileum.**

A 57-year-old Chinese woman had melena with hemoglobin of 70 g/L for a week (Fig. 10.8).

**Fig. 10.3** **a**, **b** SBCE found elevated lesions bleeding in the upper ileum, suspecting hemangioma or stromal tumors and **c**, **d** surgery confirmed venous aneurysm bleeding in the upper ileum

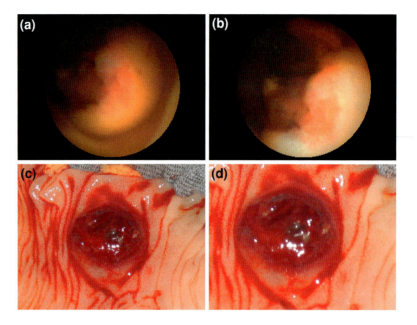

**Fig. 10.4** **a** SBCE found ileal ulcers; **b** the resected tumor was located in the jejunum–ileum junction; **c** pathological findings were that lymphoid tissue diffusely infiltrated the whole intestinal wall, suspecting lymphoma; and **d** immunohistochemical stains of resected tumor were positive for CD3, CD20, CD45RO, CD45RA, CD5, CyclinD1, and bcl-2

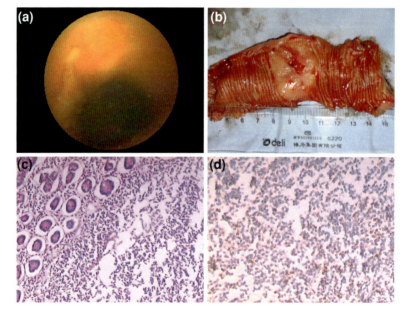

**Fig. 10.5** **a**, **b** SBCE showed a vascular lesion with blood clots in the mid–upper jejunum and **c**, **d** surgical specimen confirmed the diagnosis of vascular malformation

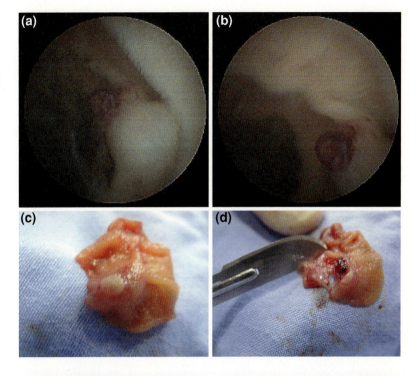

**Fig. 10.6** **a**, **b** SBCE found hookworms in the duodenum

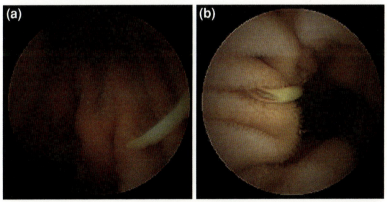

**Fig. 10.7** **a**, **b** SBCE found tapeworm in the small intestine, diagnosing Taeniasis

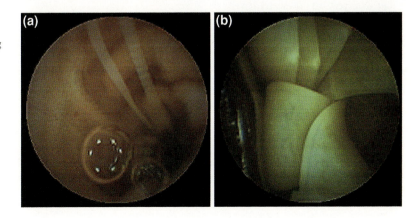

**Fig. 10.8** **a** SBCE showed an elevated lesion in mid-ileum; **b** Double-balloon enterography findings; and **c, d** pathological and Immunohistochemical stains of resected tumor confirmed the diagnosis of stromal tumor in mid-ileum

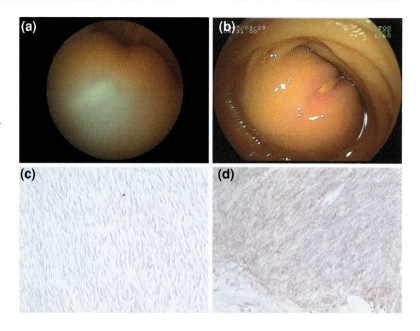

## 10.2   Small Bowel Capsule Endoscopy II

### Case 9. Small intestine carcinoma.

A Chinese patient was admitted for right lower abdominal pain and loss of weight for half a year. Fecal occult blood test was strongly positive. His hemoglobin level was 92 g/L (Fig. 10.9).

### Case 10. Crohn's disease.

The patient was admitted for left lower abdominal pain and melena for two years. Fecal occult blood test was positive. His hemoglobin level was 105 g/L (Fig. 10.10).

### Case 11. Duodenum stromal tumor.

The patient was admitted for abdominal pain and melena for a week. The hemoglobin level was 92 g/L (Fig. 10.11).

### Case 12. Colon carcinoma.

The patient presented with loss of weight and fatigue for half a year. Fecal occult blood test was strongly positive. His hemoglobin level was 82 g/L (Fig. 10.12).

**Fig. 10.9  a, b** Wide base irregular bulge in ileum, superficial erosion; **c, d** cauliflower lumps in the end of ileum, filthy moss covered, risp; and **e, f** pathological findings showed adenocarcinoma

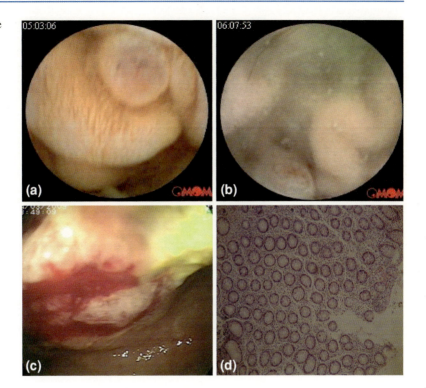

**Fig. 10.10** **a**, **b** Capsule found scattered mucosal redness and small ulcer at the end of ileum; **c** enteroscopic findings; **d** FICE revealed the intestinal mucosa locally stained and stiff; and **e**, **f** pathological findings were mucosal erosions and chronic inflammation

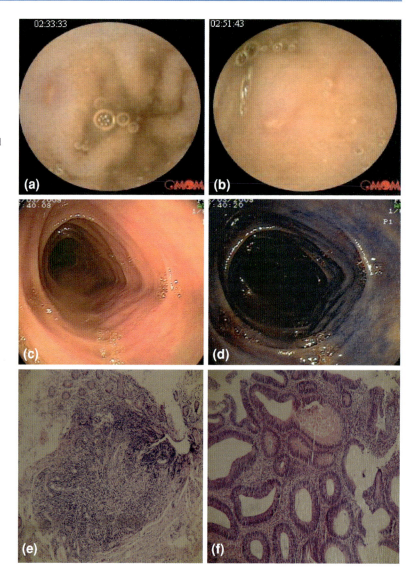

**Fig. 10.11** **a**, **b** Capsule found mucosal protrusion with the surface erosive in the jejunum and **c**, **d** pathological examination revealed lots of proliferative spinal cells in the submucosa

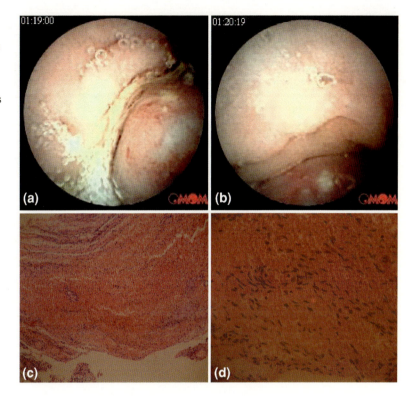

**Fig. 10.12** **a**, **b** Capsule showed the tumor was erosive and irregular bulged as a result of colonic lumen stenosis; **c**, **d** colonoscopy revealed cauliflower mass with surface erosive; and **e**, **f** pathological findings showed adenocarcinoma

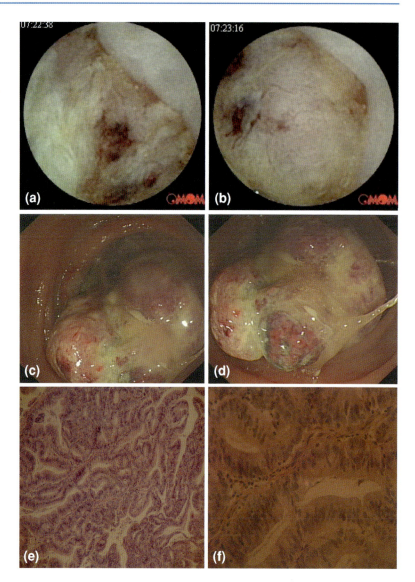

**Fig. 10.13** **a**, **b** showed a intra-luminal mass in the jejunum, showing the appearance of ulcer and necrosis. **c**, **d** GIST was further diagnosed by double-balloon enteroscopy and removed by operation, and definite diagnosis was achieved by pathological analysis and immunochemistry

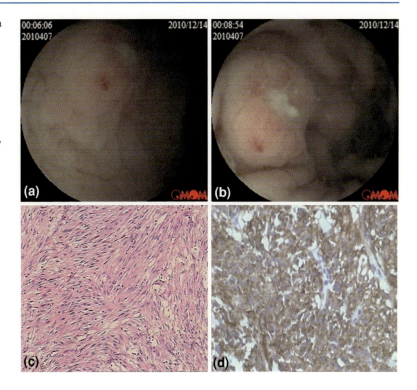

## 10.3 Small Bowel Capsule Endoscopy III

**Case 13.** A 73-year-old Chinese male complained of recurrent melena for more than 1 year. He underwent EGD and colonoscopy before CE, and unclear blood site was found. He had a history of transfusion before admission. Hemoglobin level was 65 g/L (Fig. 10.13).

**Case 14.**
A 16-year-old female underwent recurrent hematochezia and received massive transfusion because of massive blood loss (Fig. 10.14).

**Case 15.**
A 18-year-old male, who underwent endoscopic removal of cavernous hemangioma of the colon five months ago, complained of gastrointestinal re-bleeding (Fig. 10.15).

**Case 16.**
A 21-year-old male registered at our department because of recurrent abdominal pain for 2 years (Fig. 10.16).

**Case 17.**
A 32 Chinese male was admitted to hospital because of severe chronic anemia (Hb:33 g/L) (Fig. 10.17).

**Case 18.**
A female complained of intermittent abdominal distention for 3 months (Fig. 10.18).

**Case 19.**
A 20-year-old Chinese man with mucoid stool for 2 years (Fig. 10.19).

**Case 20.**
A 27-year-old Chinese man with recurrent abdominal pain for 1 year (Fig. 10.20).

The capsule failed to get through the luminal and the patient was transferred to surgery. Pathology test confirmed the diagnosis of Crohn's disease.

**Case 21.**
A 25-year-old Chinese woman with severe diarrhea for 2 months (Fig. 10.21).

**Case 22.**
A 16-year-old Chinese boy with recurrent abdominal distention for 20 days (Fig. 10.22).

**Fig. 10.14** **a**, **b** SBCE detected abnormal mucosa in the small bowel after negative upper gastrointestinal endoscopy and total colonoscopy. Suspected Meckel's diverticulum was initially diagnosed by CE. **c**, **d**, **e**, **f** Balloon-assisted enteroscopy and biopsy confirmed the diagnosis, and the abnormality was correctly verified and removed by surgical procedure

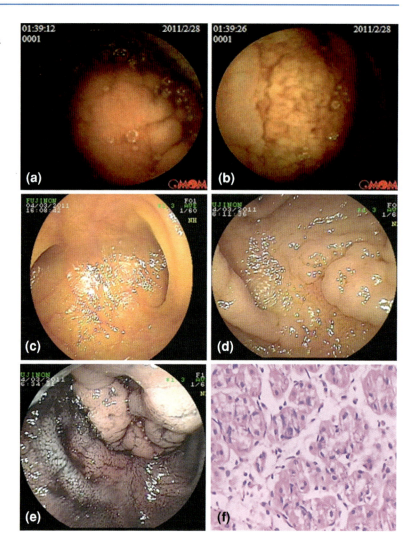

**Fig. 10.15** **a, b** CE were performed after negative DSA and repeated colonoscopy. SBCE found multiple bluish violet hemangiomas in the small intestine, and **c, d** direct view was performed by double-balloon enteroscopy, and confirmed diagnosis was obtained by postoperative pathology

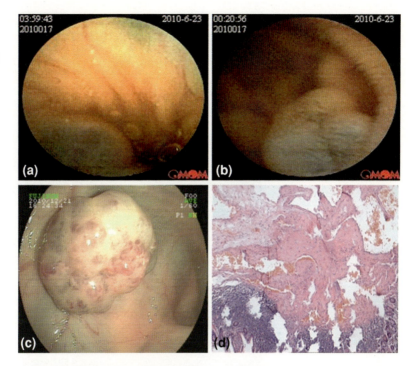

**Fig. 10.16** **a, b** SBCE found several roundworms in the small intestine, diagnosing ascariasis

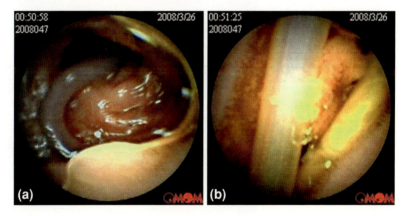

**Fig. 10.17 a–d** SBCE revealed multiple hookworms in the small bowel

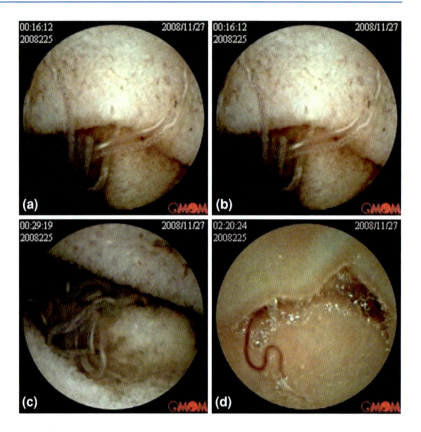

**Fig. 10.18 a, b** SBCE found the pips retention in the stomach, and subsequent EGD revealed a duodenal bulbar ulcer

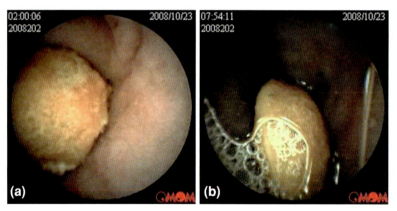

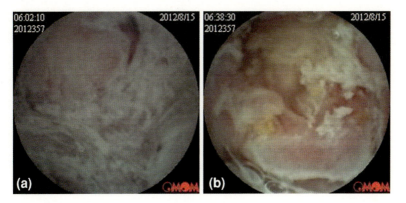

**Fig. 10.19** **a**, **b** Multiple ulcers found in ileum, considering a diagnosis of Crohn's disease or tuberculosis

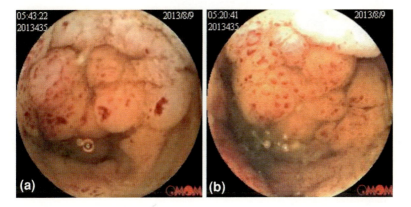

**Fig. 10.20** **a**, **b** Intestinal congestion, swelling and erosion, and nodular mucosa bulge was found in small bowel, considering a diagnosis of Crohn's disease

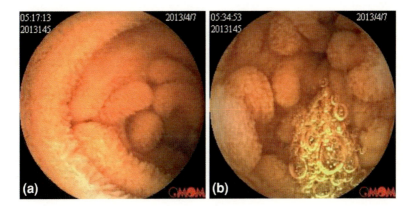

**Fig. 10.21** **a**, **b** Multiple inflammatory pseudopolyp found in ileum, considering a diagnosis of Crohn's disease. CE examination followed by a colonoscopy and multiple ulcers was found in the terminal ileum. Pathology test of the biopsy specimen confirmed the diagnosis of Crohn's disease

**Fig. 10.22** a, b A whipworm was found in the cecum, diagnosing trichuriasis

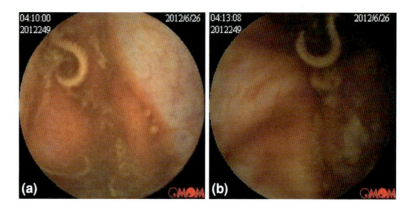

**Fig. 10.23** a, b SBCE revealed chylous exudate in the lumen due to Kaposi's sarcoma affecting the small bowel as demonstrated at double-balloon enteroscopy

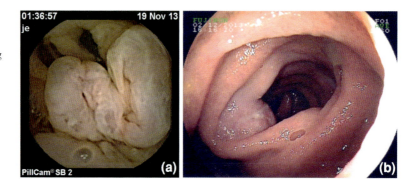

## 10.4 Small Bowel Capsule Endoscopy IV

**Case 23**.

49-year-old man with HIV infection, Kaposi's sarcoma affecting the skin, and pleuropericardial effusions referred for investigation of diarrhea, peripheral edema, and hypoalbuminemia (Fig. 10.23).

**Case 24**.

52-year-old woman with recurrent melena referred with persistent stomal bleeding following subtotal colectomy (Fig. 10.24).

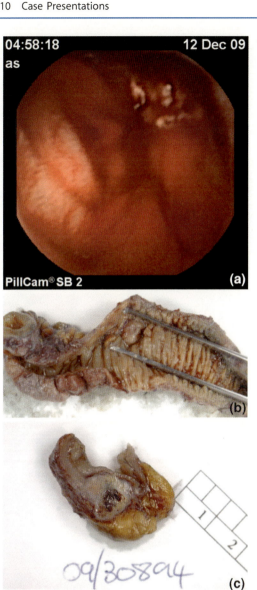

**(a)**

**(b)**

**(c)**

**(d)**

◀Fig. 10.24 **a–d** SBCE showed active small bowel bleeding but no identifiable cause. Careful palpation of the length of the small bowel at laparotomy revealed a palpable nodule which was resected. Histology was consistent with a glomus tumor

## 10.5 Small Bowel Capsule Endoscopy V

**Case 25. Small Bowel Adenocarcinoma**.

A 60-year-old patient was evaluated due to episodes of colicky abdominal pain and distention in the left lower quadrant.

CT scan of the abdomen demonstrated dilatation of several small bowel loops (Fig. 10.25a). Upper and lower endoscopies were normal.

SBCE demonstrated a single large ulceration, with partial occlusion of the mid-small bowel lumen (Fig. 10.25b). At laparotomy, a firmly ulcerated well-moderately differentiated adenocarcinoma pT3, N0, Mx was excised (Fig. 10.25c).

**Case 26. Celiac disease with ulcerative jejuno-ileitis**.

A 66-year-old male presented with severe IDA. On EGD, H. Pylori positive gastritis was found and eradicated. Ileo-colonoscopy and small bowel follow through were normal. On SBCE, the typical endoscopic features of celiac disease were found in the proximal small bowel (Fig. 10.26). Deep in the jejunum and ileum aphthous lesions and ulcerations were seen (Fig. 10.27), compatible with celiac disease complicated by ulcerative jejuno-ileitis and confirmed with biopsies (Fig. 10.28).

**Fig. 10.25** **a** Abdominal CT showed dilated small bowel loops with thickened wall and post-stenosis collapsed small bowel loops. **b** Narrowed, ulcerated small bowel on SBCE. **c** Well-moderately differentiated small bowel adenocarcinoma

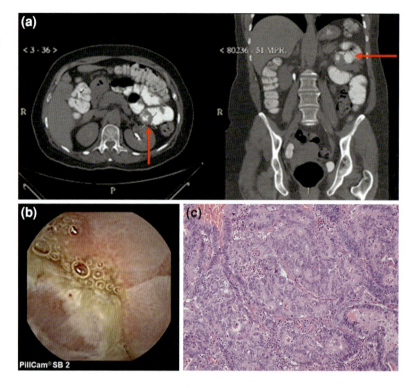

**Fig. 10.26** Proximal small bowel with shortening of villi, scalloping (**a**, **c**), and mosaic pattern (**b**)

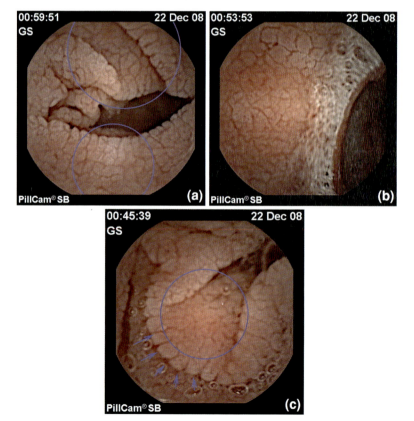

**Fig. 10.27** Mid/distal small bowel ulcerations/ aphthous lesions

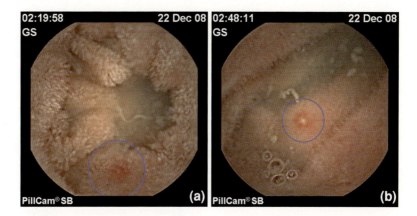

**Fig. 10.28** Histologic features of normal mucosa (**a**) or celiac (**b**)

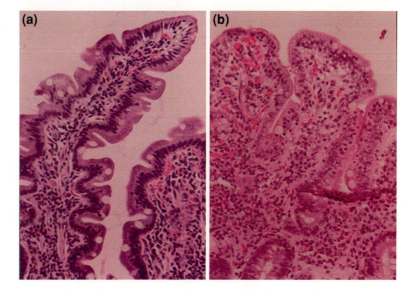

**Fig. 10.29 a–c** Esophageal capsule endoscopy (ECE) images: longitudinal furrows under *white light* (WL)—*blue arrows*—and *blue mode* (BM); FICE is not available in ECE. **d, e** Conventional endoscopy views confirming aforementioned findings (*black arrows*) and depicting multilevel cicatricial folds. Biopsies were consistent with eosinophilic esophagitis

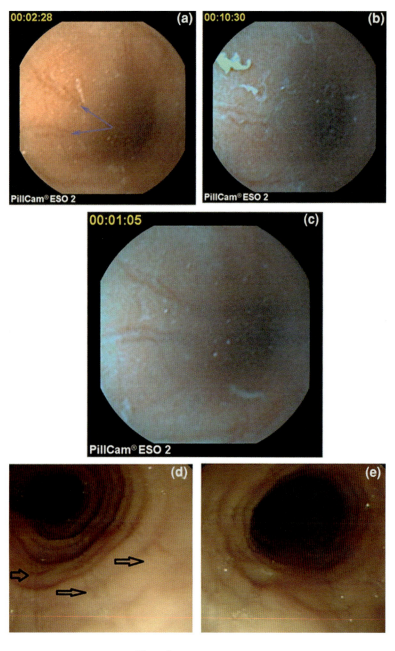

## 10.6    Esophageal Capsule Endoscopy

**Case 1.**

A 35-year-old man with severe hemophilia and recently developed dysphagia. Attends for esophageal capsule endoscopy due to 'at risk for vCJD infection' status (Fig. 10.29).

**Case 2.**

A 72-year-old woman, with primary biliary cirrhosis and intolerant to conventional endoscopy, presents for esophageal capsule endoscopy (ECE) and variceal surveillance (Fig. 10.30).

**Case 3.**

A 68-year-old man with hemophilia and "at risk of vCJD" presents for ECE and variceal surveillance (Fig. 10.31).

**Fig. 10.30**  **a–c** ECE images showing a whitish esophageal plaque (*blue mode*; BM), consistent with esophageal candidiasis or glycogenic acanthosis (*blue arrow*; **a**) and BM image of minor esophagitis and *white light* image of the palisade vessels at the GEJ (**b** and **c**)

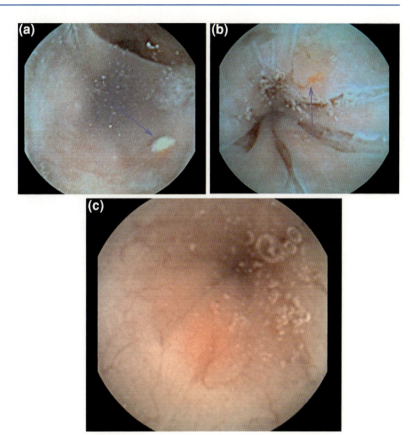

**Fig. 10.31** **a–c** C1 variceal columns under *white light* (WL) and *blue mode* (BM)

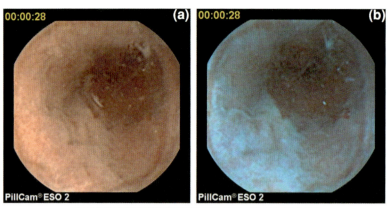

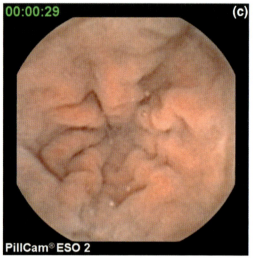

**Fig. 10.32  a–c** Magnetic-controlled capsule endoscopy (MCE) revealed multi-erosions and a polyp about 0.5 cm in size in the antrum, which were confirmed by the EGD. **d** EGD found another small polyp about 0.3 cm in the lower body (*white arrow*)

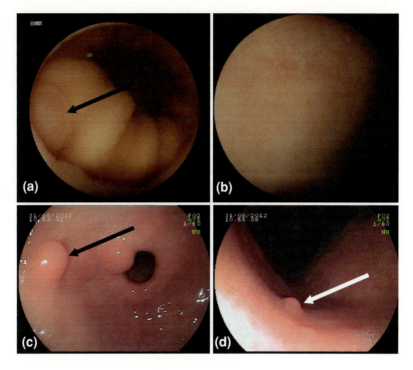

## 10.7    Gastric Capsule Endoscopy

**Case 1. Gastric polyp.**

A 66-year-old man presented with recurrent anorexia and abdominal pain for 9 months (Fig. 10.32).

**Case 2. Chronic atrophic gastritis.**

A 62-year-old woman presented with bloating for 3 years (Fig. 10.33).

**Case 3. Hemorrhagic gastritis.**

A 46-year-old woman presented with recurrent acid reflux and abdominal pain for 1 month (Fig. 10.34).

**Fig. 10.33** **a–d** Both MCE and EGD revealed diffuse nodular hyperplasia in stomach, which were consistent with chronic atrophic gastritis

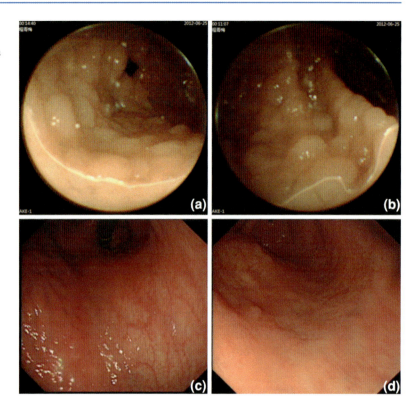

**Fig. 10.34** **a–c** MCE revealed multiple bleeding sites and a slightly elevated lesion about 0.4 cm in size in the antrum. **d, e** EGD had the similar findings with MCE. **f** Endoscopic ultrasonography showed the isoechoic elevated lesion originated from mucosa

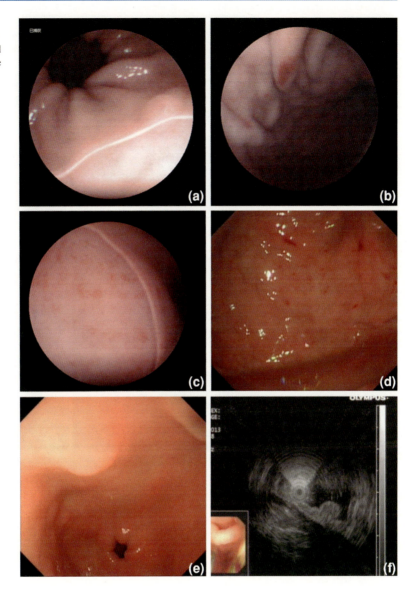

## 10.8   Colon Capsule Endoscopy

**Case 1. Polypoid hyperplasia**.

A 64-year-old female was presented with complaints of mucosanguineous feces twice daily in last 2 years. But she had no such illness as abdominal pain, bloating, or fever.

Colon capsule endoscopy displayed multiple pseudopolyps in the ascending colon, transverse colon, and descending colon (Fig. 10.35a). Mucosal edema distributed in the sigmoid colon and superficial ulcers in the rectum.

Fig. 10.35  **a** Colon
capsule endoscopy
findings; **b** Colonoscopy
findings

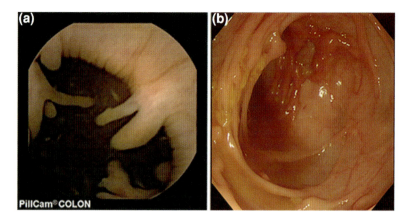

Fig. 10.36  **a** Colon
capsule endoscopy
findings; **b** Colonoscopy
findings

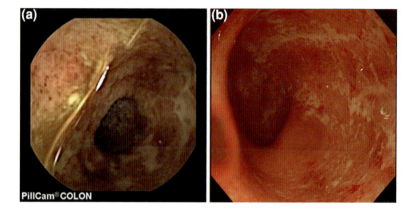

## Case 2. Mucosal edema, erosion, ulceration with effusion.

A 35-year-old man presented with 10 times bloody stool per day in last 4 months. Relative illness contained rectal tenesmus, intermittent pain in the left lower abdomen, and ten pounds of weight loss in nearly a month. He had no such illness as fever, acid reflux, or nausea. Colon capsule endoscopy displayed diffuse mucosal edema, ulcers, and erosive lesions from cecum to the rectum gradually increased (Fig. 10.36a).

# Index

Printed by Printforce, the Netherlands